Your *Clinics* subscription

You can now access the FULL TEXT of this publication online at no additional cost! Activate your online subscription today and receive...

- Full text of all issues from 2002 to the present
- Photographs, tables, illustrations, and references
- Comprehensive search capabilities
- Links to MEDLINE and Elsevier journals

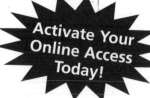

Activate Your Online Access Today!

Plus, you can also sign up for E-alerts of upcoming issues or articles that interest you, and take advantage of exclusive access to bonus features!

To activate your individual online subscription:

1. Visit our website at **www.TheClinics.com**.

2. Click on "Register" at the top of the page, and follow the instructions.

3. To activate your account, you will need your subscriber account number, which you can find on your mailing label (note: the number of digits in your subscriber account number varies from six to ten digits). See the sample below where the subscriber account number has been circled.

This is your subscriber account number

```
*************************************3-DIGIT 001
FEB00   J0167   C7   (123456-89)   10/00   Q: 1

J.H. DOE, MD
531 MAIN ST
CENTER CITY, NY  10001-001
```

4. That's it! Your online access to the most trusted source for clinical reviews is now available.

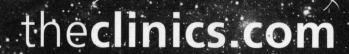

theclinics.com

ELSEVIER

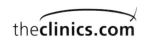

the**clinics**.com

PSYCHIATRIC CLINICS
OF NORTH AMERICA

Obesity: A Guide for Mental Health Professionals

GUEST EDITORS
Thomas A. Wadden, PhD
Albert J. Stunkard, MD, and
Robert I. Berkowitz, MD

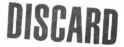
March 2005 • Volume 28 • Number 1

SAUNDERS

An Imprint of Elsevier, Inc.
PHILADELPHIA   LONDON   TORONTO   MONTREAL   SYDNEY   TOKYO

W.B. SAUNDERS COMPANY
A Division of Elsevier Inc.

The Curtis Center • Independence Square West • Philadelphia, Pennsylvania 19106

http://www.theclinics.com

THE PSYCHIATRIC CLINICS OF NORTH AMERICA
March 2005
Editor: Sarah E. Barth

Volume 28, Number 1
ISSN 0193-953X
ISBN 1-4160-2678-9

The ideas and opinions expressed in *The Psychiatric Clinics of North America* do not necessarily reflect those of the Publisher. The Publisher does not assume any responsibility for any injury and/or damage to persons or property arising out of or related to any use of the material contained in this periodical. The reader is advised to check the appropriate medical literature and the product information currently provided by the manufacturer of each drug to be administered, to verify the dosage, the method and duration of administration, or contraindications. It is the responsibility of the treating physician or other health care professional, relying on independent experience and knowledge of the patient, to determine drug dosages and the best treatment for the patient. Mention of any product in this issue should not be construed as endorsement by the contributors, editors, or the Publisher of the product or manufacturers' claims.

The Psychiatric Clinics of North America (ISSN 0193-953X) is published quarterly by the W.B. Saunders Company. Corporate and editorial offices: The Curtis Center, Independence Square West, Philadelphia, PA 19106-3399. Accounting and circulation offices: 6277 Sea Harbor Drive, Orlando, FL 32887-4800. Periodicals postage paid at Orlando, FL 32862, and additional mailing offices. Subscription prices are $170.00 per year (US individuals), $288.00 per year (US institutions), $85.00 per year (US students/residents), $205.00 per year (Canadian individuals), $349.00 per year (Canadian Institutions), $240.00 per year (foreign individuals), $349.00 per year (foreign institutions), and $120.00 per year (international & Canadian students/residents). Foreign air speed delivery is included in all *Clinics'* subscription prices. All prices are subject to change without notice. POSTMASTER: Send address changes to *The Psychiatric Clinics of North America*, W.B. Saunders Company, Periodicals Fulfillment, Orlando, FL 32887–4800. **Customer Service: 1-800-654-2452 (US). From outside of the US, call 1-407-345-4000.**

The Psychiatric Clinics of North America is covered in *Index Medicus, Current Contents/Social and Behavioral Sciences, Social Science Citation Index, Embase/Excerpta Medica,* and PsycINFO.

Printed in the United States of America.

616.89
Psy
200 5
V. 28
No. 1

GUEST EDITORS

THOMAS A. WADDEN, PhD, Professor of Psychology, Department of Psychiatry, University of Pennsylvania, School of Medicine, Weight and Eating Disorders Program, Philadelphia, Pennsylvania

ALBERT J. STUNKARD, MD, Professor, Department of Psychiatry, University of Pennsylvania, School of Medicine, Weight and Eating Disorders Program, Philadelphia, Pennsylvania

ROBERT I. BERKOWITZ, MD, Associate Professor, Department of Psychiatry, University of Pennsylvania, School of Medicine, Weight and Eating Disorders Program; and Chair, Department of Child and Adolescent Psychiatry, The Children's Hospital of Philadelphia, Philadelphia, Pennsylvania

CONTRIBUTORS

KELLY C. ALLISON, PhD, Research Assistant Professor of Psychology, Department of Psychiatry, University of Pennsylvania, School of Medicine, Weight and Eating Disorders Program, Philadelphia, Pennsylvania

ROBERT I. BERKOWITZ, MD, Associate Professor, Department of Psychiatry, University of Pennsylvania, School of Medicine, Weight and Eating Disorders Program; and Chair, Department of Child and Adolescent Psychiatry, The Children's Hospital of Philadelphia, Philadelphia, Pennsylvania

GEORGE A. BRAY, MD, Boyd Professor and Professor of Medicine, Pennington Biomedical Research Center, Louisiana State University, Baton Rouge, Louisiana

JOHANNA BROCK, BA, Department of Psychiatry, University of Pennsylvania School of Medicine, Philadelphia, Pennsylvania

KELLY D. BROWNELL, PhD, Professor and Chair of Psychology; Professor of Epidemiology and Public Health; and Director, Weight and Eating Disorders Program, Yale University, New Haven, Connecticut

KIRSTIN J. BYRNE, MS, Department of Psychiatry, University of Pennsylvania School of Medicine, Weight and Eating Disorders Program, Philadelphia, Pennsylvania

THOMAS F. CASH, PhD, Professor, Department of Psychology, Old Dominion University, Norfolk, Virginia

VICKI CATENACCI, MD, Fellow, Division of Endocrinology, Diabetes and Metabolism, University of Colorado Health Sciences Center, Denver, Colorado

CANICE E. CRERAND, PhD, Instructor of Psychology, Department of Psychiatry, University of Pennsylvania School of Medicine, Philadelphia, Pennsylvania

ANTHONY N. FABRICATORE, PhD, Weight and Eating Disorders Program, Department of Psychiatry, University of Pennsylvania, Philadelphia, Pennsylvania

GARY D. FOSTER, PhD, Associate Professor, Department of Psychiatry, University of Pennsylvania School of Medicine, Philadelphia, Pennsylvania

JAMES O. HILL, PhD, Professor, Department of Pediatrics and Medicine; and Director, Center for Human Nutrition, University of Colorado Health Sciences Center, Denver, Colorado

JOHN M. JAKICIC, PhD, Chair, Department of Health and Physical Activity; and Director, Physical Activity and Weight Management Research Center, University of Pittsburgh, Pittsburgh, Pennsylvania

ROBERT F. KUSHNER, MD, Professor, Department of Medicine, Northwestern University Feinberg School of Medicine; and Medical Director, Wellness Institute, Northwestern Memorial Hospital, Chicago, Illinois

ANGELA P. MAKRIS, PhD, RD, Instructor, Department of Psychiatry, University of Pennsylvania School of Medicine, Philadelphia, Pennsylvania

JAMES E. MITCHELL, MD, Neuropsychiatric Research Institute and the Department of Neuroscience, University of North Dakota School of Medicine and Health Sciences, Fargo, North Dakota

TRICIA COOK MYERS, PhD, Neuropsychiatric Research Institute and the Department of Neuroscience, University of North Dakota School of Medicine and Health Sciences, Fargo, North Dakota

AMY D. OTTO, PhD, RD, LDN, Assistant Professor, Department of Health and Physical Activity; and Assistant Director, Physical Activity and Weight Management Research Center, University of Pittsburgh, Pittsburgh, Pennsylvania

JOHN R. PENDER, MD, Clinical Associate Professor, Department of Surgery, Brody School of Medicine, East Carolina University, Greenville, North Carolina

WALTER J. PORIES, MD, FACS, Professor, Department of Surgery, Brody School of Medicine, East Carolina University, Greenville, North Carolina

KARINE PROULX, MS, PhD candidate, Neuroscience Graduate Program, University of Cincinnati College of Medicine, Cincinnati, Ohio

JULIE L. ROTH, MD, Assistant Professor of Medicine, Northwestern University Feinberg School of Medicine, Chicago, Illinois

DAVID B. SARWER, PhD, Associate Professor, Departments of Psychiatry and Surgery; The Edwin and Fannie Gray Hall Center for Human Appearance, University of Pennsylvania School of Medicine, Philadelphia, Pennsylvania

RANDY J. SEELEY, PhD, Professor, Department of Psychiatry; and Associate Director, Obesity Research Center, University of Cincinnati College of Medicine, Cincinnati, Ohio

ALBERT J. STUNKARD, MD, Professor, Department of Psychiatry, University of Pennsylvania, School of Medicine, Weight and Eating Disorders Program, Philadelphia, Pennsylvania

J. KEVIN THOMPSON, PhD, Professor, Department of Psychology, University of South Florida, Tampa, Florida

ADAM GILDEN TSAI, MD, Department of Psychiatry, University of Pennsylvania School of Medicine, Weight and Eating Disorders Program, Philadelphia, Pennsylvania

THOMAS A. WADDEN, PhD, Professor of Psychology, Department of Psychiatry, University of Pennsylvania, School of Medicine, Weight and Eating Disorders Program, Philadelphia, Pennsylvania

SHIRLEY S. WANG, MS, Department of Psychology, Yale University, New Haven, Connecticut

LESLIE G. WOMBLE, PhD, Department of Psychiatry, University of Pennsylvania School of Medicine, Weight and Eating Disorders Program, Philadelphia, Pennsylvania

HOLLY R. WYATT, MD, Assistant Professor, Division of Endocrinology, Diabetes and Metabolism, University of Colorado Health Sciences Center; and Program Director, Centers for Obesity Research and Education, Denver, Colorado

CONTRIBUTORS – SPECIAL ARTICLES

KAREN E. ANDERSON, MD, Assistant Professor, Psychiatry and Neurology, Department of Psychiatry, Maryland Parkinson's and Movement Disorders Center, Movement Disorders Division, University of Maryland, School of Medicine, Baltimore, Maryland

PERMINDER S. SACHDEV, MD, PhD, FRANZCP, Professor of Neuropsychiatry, School of Psychiatry, University of New South Wales, Sydney, Australia; and Director, Neuropsychiatric Institute, Prince of Wales Hospital, Randwick, Australia

CONTENTS

> Obesity has reached epidemic proportions in the United States, with 31% of adults and at least 15% of children obese. Obesity affects every segment of the US population. Obesity increases the risk of many other chronic diseases and decreases overall quality of life. The epidemic of obesity arose gradually over time, apparently from a small, consistent positive energy balance. There is no indication that the prevalence of obesity is decreasing, and substantial public health efforts will be required to reverse the epidemic. Because of the complexity of obesity, it is likely to be one of the most difficult public health issues society has faced.

> Mammals are designed to carefully regulate the amount of stored energy in the body with most of that energy stored as lipid in adipose tissue. To maintain energy balance requires that significant deviations in the amount of stored fuel be detected, and this triggers error correction mechanisms to bring the levels of stored fuel back to the defended level. Evidence suggests that specific pathways located within the arcuate nucleus of the hypothalamus integrate several signals from stored fuel that in turn regulate food intake and energy expenditure.

> Obesity is associated with several psychiatric disorders. There is an association with depression and weight gain for women, but there

is less of an association for men. Obesity also is associated with bipolar disorder and schizophrenia. Several second-generation antipsychotic medications, antidepressant medications, and mood stabilizers are associated with weight gain and increased risk for type 2 diabetes mellitus and lipid disorders. This article reviews medical monitoring of patients treated with drugs related to weight gain.

dietary approaches to obesity treatment, with an emphasis on the relative roles of fat, carbohydrate and protein on hunger and satiety and the efficacy of various macronutrient-based strategies for weight loss.

This article highlights appropriate recommendations for physical activity for treating obesity.

This article reviews the behavioral treatment of obesity, its short- and long-term results, and methods to improve long-term weight loss. The terms "behavioral treatment," "lifestyle modification," and "behavioral weight control" are often used interchangeably.

Each year, millions of Americans participate in commercial and self-help weight loss programs. Health care providers, including psychiatrists, need information about these programs so that they can advise patients appropriately. This article describes the components, costs, and efficacy of the major commercial (nonmedical, medically supervised, and Internet-based) and organized self-help programs.

As new drugs are developed for treatment of obesity, a framework is needed to describe them. The framework used in this article divides them into three groups: those that reduce food intake, those that alter metabolism, and those that increase thermogenesis. Monoamines acting on noradrenergic receptors, serotonin receptors, dopamine receptors, and histamine receptors can reduce food intake. Several peptides also modulate food intake. The noradrenergic drugs phentermine, diethylpropion, benzphetamine, and phendimetrazine are approved only for short-term use. Sibutramine, a norepinephrine—serotonin reuptake inhibitor, is approved for long-term use. Also approved for long-term use is orlistat, which inhibits pancreatic lipase and can block hydrolysis of 30% of the dietary triglyceride in subjects eating a 30% fat diet. The thermogenic combination of ephedrine and caffeine has not been approved by regulatory agencies. Several new drugs, including axokine, topiramate, and rimonabant, are being evaluated in clinical trials. Medications for obesity treatment should be viewed as useful adjuncts to diet and physical activity that may help selected patients achieve and maintain weight loss. Thus, physicians must be knowledgeable regarding the efficacy and safety profiles of medications.

The increase in prevalence of obesity in America has become an epidemic. Obesity is not just a problem of girth and weight. The disabilities caused by obesity are physiologic and psychosocial. The mortality rate of an obese individual is 2.5 times higher than that of the nonobese patient. Although performed since the 1950s, there has been a recent surge in the popularity of obesity reducing surgery. Several options are available, but there is significant variability in the weight reduction, morbidity, and mortality of these procedures.

This article addresses the causes of obesity. Biased by misattributions of cause, the nation has sidestepped the need for changes in the environment and instead has focused on the individual, typically by assigning blame to individuals and calling for personal responsibility. The article discusses medical versus public health models as they relate to obesity issue, and ends by proposing changes in public policy the authors believe may help advance the field.

SPECIAL ARTICLES

This article provides an overview of neuroleptic-induced movement disorders.

This article provides an overview of conditions affecting movement, focusing on behavioral symptoms, along with review of other pertinent clinical data.

FORTHCOMING ISSUES

RECENT ISSUES

PSYCHIATRIC
CLINICS
OF NORTH AMERICA

ELSEVIER
SAUNDERS

Psychiatr Clin N Am 28 (2005) xiii–xvi

Preface

Obesity: A Guide for Mental Health Professionals

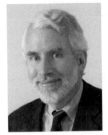
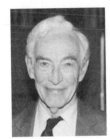
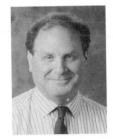

Thomas A. Wadden, PhD   Albert J. Stunkard, MD   Robert I. Berkowitz, MD

Guest Editors

Hardly a day passes without another report of America's epidemic of obesity. Despite increased awareness of the problem, and greater attention from the National Institutes of Health and other public agencies, the epidemic shows no signs of abating. Most recent data from the National Health and Nutrition Examination Survey (NHANES-IV) indicate that 34% of adults now are overweight, defined by a body mass index (BMI) of 25.0 to 29.9 kg/m^2, and 31% are obese (BMI $\geq$ 30 kg/m^2). Obesity is associated with approximately 325,000 deaths a year and costs our nation more than $100 billion per year. These figures say nothing of the personal suffering–both physical and emotional–that obese individuals endure.

The epidemic of obesity has generated a host of books, including this one, on the etiology, prevention, and treatment of this disorder. This compilation differs from previous ones principally in its intended audience: psychiatrists, psychologists, and other mental health professionals. As such, it examines the psychiatric status of obese individuals, including the frequently encountered problems of depression, binge eating, and body image disturbance. Several articles provide practical suggestions intended to guide treatment. The editors, however, recognize that some practitioners will not wish to provide weight reduction therapy, often because of competing therapeutic demands. However, after finishing this compilation, these practitioners should be able refer obese patients to appropriate programs and to support their progress during weight reduction.

doi:10.1016/j.psc.2004.12.001   *psych.theclinics.com*

This issue of *Psychiatric Clinics of North America* includes 14 articles that have been prepared by an exceptional group of investigators. All are experts in their areas of study and practice, and we are grateful for their contributions. The articles are not formally divided into sections but fall into six groupings: (1) prevalence, etiology, and physical consequences of obesity; (2) psychiatric complications associated with obesity; (3) medical and behavioral assessment of the obese patient; (4) lifestyle approaches to weight management, including diet, exercise, behavior therapy, and commercial programs; (5) pharmacologic and surgical interventions; and (6) the prevention of obesity through public policy. The articles are briefly introduced according to these groupings.

James Hill and colleagues provide a thorough overview of the epidemic of obesity. In addition to describing the prevalence and complications of this disorder, they discuss the relative contributions of genetic and environmental factors to obesity. They show how ancient genes that promoted survival in times of scarcity make losing weight so difficult in times of abundance. In the article that follows, Karine Prolux and Randy Seeley illuminate the basic mechanisms of body weight regulation. This is a fascinating story that received a major boost in 1994 with the discovery of leptin, a hormone that signals the brain concerning the status of the body's energy stores. The past decade has revealed that energy intake and expenditure are regulated by an elaborate neuroendocrine system that has multiple targets in the arcuate nucleus of the hypothalamus. Mental health practitioners will already know the important functions that the hypothalamus plays in the regulation of emotion, sleep, and other basic functions.

Robert Berkowitz and Anthony Fabricatore carefully examine the psychosocial status of obese individuals and arrive at some surprising conclusions. Foremost among these is that the majority of overweight and obese individuals (in the general population) have essentially normal psychological functioning. Obesity, however, presents a greater risk of depression in women than men, and the risk in persons with extreme obesity (BMI $> 40 \text{ kg/m}^2$) is increased fivefold. The authors also tackle the problem of weight gain associated with psychiatric medications and identify the agents least likely to increase body weight. Kelly Allison and Albert Stunkard discuss the prevalence, etiology, and treatment of two eating disorders frequently encountered in obese individuals: binge eating and night eating. Both conditions are associated with increased levels of depression, and both have been treated with antidepressant medications. Although these agents may be useful with both conditions, behavioral weight control methods appear more effective in treating the obese individual with binge eating. David Sarwer and colleagues discuss body image dissatisfaction in obese individuals. Although such dissatisfaction is almost universal, even in women of average weight, the most severe form of this problem, body dysmorphic disorder, occurs in fewer than 10% of obese women. The cognitive behavioral interventions reviewed by the authors reduce body image dissatisfaction even in the absence of weight loss.

Before undertaking a significant weight loss effort, obese individuals should undergo a medical evaluation to identify possible contraindications to treatment, as well as to fully assess physical complications of excess weight. Robert Kushner and Julie Roth provide a simple but thorough guide to this evaluation. Although psychiatrists are unlikely to perform the physical examination, they should be aware of frequently overlooked complications, including obstructive sleep apnea, polycystic ovarian syndrome, and nonalcoholic fatty liver disease. James Mitchell and Trisha Myers provide welcome guidance for assessing possible behavioral complications of obesity, described in the previous articles, and for determining the contribution of eating and activity habits to the patient's weight problem. The authors share with readers an extensive questionnaire (ie, EDQ) they have developed to assess behavioral factors. Patients' completion of this questionnaire, before meeting with the practitioner, expedites the conduct of the behavioral assessment.

Results of the behavioral assessment should yield suggestions for intervention, as does an algorithm proposed by an expert panel convened by the National Heart Lung and Blood Institute (of the National Institutes of Health). The algorithm recommends that all obese individuals initially be treated by a comprehensive program of diet, exercise, and behavior therapy (often referred to as *lifestyle modification*). In this issue, Angie Makris and Gary Foster review principles of sound nutrition, as well as controversies concerning the optimal macronutrient composition of reducing diets. Readers will appreciate their balanced, evidence-based evaluation of low-carbohydrate diets and other popular approaches. John Jakicic and Amy Otto similarly examine recommendations for increasing physical activity in obese individuals and for facilitating the maintenance of weight loss. They review recent finings that multiple short bouts (ie, 10 minutes) of physical activity are as beneficial to weight management and health as is one long bout (ie, 40 minutes). Wadden and colleagues review principles of behavior therapy that are used to facilitate patients' adoption of a new eating and activity habits. Behavioral treatment can be provided in either group or individual sessions and induces a loss of approximately 8% to 10% of initial weight in 4 to 6 months. Practitioners who do not wish to provide such therapy themselves will benefit from the article by Adam Gilden Tsai and colleagues, which discusses commercial and self-help programs for obesity. Several of these programs, including Weight Watchers, provide sensible recommendations for modifying diet and activity, along with valuable group social support.

Pharmacotherapy is an option for patients with a BMI of 30 kg/m^2 or more who are unable to achieve a 10% weight loss with lifestyle modification alone. George Bray provides a thorough consideration of current FDA-approved medications for obesity, as well as those on the horizon. Pharmacotherapy should improve significantly over the next 10 to 20 years as the neuroendocrinological basis of body weight regulation is further elucidated. John Pender and Walter Pories complete the examination of obesity therapies with their review of surgical options, which are appropriate for persons with a BMI of 40 kg/m^2 or more. The authors report that the gastric bypass induces a loss of 25% to 30% of initial weight in 12 to 18 months, with excellent maintenance of weight loss 10 years later. These benefits, however, must be weighed against the risks of the procedure.

Space limitations prevented us from examining the treatments of obesity in children and adolescents. Shirley Wang and Kelly Brownell, however, argue persuasively that treatment is not the answer to the epidemic of obesity in either children or adults. Instead, far greater attention must be devoted to the prevention of obesity by tackling the environment that lies at the heart of the epidemic. Such efforts call for public health campaigns and bold policy initiatives, as used to address cigarette smoking, drunk driving, and the AIDs epidemic. We could not agree more. We must improve treatments for individuals who already are obese, but our greater need is to prevent the development of this disorder, particularly in our children.

We hope this issue of the *Psychiatric Clinics of North America* will help mental health professionals do their part to confront obesity, a disease with profound health and economic consequences. We thank Sarah Barth of Elsevier for her able assistance in guiding the development of this issue, as well as Kirstin Byrne, Johanna Brock, and Lauren Paster for their editorial assistance. Douglas Whitaker and Andrew Swinney also are acknowledged for their inspiring contributions.

Thomas A. Wadden, PhD
Albert J. Stunkard, MD
Robert I. Berkowitz, MD
Department of Psychiatry
University of Pennsylvania
School of Medicine
Weight and Eating Disorders Program
3535 Market Street, Suite 3108
Philadelphia, PA 19104, USA

E-mail addresses: wadden@mail.med.upenn.edu (T.A. Wadden);
stunkard@mail.med.upenn.edu (A.J. Stunkard);
Rberk@mail.med.upenn.edu (R.I. Berkowitz)

ELSEVIER
SAUNDERS

PSYCHIATRIC
CLINICS
OF NORTH AMERICA

Psychiatr Clin N Am 28 (2005) 1–23

Obesity: Overview of an Epidemic

James O. Hill, PhD[a], Vicki Catenacci, MD[b], Holly R. Wyatt, MD[b,c,*]

[a]*Department of Pediatrics and Medicine, Center for Human Nutrition, University of Colorado Health Sciences Center, 4200 East 9th Avenue, Campus Box C263, Denver, CO 80262, USA*
[b]*Division of Endocrinology, Diabetes and Metabolism, University of Colorado Health Sciences Center, 4200 East 9th Avenue, Campus Box C263, Denver, CO 80262, USA*
[c]*Centers for Obesity Research and Education, 4200 East 9th Avenue, Campus Box C263, Denver, CO 80262, USA*

A recent report suggests that obesity, caused by poor diet and physical inactivity, likely soon will overtake tobacco smoking as the leading cause of preventable deaths in the United States [1]. This report states that in 2000, it was estimated that obesity, was responsible for about 400,000 preventable deaths. This compares to an estimated 435,000 preventable deaths caused by tobacco smoking. The International Food Information Council (IFIC) tracks media coverage of issues related to nutrition and obesity. It found [2] that in the third quarter of 1999 there were about 50 print media articles on obesity. In the second quarter of 2003, this had risen to over 1300. In 1999, obesity was absent from most lists of the most serious public health problems facing Americans, yet today it is first or second on most lists. There is general consensus that obesity has reached epidemic proportions in the United States [3,4] and will soon reach epidemic proportions globally [5]. How did this obesity epidemic arise so quickly, and what will it take to successfully reverse it?

Prevalence of obesity

Overweight and obesity are defined based on body mass index (BMI), which is determined as weight (kg) divided by height^2 (m). Table 1 shows the categories of BMI. A healthy BMI range is 18.5 to 24.9 kg/m^2. Overweight is

---

This work was supported by grants # DK02703, DK42549, DK48520 from the National Institutes of Health.
* Corresponding author.
E-mail address: holly.wyatt@uchsc.edu (H.R. Wyatt).

0193-953X/05/$ - see front matter © 2005 Elsevier Inc. All rights reserved.
doi:10.1016/j.psc.2004.09.010
psych.theclinics.com

Table 1
Categories of body mass index and disease risk* relative to normal weight and waist circumference

	BMI kg/m^2	Obesity class	Men ≤ 102 cm (≤ 40 in) women ≤ 88 cm (≤ 35 in)	> 102 cm (> 40 in) >88 cm (> 35 in)
Underweight	< 18.5		–	–
Normal**	18.5–24.9		–	–
Overweight	25.0–29.9		Increased	High
Obesity	30.0–34.9	I	High	Very high
	35.0–39.9	II	Very high	Very high
Extreme obesity	≥ 40	III	Extremely high	Extremely high

* Disease risk for type 2 diabetes, hypertension, and cardiovascular disease.

** Increased waist circumference can also be a marker for increased risk even in persons of normal weight.

(*Data from* National Heart, Lung, and Blood Institute Obesity Education Initiative Expert Panel: clinical guidelines on the identification, evaluation, and treatment of overweight and obesity in adults: the evidence report. Obes Res 1998;6(Suppl 2):51S–210S.)

defined as a BMI from 25 to 29.9 kg/m^2, and obesity is defined as BMI of at least 30 kg/m^2 [6]. Obesity can be subdivided further based on subclasses of BMI as shown in Table 1. Waist circumference also can be used in combination with a BMI value to evaluate health risk for individuals.

The strongest data on obesity prevalence rates over time in the US come from results of the National Health and Nutrition Examination Surveys (NHANES). NHANES periodically collect measured heights and weights in representative samples of the population. The most recent NHANES data were collected during from 1999 to 2000 [7,8]. As shown in Fig. 1, obesity rates in adults have been increasing gradually over the past 30 years, with the latest statistics showing that from 1999 to 2000, approximately 65% of adults were overweight or obese, and approximately 31% were obese. Obesity rates in the US have more than doubled in the last 30 years.

It further appears that increasing BMI and increasing obesity prevalence rates are affecting the entire adult population, with no group being immune. Increases in obesity rates are being seen among men and women of all ethnic groups, of all ages, and of all educational and socioeconomic levels [8,9]. Although the entire population seems to be getting heavier each year, there is evidence that obesity affects some subgroups in the population to a greater extent than others. For example African-American and Hispanic women have had a higher prevalence of obesity (BMI greater than 30) than Caucasian women, or men of any ethnic background (Fig. 2). Obesity prevalence rates increased over time in all gender–ethnic groups (Figs. 3–6). Further, obesity rates consistently have been higher in those of a low socioeconomic status (SES) and in those with lower education level [10,11]. As shown in Figs. 7 and 8, however, similar weight gain seems to be occurring in all income and educational levels [12].

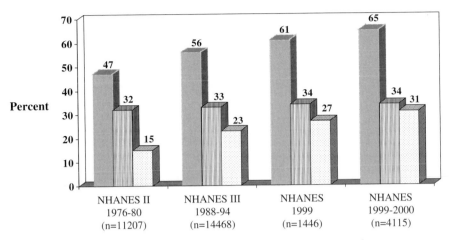

Fig. 1. Age-adjusted prevalence rates of overweight and obesity in US adults over time. (*Data from* National Center for Health Statistics Website. Available at: www.cdc.gov/nchs/products/pubs/pubd/hestats/obese/obse99.htm. Accessed April 2004. and Flegal KM, Carroll MD, Ogden CL, et al. Prevalence and trends in obesity among US adults, 1999–2000. JAMA 2002;288:1723–7.)

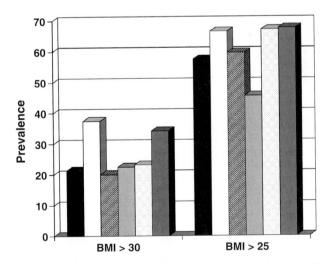

Fig. 2. Age-adjusted prevalence rates of overweight and obesity broken down by race–ethnic groups for men and women. Black bars indicate black men, white bars black women, diagonal bars white men, gray bars white women, dotted bars Mexican American men, dark gray bars Mexican American women. (*Data from* Flegal KM, Carroll MD, Kuczmarski RL, Johnson CL. Overweight and obesity in the United States: prevalence and trends, 1960–1994. Int J Obes 1998;22:39–47.)

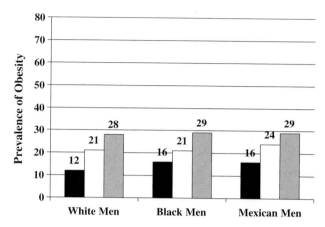

Fig. 3. Prevalence rates of obesity in men over time. Black bars indicate 1976 to 1980; white bars indicate 1988 to 1994, and gray bars indicate 1999 to 2001. (*Data from* the National Center for Health Statistics Website. Available at: www.cdc.gov/nchs/products/pubs/pubd/hestats/obese/obse99.htm. Accessed April 2004.)

The fact that minority and low SES individuals are affected by obesity disproportionately may not be surprising, because the cheapest foods are those containing high levels of fat and sugar [13]. This means that the way to get the most calories for the least money is to eat a diet that is high in fat and sugar. This illustrates the interaction of biology and economics in supporting the obesity epidemic. Those foods for which people have a high biological preference (ie, foods high in sugar and high in energy

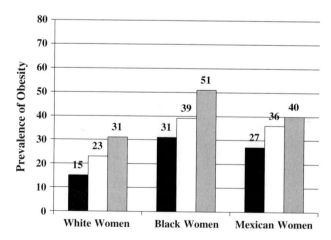

Fig. 4. Prevalence rates of obesity in women over time. Black bars indicate 1976 to 1980; white bars indicate 1988 to 1994, and gray bars indicate 1999 to 2001. (*Data from* the National Center for Health Statistics Website. Available at: www.cdc.gov/nchs/products/pubs/pubd/hestats/obese/obse99.htm. Accessed April 2004.)

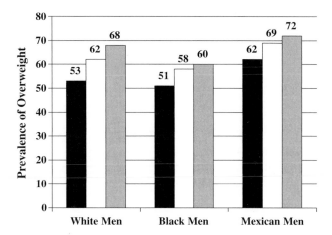

Fig. 5. Prevalence rates of overweight in men over time. Black bars indicate 1976 to 1980; white bars indicate 1988 to 1994, and gray bars indicate 1999 to 2001. (*Data from* the National Center for Health Statistics Website. Available at: www.cdc.gov/nchs/products/pubs/pubd/hestats/obese/obse99.htm. Accessed April 2004.)

density) and that contribute to overeating are the cheapest and most accessible [13,14]. Further, minority and low SES individuals may engage in less physical activity than people from other sectors of the population. In low SES populations, there are often issues of neighborhood safety, so that children are not allowed to go outside and play. People who have more financial resources combat these circumstances more easily, and

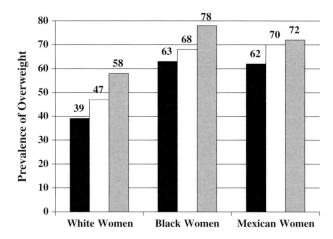

Fig. 6. Prevalence rates of overweight in women over time. Black bars indicate 1976 to 1980; white bars indicate 1988 to 1994, and gray bars indicate 1999 to 2001. (*Data from* the National Center for Health Statistics Website. Available at: www.cdc.gov/nchs/products/pubs/pubd/hestats/obese/obse99.htm. Accessed April 2004.)

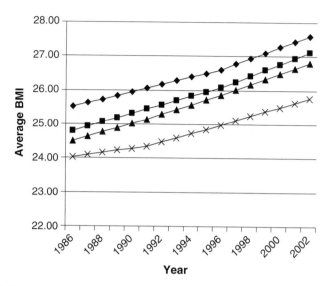

Fig. 7. Weight gain by education level over time. Diamonds indicate no college; squares indicate high school. Triangles indicate some college, and × indicates college. (*Data from* the Behavioral Risk Factor Surveillance System.)

consequently are more physically active and less obese than those with fewer resources.

Those individuals who are already overweight or obese also may be gaining weight at a more rapid rate than those with a BMI in the healthy range. For example, a recent report from the Rand Institute shows that it is

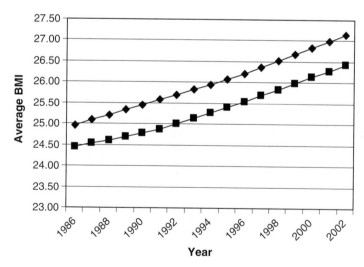

Fig. 8. Weigh gain by income level over time. Diamonds indicate lowest income, and squares indicate highest income. (*Data from* the Behavioral Risk Factor Surveillance System.)

not just that more Americans are becoming obese, and severe obesity is increasing the most in relative terms. The greatest relative increase has been in the proportion of individuals above a BMI of 50 kg/m² [15] (Fig. 9).

Obesity rates are high in most age groups. Figs. 10 & 11 show obesity and overweight prevalence rates for different age groups for men and women (from NHANES III). Obesity rates, in general, increase with age until approximately age 75, when rates decline. This could be because of increasing mortality from obesity-related conditions.

Children have not been immune from the obesity epidemic. Fig. 12 shows the prevalence over time of overweight in children. In this figure, based on NHANES III data [16], overweight is defined from age- and gender-specific growth charts developed by Cole et al [17]. At least 15% of US children are overweight and, just as with adults, the prevalence of overweight has increased over time. Further, just as with adults, overweight appears to be increasing more rapidly in minority children than in Caucasian children of all ages (Figs. 13, 14). A recent report from the Foundation for Child Development [18] has found that when considering overall health, children today are faring only slightly better than they did 30 years ago. Increasing childhood obesity was suggested as a major reason for such small progress.

The gradual fattening of Americans

Hill et al [19] examined the trends in the increase of obesity in the United States. Their analysis suggests that the obesity epidemic arose from gradual

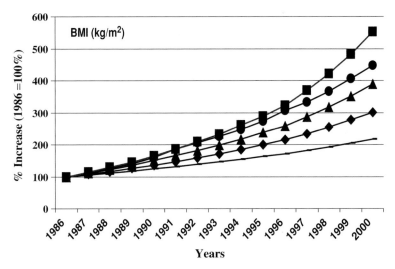

Fig. 9. Relative increase in the proportion of individuals above a BMI of 50 kg/m². Lines indicate BMI > 30; diamonds indicate BMI > 35. Triangles indicate BMI > 40; circles indicate BMI > 45, and squares indicate BMI > 50. (*Data from* Sturm R. Increases in clinically severe obesity in the United States, 1986–2000. Arch Intern Med 2003;163(18):2146–8.)

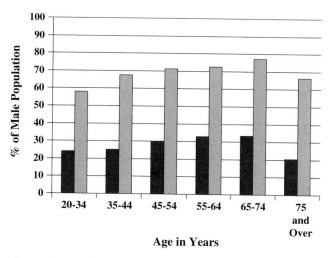

Fig. 10. Prevalence of overweight and obesity in men for different age groups. Black bars indicate obese, and gray bars indicate overweight. (*Data from* the National Center for Health Statistics Website. Available at: www.cdc.gov/nchs/products/pubs/pubd/hestats/obese/obse99. htm. Accessed April 2004.)

yearly weight gain in the population produced from a slight, consistent degree of positive energy balance (ie, energy intake exceeding energy expenditure). Using longitudinal and cross-sectional data sets, they found that the average US adult has gained 1 to 2 pounds per year for the last 20 to 30 years. Fig. 15, from NHANES data, shows how the BMI distribution has moved to the right over the past several years. This figure also shows the projected BMI distribution in 2008 if weight gain continues at its current rate. In Fig. 15, the authors show the distribution of weight gain over an 8-year period, using data from the CARDIA [9] and NHANES [7] studies. In the lower panel, they show this distribution in excess energy stored per day, assuming an excess of 14,700 kJ produces 1 pound of weight gain. Finally, the authors assumed that excess energy was stored with an efficiency of 50% (a very conservative assumption). They concluded that that weight gain in 90% of the adult population is caused by a positive energy balance of 420 kJ/ per day or less (Fig. 16). Thus, it appears that the obesity epidemic arose very gradually over a long period of time because of a very slight but consistent degree of positive energy balance.

Health risks associated with obesity

Obesity is linked to the most prevalent and costly medical problems seen in this country, including type 2 diabetes, hypertension, coronary artery disease (CAD), and many forms of cancer. Box 1 lists the symptoms and diseases that are related to obesity directly or indirectly.

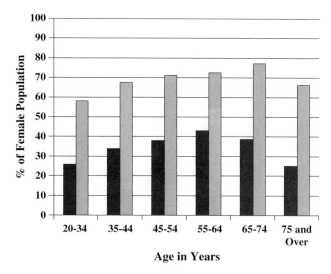

Fig. 11. Prevalence of overweight and obesity in women for different age groups. Black bars indicate obese, and gray bars indicate overweight. (*Data from* the National Center for Health Statistics Website. Available at: www.cdc.gov/nchs/products/pubs/pubd/hestats/obese/obse99. htm. Accessed April 2004.)

Type 2 diabetes and impaired glucose tolerance

Body mass index, abdominal fat distribution, and weight gain are important risk factors for the development of type 2 diabetes. It is estimated that 90% of individuals with type 2 diabetes are obese [20]. Data from

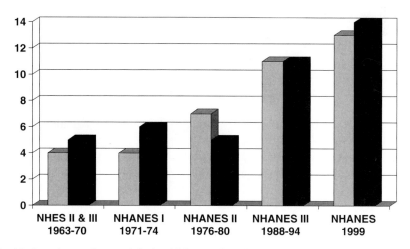

Fig. 12. Prevalence of overweight in children and adolescents over time. Gray bars indicate children between the ages of 6 and 12; black bars indicate adolescents between the ages of 12 and 19. (*Data from* Ogden CL, Flegal KM, Carroll MD, et al. Prevalence and trends in overweight among US children and adolescents, 1999–2000. JAMA 2002;288(14):1728–32.)

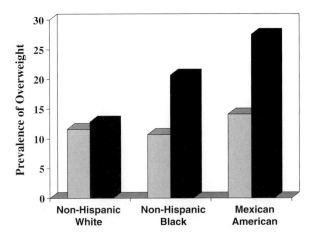

Fig. 13. Overweight prevalence by race/ethnicity for adolescent boys aged 12 to 19 years. Gray bars indicate NHANES 1988 to 1994; black bars indicate NHANES 1999 to 2000. (*Data from* Ogden CL, Flegal KM, Carroll MD, et al. Prevalence and trends in overweight among US children and adolescents, 1999–2000. JAMA 2002;288(14):1728–32.)

NHANES III found that almost 70% of adult men and women in the US with type 2 diabetes have a BMI of 27 or greater, and the risk of diabetes increases linearly with BMI [21]. Data from 8 years of follow-up of a cohort of over 113,000 US women aged 30 to 55 years in the Nurses Health Study found that among women with BMI 23 to 23.9 kg/m^2, the relative risk of diabetes was 3.6 times that of women having a BMI less than 22 kg/m^2 [22].

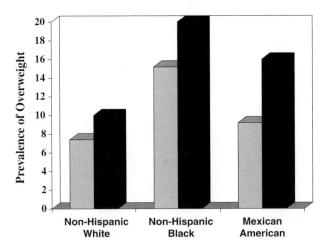

Fig. 14. Overweight prevalence by race/ethnicity for adolescent girls aged 12 to 19 years. Gray bars indicate NHANES 1988 to 1994; black bars indicate NHANES 1999 to 2000. (*Data from* Ogden CL, Flegal KM, Carroll MD, et al. Prevalence and trends in overweight among US children and adolescents, 1999–2000. JAMA 2002;288(14):1728–32.)

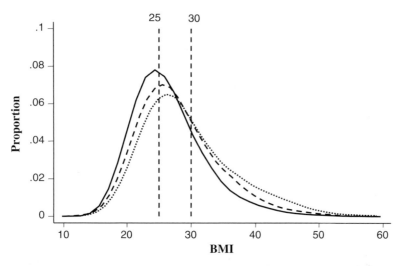

Fig. 15. Projected BMI distribution over time. Solid line indicates NHANES III 1988 to 1994; dashed line indicates NHANES 1999 to 2000; dotted line indicates projected 2008. (*From* Hill JO, Wyatt HR, Reed GW, et al. Obesity and the environment: where do we go from here? Science 2003;299:853–5; with permission.)

Dyslipidemia

Visceral obesity is associated with elevated triglycerides, low high-density lipoprotein (HDL) cholesterol, and increased small, dense low-density lipoprotein (LDL) particles [23]. Data from NHANES III suggest that prevalence of hypercholesterolemia (total cholesterol greater than 240 mg/ dL) increased progressively with BMI in men. In women, the prevalence was highest at a BMI of 25 to 27 kg/m^2, and did not increase further with increasing BMI [24].

Metabolic syndrome

Metabolic syndrome, also known as syndrome X, is a specific body phenotype of abdominal obesity associated with a group of metabolic disorders that are risk factors for CAD. Characteristics of this syndrome include abdominal obesity (waist circumference greater than 40 inches in men and greater than 35 inches in women), hypertension, high triglycerides, low HDL cholesterol, and impaired glucose tolerance. Many studies have pointed to an association between insulin resistance and intra-abdominal fat accumulation (visceral obesity). There is no clear proof, however, of a causal link between visceral fat accumulation and insulin resistance. It is not known whether visceral fat is involved in the pathogenesis of metabolic syndrome, or whether it is a marker for people who are at increased risk of the metabolic complications of obesity [25].

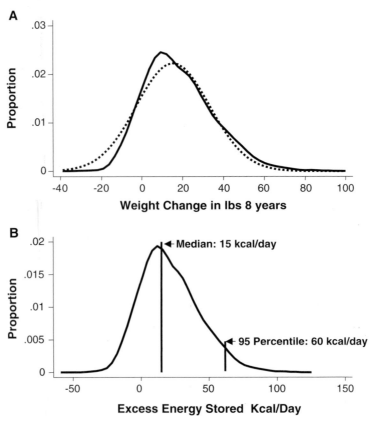

Fig. 16. (*A*) Distribution of weight gain over an 8-year period using data from NHANES and CARDIA studies. Solid line indicates NHANES ages 20 to 40; dotted line indicates CARDIA. (*B*) Distribution of excess energy stored per day accounting for predicted weight gain. (*From* Hill JO, Wyatt HR, Reed GW, et al. Obesity and the environment: where do we go from here? Science 2003;299:853–5; with permission.)

Coronary artery disease

Obese persons, particularly those with abdominal fat distribution, are at increased risk for CAD. The risk of CAD begins to increase at a BMI of 23 kg/m² for men and 22 kg/m² for women [26]. It previously was thought that most of the increased risk was mediated by obesity-related increases in risk factors, particularly hypertension, dyslipidemia, impaired glucose tolerance/diabetes, and metabolic syndrome. Several long-term epidemiologic studies, however, including the Nurses Health Study and the Framingham Study have shown that overweight and obesity-increased the risk for CAD even after correction for other known risk factors [27,28]. The American Heart Association recently added obesity to its list of major risk factors for CAD [29].

Box 1. Comorbidities and complications of obesity

Cardiovascular
Atherosclerotic cardiovascular disease
Dyslipidemia
Hypertension
Congestive heart failure
Stroke
Varicose veins
Pulmonary embolism

Pulmonary
Sleep apnea
Hypoventilation syndrome

Psychological
Depression
Poor self-image
Poor quality of life

Gastrointestinal
Gallbladder disease
Gastroesophageal reflux disease
Nonalcoholic fatty liver disease

Dermatological
Acanthosis nigricans
Hirsutism
Venous stasis
Cellulitis

Orthopedic
Degenerative osteoarthritis
Restrictive mobility

Reproductive
Polycystic ovary syndrome
Menstrual abnormalities
Infertility

Metabolic
Type 2 diabetes
Impaired glucose tolerance
Gout
Insulin resistance
Metabolic syndrome

Cancer
Breast
Colon
Prostate

Sleep apnea

Obese men and women are also at high risk for sleep apnea, in which partial or complete upper airway obstruction during sleep leads to episodes of apnea or hypopnea. The interruption in night-time sleep and repeated episodes of hypoxemia lead to daytime somnolence, morning headache, systemic hypertension, and eventually can result in pulmonary hypertension and right heart failure. In a study of 200 obese women and 50 obese men (mean BMI 45.3 kg/m^2) and 128 controls matched for age and sex, 40% of obese men and 3% of obese women demonstrated sleep apnea warranting therapeutic intervention. Another 8% of men and 5.5% of women showed sleep apneic activity that warranted recommendation for evaluation in the sleep laboratory. In contrast, none of the 128 controls demonstrated sleep apneic activity severe enough for therapeutic intervention [30].

Nonalcoholic fatty liver disease

Obesity is associated with a spectrum of liver disease known as nonalcoholic fatty liver disease (NAFLD) or nonalcoholic steatohepatitis (NASH). Manifestations of this disorder include hepatomegaly, abnormal liver function tests, and abnormal liver histology, including macrovesicular steatosis, steatohepatitis, fibrosis, and cirrhosis [31,32]. The exact prevalence of this disorder in obese patients is not known fully; however, data from autopsy studies suggest that steatohepatitis occurs in approximately 20% of obese patients [33]. NAFLD progresses to cirrhosis in approximately 10% of patients; however, the high prevalence of obesity and obesity-related liver disease makes NAFLD an important cause of cirrhosis.

Cancer

Overweight and obesity are associated with increased risk of esophageal, pancreatic, renal cell, postmenopausal breast, endometrial, cervical, and prostate cancers [34–38]. Several studies also have found a direct link between BMI and colon cancer in men and women [39,40]. A recent prospective study of more than 900,000 US adults found that increased body weight and obesity were associated with increased death rates for all cancers combined [41]. They estimated that overweight and obesity could account for about 14% of all cancer deaths in men and 20% of cancer deaths in women.

Health risks of obesity in children and adolescents

It is not just adults whose health is being impacted by obesity. As more and more children and adolescents are becoming obese, they are beginning to develop chronic diseases usually seen much later in life. For example, many obese children and adolescents are being diagnosed with type 2 diabetes [42], a disease that was virtually nonexistent in this population a few generations ago. Similarly, there is evidence that obesity in children and adolescents facilitates progression of cardiovascular disease [43].

Quality of life and function

Obesity has been associated with impaired quality of life. A 1998 study measured the impact of obesity on functional health status and subjective well-being. Health-related quality of life (HRQL), measured by the Medical Outcomes Study Short Form-36 Health Survey (SF-36), of over 300 obese patients seeking treatment for obesity at a university-based weight management center, was compared with that of the general population and with other patients with chronic medical conditions. Obese participants (mean BMI of 38.1 kg/m^2) reported significantly lower scores (more impairment) on all eight quality-of-life domains, especially bodily pain and vitality. The morbidly obese (mean BMI 48.7 kg/m^2) reported significantly worse physical, social, and role functioning, worse perceived general health, and greater bodily pain than did either the mildly (mean BMI 29.2 kg/m^2) or moderately to severely obese (mean BMI 34.5 kg/m^2). The obese also reported significantly greater disability caused by bodily pain than did patients with other chronic medical conditions [44].

Bias and discrimination against the obese have been documented [45,46]. Discrimination has been shown in employment, education, and health care [45]. Social stigmatization of obese children is present [46] and could represent one of the most serious consequences of obesity in children.

How did the epidemic arise?

To understand why the obesity epidemic arose, it is necessary to examine how body weight is regulated. The key to understanding body weight regulation is understanding energy balance. The body's state of energy balance is determined by the amount of energy ingested in food in relation to the amount of energy expended in metabolism and physical activity [47,48]. To maintain a stable body weight, energy intake must, over time, exactly equal energy expenditure. Negative energy balance (where energy expenditure exceeds energy intake) results in weight loss, and positive energy balance (where energy intake exceeds energy expenditure) results in weight gain.

There is considerable debate as to whether and to what extent, the body has physiological processes that serve to maintain energy balance. It does appear that there is some physiological regulation of energy balance, since changes on one or the other side (ie, energy intake or energy expenditure) of the energy balance equation do produce changes on the other side. For example, chronic changes in the amount of food consumed lead to changes in metabolism that serve to oppose a change in body weight [49]. Similarly, chronic changes in physical activity appear to have some impact on food intake [50,51]. Such compensatory physiological changes, however, are not sufficient to completely prevent changes in body weight in the face of positive or negative energy balance [50,51] suggesting a relatively weak physiological regulation of energy balance. Further, the physiological system may be biased to protect more against body weight loss than against body weight gain. This makes some sense in that for most of mankind's history, starvation was a much more serious problem than obesity [52].

The components of energy balance can be influenced by genetic and environmental factors. It is known, for example, that genes can impact each component of energy balance [53] and can explain much of the differences between individuals in body weight and body composition. Although one can conclude that genes are permissive for weight gain, the gradual weight gain of the population is not primarily caused by genetic factors.

The extent to which the body's physiological regulatory mechanisms serve to maintain a healthy weight depends on the environment. In an environment where high levels of physical activity are necessary for securing food and shelter and for transportation and where food is inconsistently available, the body's physiological regulatory mechanisms work well and serve to help facilitate sufficient food intake to avoid loss of body mass. As the environment gradually has changed to one where high levels of physical activity are not required in daily life and where food is abundant, inexpensive, and served in large portions, however, the physiological regulation of body weight appears to be insufficient to oppose weight gain and obesity.

Obesity researchers increasingly are looking to the environment for an explanation for the gradual weight gain of the population. Brownell was among the first to point out the potential role that environmental factors play in facilitating food intake and in discouraging physical activity, and he describes these factors elsewhere in this issue. The current food environment is one where food is inexpensive, abundant, and served in very large portions [19]. Similarly, there is only a rare need for physical activity for food, shelter, and transportation [19]. These environmental influences serve to reduce physical activity (which reduces energy intake) and to increase energy intake. The body's physiological system for regulating energy balance is not sufficiently strong in most people to completely oppose these environmental influences, and the result is that most Americans seem to be in a state of gradual positive energy balance over time, producing gradual weight gain over time and obesity. It is important to realize that changes in the environment occurred gradually over time, and only recently has society realized that the obesity epidemic arose as an unintended consequence of societal progress. The environment is one to which our ancestors aspired, and includes a consistent supply of good-tasting, inexpensive, available food and the ability to not have to work hard physically to secure food, shelter, and transportation.

With the realization that the environment is facilitating obesity has come interest in modifying the environment to help address the obesity epidemic.

Although research in this area is only beginning, it represents an exciting new approach to obesity. There are, however, some cautions. First, it is unlikely that modifying the environment alone will solve the problem with obesity. The problem is that so many things that have contributed to obesity are things that enrich lives in other ways. For example, there is instant access to information throughout the world through televisions, computers, and personal digital assistants. The fact that these tools contribute to reduced physical activity and thus promote weight gain only recently has been realized. Similarly, the increase in families where both parents work has increased and contributed to the rise of fast food restaurants, because few people have the time or energy to come home from work and prepare home cooked meals. It is unlikely that people can go back in time by giving up these things. It is more likely that people will learn how to modify the environment to support and sustain specific behavioral changes in the population to help people maintain healthy weights. The need to deal with environment and behavior is illustrated in Fig. 17. Human biology developed to work best in a different environment, one where food was inconsistent, and high levels of physical activity were required to secure food, shelter, and for transportation. In previous environments, physical activity was the driver for achieving energy balance, and food intake was pulled along [47]. People developed multiple physiological systems to facilitate eating with no need for physiological systems for food restriction,

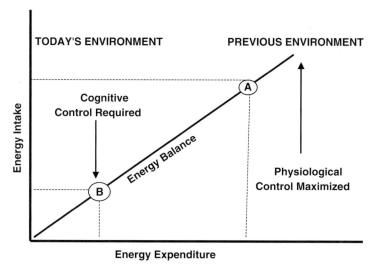

Fig. 17. The past environment (A) required high levels of activity and allowed energy balance and a stable body weight to be achieved under physiological control. Activity was the driver and pulled along food intake. The current environment (B) has created a different situation where very little physical activity is required for daily activities. Energy balance is achieved through conscious efforts to eat less to match the low levels of expenditure.

and no need to develop a biological preference to be physically active when physical activity was not required. Essentially, human biology tells people to eat whenever food is available and rest whenever physical activity is not required. In previous environments, this biology was adequate to allow most people to maintain a healthy weight without conscious effort. Body weight regulation was achieved for most with simple physiological control.

Fig. 16 also illustrates how the situation is different in today's environment. Today's environment requires very little physical activity. Securing food and shelter and moving around the environment do not require the high levels of physical activity required in the past [19]. Technology has made it possible to be productive while being largely sedentary. Under such conditions, weight gain can be prevented only with conscious efforts to eat less or to be physically active. The minority of Americans who are maintaining a healthy weight likely are exercising cognitive control of eating and physical activity patterns to eat less than they would otherwise and to be physically active without the necessity to be physically active. In today's environment, maintaining a healthy body weight cannot be left to physiological processes but requires cognitive effort. This does not mean that one should not look for ways to modify the environment to make it easy for people to avoid overeating and a sedentary lifestyle. It does mean that the focus cannot be exclusively on changing individual behavior or on changing the environment, but on the combination. The environment must be changed to facilitate and sustain the behavior changes required to avoid obesity.

Dealing with the complexity of obesity

The more that is understood about the etiology of obesity, the more complex it appears. Obesity involves interaction among human biology, behavior, and the environment. Major efforts are underway that focus on each of the major issues, but few, if any, focus on how the issues interact. Focusing only on one of these major areas is likely to be incomplete. The biology of obesity needs to be understood, but only in rare cases is obesity the result of a biological defect. Similarly, one needs to understand better how to change behavior, but to do this one has to appreciate our biology and the environment. Figuring out how to change the environment to make a difference in obesity also will require appreciation of biology and behavior. Finally, obesity even involves the ways people constructed society, the shared collective worldview, and the material base of this worldview. For example, a recent analysis of economics and lifestyle [14,54,55] suggests the need to better understand the complex economic factors that are supporting current diet and physical activity patterns, and to think about how these could be changed to support a healthier lifestyle. Researchers must begin to examine ways that to replace those aspects of society that support obesity with those that support healthier lifestyles. There is a need to begin to construct a vision of what society would look like if it supported maintenance of a healthy body weight and supported obesity prevalence rates that were acceptable.

Strategies for getting out of the obesity epidemic

It is important to begin to craft strategies that could get society out of the obesity epidemic. Fig. 18, adopted from the work of Rossner, illustrates some possibilities. If nothing is done, the weight of the population will continue to increase until a time when all of those who are not protected genetically will be overweight or obese. How might obesity prevalence rates be reduced to acceptable levels over time?

One possibility is to reduce weight in many of those people who are already overweight or obese. The problem is that the ability to produce and maintain substantial weight loss is not good [56–58]. Most people who lose large amounts of weight regain this weight completely within a few years [56–58]. Rarely does anyone go permanently from the obese category to the healthy weight category. Health care professionals recommend that weight loss goals of 5% to 10% of initial weight can be achieved and maintained in many people [6]. The bottom line is that there is not a good ability to produce and maintain significant amounts of weight loss in large numbers of overweight and obese individuals. Although obesity treatment strategies will improve over time, this strategy cannot be relied upon to reverse the obesity epidemic.

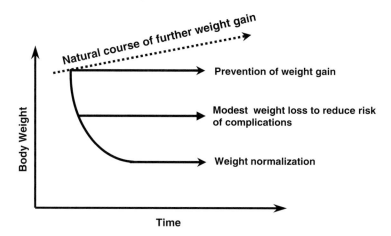

Fig. 18. Possible outcomes of obesity treatments. (*From* Rossner S. Factors determining the long-term outcome of obesity treatment. In: Bjorntorp P, Brodoff BN, editors. Obesity. Philadelphia: J.B. Lippincott; 1992. p. 712–9; with permission.)

One possible way to reverse the obesity epidemic is through prevention. This could begin with stopping the gradual weight gain in the adult population and identifying and stopping excessive weight gain in children. It previously has been demonstrated that weight gain in most adults can be prevented with small changes in energy balance of 100 420 kJ per day or less [47]. Preventing further weight gain in the population could have significant positive impacts on health and health care costs of the population, since increasing BMI is associated with increasing risk of chronic disease and with increasing health care costs [15]. The extent of changes in energy balance required for children and adolescents has not been quantified, but should be less than that required for significant weight loss. By using a strategy of stopping excessive weight gain, the prevalence of obesity would decrease with each successive generation. Although it may take decades to reverse the obesity epidemic using this strategy, the positive is that the behavior changes required to stop excessive weight gain may be produced and maintained. This can be done by focusing on specific behavior change and modifying the environment in ways to support and sustain the desired behavior changes.

Summary

In pursuing the good life people have created an environment and a society that unintentionally promote weight gain and obesity, given people's genetic and biological make-up. The consequences of the obesity epidemic are severe, affecting the health, quality of life, and economics of the nation. Dealing with the epidemic of obesity is likely to be one of the greatest challenges society has faced. To reverse the obesity epidemic, specific strategies need to be developed that recognize the complexity of the issue. Obesity involves biology, behavior, and the environment. The ways society currently promotes obesity must be re-examined, and what things can be changed must be determined. The ways communities are built need to be re-examined, along with the ways foods are produced and marketed and the ways sedentary behavior is promoted inadvertently.

There is a growing realization that it is time to get serious about public health efforts to reverse the obesity epidemic. Although obesity prevalence rates have been rising since the 1980s it is only within the past 5 years that the issue has risen to a high priority for the public health community and policy makers. Thus, it is not surprising that no large-scale national initiatives exist to deal with the problem. The need to develop such initiatives is apparent, but there is no clear strategy for doing so.

There is some reason to be optimistic about dealing with obesity. Many previous threats to public health have been addressed successfully. It was probably inconceivable in the 1950s to think that major public health initiatives could have such a dramatic effect on reducing the prevalence of smoking in the United States. Yet, this serious problem was addressed by a combination of strategies involving public health, economics, political advocacy, behavior change, and environmental change. Similarly, Americans have been persuaded to use seat belts and recycle, addressing two other challenges to public health [59].

But, there is also reason to be pessimistic. The challenge with obesity may be greater than past challenges. In the other examples cited, clear goals existed: to stop smoking, increase the use seatbelts, and increase recycling. The difficulty of achieving these goals should not be minimized, but they were clear and simple goals. With obesity, there is no clear agreement about goals. There is no agreement among experts as to which strategies should be implemented on a widespread basis to achieve the behavioral changes in the population needed to reverse the high prevalence rates of obesity. Success models are needed that will help people understand what to do to address obesity. But, while success models are needed, there is a great deal of urgency in responding to the obesity epidemic. Once people get serious about addressing obesity, it will likely take decades to reverse obesity rates to levels seen 30 years ago. Meanwhile, the prevalence of overweight and obesity increases yearly, and the opportunity to prevent obesity in most people is being lost rapidly.

References

[1] Mokdad AH, Marks JS, Stroup DF, et al. Actual causes of death in the United States, 2000. JAMA 2004;291(10):1238–45.
[2] Data from International Food Information Council (IFIC). Available at: http://ific.org/foodinsight/2004/jf/fftfi104.cfm. Accessed April 2004.
[3] Mokdad AH, Bowman BA, Ford ES, et al. The continuing epidemics of obesity and diabetes in the United States. JAMA 2001;286:1195–200.
[4] US Department of Health and Human Services. The Surgeon General's call to action to prevent and decrease overweight and obesity. Rockville, MD: US Department of Health and Human Services, Public Health Service. Office of the Surgeon General. 2001.
[5] World Health Organization. Obesity: preventing and managing the global epidemic. Report of a WHO Consultation on Obesity, Geneva 3–5 June 1997. Geneva (Switzerland): World Health Organization; 1998.
[6] National Heart, Lung, and Blood Institute Obesity Education Initiative Expert Panel. Clinical guidelines on the identification, evaluation, and treatment of overweight and obesity in adults: the evidence report. Obes Res 1998;6(Suppl 2):51S–210S.
[7] Flegal KM, Carroll MD, Ogden CL, et al. Prevalence and trends in obesity among US adults, 1999–2000. JAMA 2002;288:1723–7.
[8] Data from National Center for Health Statistics Website. Available at: www.cdc.gov/nchs/products/pubs/pubd/hestats/obese/obse99.htm Accessed April 2004.
[9] Lewis CE, Jacobs DR, McCreath H, et al. Weight gain continues in the 1990s: 10-year trends in weight and overweight from the CARDIA study. Am J Epidemiol 2000;151:1172–81.
[10] Molarius A, Seidell JC, Sans S, et al. Educational level, relative body weight, and changes in their association over 10 years: an international perspective from the WHO MONICA Project. Am J Public Health 2000;90(8):1260–8.
[11] Sobal J, Stunkard A. Socioeconomic status and obesity: a review of the literature. Psychol Bull 1989;105:260–75.

[12] Truong K, Sturm R. Does the obesity epidemic widen socioeconomic health disparities in the US? Working paper. Rand Institute; 2004.

[13] Drewnowski A, Specter SE. Poverty and obesity: the role of energy density and energy costs. Am J Clin Nutr 2004;79(1):6–16.

[14] Cawley J. An economic framework for understanding physical activity ad eating behaviors. Am J Prev Med, in press.

[15] Sturm R, Ringel JS, Andreyeva T. Increasing obesity rates and disability trends. Health Aff 2004;23(2):199–205.

[16] Ogden CL, Flegal KM, Carroll MD, et al. Prevalence and trends in overweight among US children and adolescents, 1999–2000. JAMA 2002;288(14):1728–32.

[17] Cole TJ, Bellizzi MC, Flegal KM, et al. Establishing a standard definition for child overweight and obesity worldwide: international survey. BMJ 2000;320(7244):1240–3.

[18] Data from Foundation for Child Development Web site. Available at: http://www.fcd-us.org/news/fact_sheet68910882.html. Accessed April 2004.

[19] Hill JO, Wyatt HR, Reed GW, et al. Obesity and the environment: where do we go from here? Science 2003;299:853–5.

[20] Allison DB, Saunders SE. Obesity in North America: an overview. Med Clin North Am 2000;84(2):305–33.

[21] National Task Force on the Prevention and Treatment of Obesity. Overweight, obesity and health risk. Arch Intern Med 2000;160:898–904.

[22] Colditz GA, Willett WC, Stampfer MJ, et al. Weight as a risk factor for clinical diabetes in women. Am J Epidemiol 1990;132(3):501–13.

[23] Terry RB, Wood PD, Haskell WL, et al. Regional adiposity patterns in relation to lipids, lipoprotein cholesterol, and lipoprotein subfraction mass in men. J Clin Endocrinol Metab 1989;68(1):191–9.

[24] Brown CD, Higgins M, Donato KA, et al. Body mass index and the prevalence of hypertension and dyslipidemia. Obes Res 2000;8(9):605–19.

[25] Frayn KN. Visceral fat and insulin resistance—causative or correlative? Br J Nutr 2000; 83(Suppl 1):S71–7.

[26] Stamler J, Wentworth D, Neaton JD. Is relationship between serum cholesterol and risk of premature death from coronary disease continuous or graded? Findings in 356,222 primary screenees of the Multiple Risk Factor Intervention Trial (MRFIT). JAMA 1986;256(20): 2823–8.

[27] Manson JE, Willett WC, Stampfer MJ, et al. Body weight and mortality among women. N Engl J Med 1995;333(11):677–85.

[28] Hubert HB, Feinleib M, McNamara PM, et al. Obesity as an independent risk factor for cardiovascular disease: a 26-year follow-up of participants in the Framingham Heart Study. Circulation 1983;67(5):968–77.

[29] Eckel RH, Krauss RM. American Heart Association call to action: obesity as a major risk factor for coronary heart disease. AHA Nutrition Committee. Circulation 1998;97(21): 2099–100.

[30] Vgontzas AN, Tan TL, Bixler EO, et al. Sleep apnea and sleep disruption in obese patients. Arch Intern Med 1994;154(15):1705–11.

[31] Matteoni C, Younossi ZM, McCullough A. Nonalcoholic fatty liver disease: a spectrum of clinical pathological severity. Gastroenterology 1999;116(6):1413–9.

[32] Adler M, Schaffner F. Fatty liver hepatitis and cirrhosis in obese patients. Am J Med 1979; 67(6):811–6.

[33] Wanless IR, Lentz JS. Fatty liver hepatitis (steatohepatitis) and obesity: an autopsy study with analysis of risk factors. Hepatology 1990;12(5):1106–10.

[34] Romero Y, Cameron AJ, Locke GR III, et al. Familial aggregation of gastroesophageal reflux in patients with Barrett's esophagus and esophageal adenocarcinoma. Gastroenterology 1997;113(5):1449–56.

[35] Michaud DS, Giovannucci E, Willett WC, et al. Physical activity, obesity, height, and the risk of pancreatic cancer. JAMA 2001;286(8):921–9.

[36] Chow WH, Gridley G, Fraumeni JF, et al. Obesity, hypertension, and the risk of kidney cancer in men. N Engl J Med 2000;343(18):1305–11.

[37] Huang Z, Hankinson SE, Colditz GA, et al. Dual effects of weight and weight gain on breast cancer risk. JAMA 1997;278(17):1407–11.

[38] Schottenfeld D, Fraumeni JF. Cancer epidemiology and prevention. New York: Oxford Press; 1996.

[39] Giovannucci E, Ascherio A, Rimm EB, et al. Physical activity, obesity, and risk for colon cancer and adenoma in men. Ann Intern Med 1995;122(5):327–34.

[40] Giovannucci E, Colditz GA, Stampfer MJ, et al. Physical activity, obesity, and risk of colorectal adenoma in women (United States). Cancer Causes Control 1996;7(2):253–63.

[41] Calle EE, Rodriguez C, Walker-Thurmond K, et al. Overweight, obesity, and mortality from cancer in a prospectively studied cohort of US adults. N Engl J Med 2003;348(17):1625–38.

[42] Fagot-Campagna A, Pettitt DJ, Engelgau MM, et al. Type diabetes among North American children and adolescents: an epidemiological review and public health perspective. J Pediatr 2000;136(5):664–72.

[43] Freedman DS, Dietz WH, Srinivasan SR, et al. The relation of overweight to cardiovascular risk factors among children and adolescents: the Bogalusa Heart Study. Pediatrics 1999;103: 1175–82.

[44] Burton WN, Chen CY, Schultz AB, et al. The economic costs associated with body mass index in the workplace. J Occup Environ Med 1998;40(9):786–92.

[45] Puhl R, Brownell KD. Bias, discrimination, and obesity. Obes Res 2001;9(12):788–805.

[46] Schwartz MB, Puhl R. Childhood obesity: a societal problem to solve. Obes Rev 2003;4(1): 57–71.

[47] Peters JC, Wyatt HR, Donahoo WT, Hill JO. From instinct to intellect: the challenge of maintaining healthy weight in the modern world. Obes Rev 2002;3(2):69–74.

[48] Hill JO, Wyatt HR, Melanson EL. Environmental and genetic contributions to obesity. Med Clin North Am 2000;84(2):333–46.

[49] Horton TJ, Drougas H, Brachey A, et al. Fat and carbohydrate overfeeding in humans: different effects on energy storage. Am J Clin Nutr 1995;62(1):19–29.

[50] Blundell JE, Stubbs RJ, Hughes DA, et al. Cross talk between physical activity and appetite control: does physical activity stimulate appetite? Proc Nutr Soc 2003;62(3):651–61.

[51] Epstein LH, Paluch RA, Consalvi A, et al. Effects of manipulating sedentary behavior on physical activity and food intake. Journal of Pediatrics 2002;140(3):334–9.

[52] Prentice AM. Fires of life: the struggles of an ancient metabolism in a modern world. British Nutrition Foundation, Nutrition Bulletin 2001;26:13–27.

[53] Bouchard C, Perusse L, Rice T, et al. Genetics of human obesity. In: Bray GA, Bouchard C, editors. Handbook of obesity. New York: Marcel Dekker; 2004. p. 157–200.

[54] Sturm R. The economics of physical activity: societal trends and rationale for Interventions. Am J Prev Med, in press.

[55] Hill JO, Peters JC, Sallis JF. An economic analysis of eating and physical activity: a next step for research and policy change. Am J Prev Med, in press.

[56] Wing RR, Hill JO. Successful weight loss maintenance. Annu Rev Nutr 2001;21:323–41.

[57] Brownell KD. Diet, exercise and behavioural intervention: the nonpharmacological approach. Eur J Clin Invest 1998;28(Suppl 2):19–21 [discussion 22].

[58] Wadden TA, Foster GD, Letizia KA. One-year behavioral treatment of obesity: comparison of moderate and severe caloric restriction and the effects of weight maintenance therapy. J Consult Clin Psychol 1994;62:165–71.

[59] Economos CD, Brownson RC, DeAngelis MA, et al. What lessons have been learned from other attempts to guide social change? Nutr Rev 2001;59:S40–56 [discussion S57–65].

ELSEVIER
SAUNDERS

PSYCHIATRIC
CLINICS
OF NORTH AMERICA

Psychiatr Clin N Am 28 (2005) 25–38

The Regulation of Energy Balance by the Central Nervous System

Karine Proulx, MS[a], Randy J. Seeley, PhD[b],*

[a]Department of Neuroscience, University of Cincinnati College of Medicine, 2170 East Galbraith Road, ML 0506, Building 43, Room 312, Cincinnati, OH 45237, USA
[b]Department of Psychiatry, University of Cincinnati College of Medicine, 2170 East Galbraith Road, ML 0506, Building 43, Room 312, Cincinnati, OH 45237, USA

Obesity is the result of a sustained mismatch in which caloric intake exceeds caloric expenditure. In fact, despite what the growing obesity epidemic might argue, under most circumstances the energy balance equation is regulated with tremendous precision over time. Such profound accuracy implies that body weight, or more precisely body adipose mass, is a biologically regulated variable, and that evolution has selected for mechanisms by which caloric intake can be matched to caloric expenditure. Although obesity is increasingly common, it is even more common in those suffering from serious psychiatric disorders [1]. Although many of the drugs used to treat psychiatric disorders can produce weight gain, it would appear that the relationship between obesity and mental health problems exists independent of medication. Epidemiological studies have demonstrated that mood and binge-eating disorders coexist with obesity in a significant minority of individuals [2,3]. The comorbidity of psychiatric disorders with obesity suggests the existence of common biological underpinnings that may influence the regulation of normal cognition and mood, on the one hand, and the central nervous system (CNS) circuits that regulate energy balance on the other. Thus the purpose of this article is to review a handful of the neurochemical systems implicated in the regulation of energy homeostasis. Where possible, the authors speculate about how some of these neurochemical systems have been linked to psychiatric disorders.

This article was supported by grants from the NIH (DK54890) and funds from the Procter & Gamble Company.
* Corresponding author.
E-mail address: randy.seeley@uc.edu (R.J. Seeley).

The regulation of body weight

Much evidence supports the notion that mammals are designed to carefully regulate the amount of stored energy in the body with most of that energy stored as lipid in adipose tissue [4]. To regulate energy balance requires that significant deviations in the amount of stored fuel must be detected, and this triggers error correction mechanisms that alter food intake, energy expenditure or both to bring the levels of stored fuel back to the defended level. So when an individual goes on a diet and voluntarily moves into negative energy balance, stores of fat are catabolized to provide energy. What also occurs is the recruitment of a complex and redundantly wired neuroendocrine system that serves to make the individual prone to consume additional calories and increase energy efficiency, reducing the energy expended in daily activity. The combination of increased calorie intake and decreased calorie expenditure biases the individual toward being in positive energy balance, which in turn restores the level of stored fuel to its defended levels.

Leptin

Several lines of evidence point to a crucial role for circulating hormones as critical to the detection of the levels of stored fuel in adipose mass. One of these hormones has been termed leptin from the Greek "leptos" for thin [5]. Leptin is the product of the ob gene and is made primarily in adipocytes [6]. Circulating levels of leptin are proportional to body fat and are reduced in times of negative energy balance in rodents and people [7,8]. Mice that do not make a biologically active form of leptin, ob/ob mice, overeat and gain tremendous amounts of weight [5]. Leptin replacement in ob/ob mice reverses this phenotype, resulting in significant weight loss [5]. Although most obese individuals have elevated levels of leptin, a handful of individuals have been identified with mutations similar to that found in ob/ob mice. Like the mice, these individuals show ravenous appetites and profound obesity that can be potently treated by exogenous leptin treatment [9]. Although leptin treatment works very well in leptin-deficient patients, use of leptin in obese patients with already high levels of leptin has shown limited efficacy [10].

Some controversy surrounds the relative contribution of peripheral and CNS leptin receptors to the control of energy balance; however, it is clear that the CNS is an important target of leptin's actions [11]. Leptin acts in the CNS by means of the long form of its receptor that is found in several regions of the brain, including prominently in the arcuate nucleus of the hypothalamus [11]. Central administration of leptin recapitulates much of the effect of peripherally administered leptin at lower doses, indicating that the CNS is an important target for leptin's actions [12]. Selective deletion of leptin receptors in the CNS leads to increased food intake and obesity [13].

Recently, also leptin has been described to have powerful effects to change the very wiring of the CNS circuits that control food intake and body weight. Thus, leptin acts to change several properties of critical homeostatic circuitry that project from the arcuate to other key hypothalamic regions [14].

Insulin

When people or animals consume nutrients, blood glucose levels rise, and in turn, insulin is secreted to facilitate the uptake of glucose into several peripheral tissues, where it can be burned or stored. In addition to this critical peripheral action, insulin shares many properties with leptin. Like leptin, circulating insulin levels reflect the amount of stored body fat [15,16]. Insulin also has specific receptors in the CNS located in some of the same regions as leptin receptors (including high concentrations in the arcuate) [17]. Administration of insulin directly into the CNS reduces food intake and produces sustained body weight loss [18–20]. Targeted disruption of CNS insulin receptors leads to increases in body weight [21]. So while peripheral administration of insulin can produce weight gain by means of its actions on adipocytes, in the CNS, insulin causes weight loss [4,22]. This dichotomy can be highlighted by insulin mimetic molecules that are more lipid soluble than insulin and therefore cross the blood-brain barrier at a much higher rate [23]. Either central or peripheral administration of such molecules results in decreased weight gain over time [24]. Taken together, these data make a compelling case that similar to leptin, insulin acts as a signal to the CNS about the status of peripheral energy stores.

Ghrelin

Leptin and insulin are negative feedback signals. They increase when there are sufficient calorie stores, and their presence inhibits further food intake. This is not the only way to design the system. A positive feedback signal would be one that increased when calorie stores were dwindling and produced an increase in food intake. One hormone has been hypothesized to be such a positive signal: ghrelin. This is the only peripheral hormone identified that increases food intake [25–27].

Circulating peripheral ghrelin is produced primarily in the stomach [28], and levels are increased after periods of negative energy balance that result in decrease calorie stores [29–31]. Ghrelin acts on the growth hormone secretagogue receptor (GHS-R) to increase growth hormone levels [32,33]. Independent of this action, however, ghrelin can produce increased food intake and sustained increases in body weight [26,27,34,35]. Like insulin and leptin, ghrelin appears to have peripheral and central actions. Ghrelin's receptor is found in key regions of the hypothalamus such as the arcuate

[36], and central administration of ghrelin results in potent increases in food intake [27]. Ghrelin also appears to be made in the CNS [37], and whether peripherally derived ghrelin acts directly upon the arcuate nucleus remains controversial. Some data would indicate that peripheral ghrelin acts by means of changes in vagal nerve activity [38], and the relationship between peripheral and central ghrelin regulation remains unclear.

Hypothalamic targets of peripheral signals

The arcuate nucleus of the hypothalamus has dense receptor populations for leptin, insulin, and ghrelin. As a consequence, this particular nucleus makes a logical starting place to identify critical neurochemical targets for these important peripheral signals. Within the arcuate, there are at least two distinct populations of cells that are regulated reciprocally by the peripheral hormones. One population of cells synthesizes the large precursor peptide proopiomelanocortin (POMC). Although this precursor can be cleaved into a number of biologically active peptides, several of its products are agonists for one or more of the five identified melanocortin receptors (MC-R) [39]. One of these ligands is corticotropin (ACTH), which acts as an agonist for MC2-R found almost exclusively in the adrenal gland, where it stimulates glucocorticoid secretion [39]. Another important ligand cleaved from POMC is α-melanocyte stimulating hormone (α-MSH). α-MSH is an agonist at peripheral MC1-R that controls skin and hair pigmentation [39].

In the CNS, α-MSH is an agonist at MC3-R and MC4-R. α-MSH and various synthetic analogs can reduce food intake potently and produce body weight loss when delivered directly in the CNS [40–42]. Presumably the potent effect on food intake is mediated by α-MSH acting on MC4-R, since mice with targeted genetic disruption of MC4-R show increased food intake and body fat [43]. Mice with genetic disruption of MC3-R show a small increase in body fat that is not attributable to changes in food intake [44]. Arcuate POMC neurons project to several other hypothalamic regions but also have monosynaptic projections to the spinal cord, where they can influence sympathetic activity directly [45].

The second set of neurons in the arcuate synthesizes agouti-related protein (AgRP) and neuropeptide Y (NPY) [46,47]. AgRP is a unique peptide, because it acts as an endogenous competitive antagonist/inverse agonist at MC3-R and MC4-R [48,49]. Thus in the presence of α-MSH, AgRP can lower MC4-R activity by reducing the ability of α-MSH to bind and activate MC4-R 49. Even in the absence of α-MSH, however, AgRP can act to reduce constitutive activity of MC4-R [48]. As would be predicted from this dual action of AgRP to reduce MC4-R activity, central administration of AgRP produces potent increases in food intake and subsequent body weight gain [50]. In fact, the effects of AgRP are incredibly long-lived, with a single injection capable of increasing food intake for periods as long as 6 days [51].

Coproduced with AgRP in arcuate neurons is NPY, a member of the pancreatic polypeptide family with very potent orexigenic properties [52]. Although NPY interacts with at least five distinct NPY receptor subtypes (NPY-Y1, Y2, Y4, Y5, Y6) to mediate a wide spectrum of central and peripheral actions that include anxiolysis, memory, and circadian rhythms [53], NPY's potent effects on feeding occur specifically through coordinated activation of NPY-Y1 and NPY-Y5 [54]. This hyperphagia, together with a concomitant reduction in brown adipose tissue thermogenesis, leads to potent weight gain when the peptide is administered chronically [55].

Regulation of proopiomelanocortin and neuropeptide Y/Agouti-related protein neurons by peripheral signals

Proopiomelanocortin and NPY/AgRP neurons detect changes in energy balance conveyed by the peripheral hormones (Fig. 1). In the case of POMC, one would predict that leptin and insulin should activate POMC neurons. Leptin has been shown to increase the firing rate of POMC neurons [14], and both leptin and insulin stimulate POMC gene expression [56–58]. Moreover, the effects of leptin and insulin to suppress food intake can be blocked by melanocortin receptor antagonists [59–61]. Leptin and insulin also appear to inhibit AgRP/NPY neurons, since both inhibit gene expression of AgRP/NPY in the arcuate nucleus [62–65]. Taken together, these data implicate an important role for the melanocortin/NPY system to mediate the effects of leptin and insulin to suppress food intake.

The prediction for ghrelin should be just the opposite of leptin and insulin. Because ghrelin levels are elevated during negative energy balance, ghrelin should activate AgRP/NPY neurons while suppressing POMC neurons. Several lines of evidence indicate that ghrelin increases neuronal firing of AgRP/NPY neurons [37] and increases AgRP and NPY gene expression [28]. Moreover, blocking of AgRP or NPY with antagonists or immunoneutralizing antibodies blocks ghrelin's ability to increase food intake [27,66]. In mice with targeted genetic disruption of both AgRP and NPY, ghrelin appears to be ineffective to increase food intake [67]. Finally, ghrelin inhibits the neuronal firing of POMC neurons [37]. Thus, in several meaningful ways, ghrelin acts in opposition to the arcuate nucleus actions of leptin and insulin.

These two populations of neurons appear to be regulated reciprocally by peripheral hormone levels. This is not the only mechanism, however, that coordinates the activity of AgRP/NPY neurons with their POMC neighbors. AgRP/NPY neurons have collaterals that synapse on POMC neurons within the arcuate [14]. Colocalized in these terminals is the inhibitory neurotransmitter γ-aminobutyric acid (GABA), such that when AgRP/NPY neurons are activated, they also release GABA onto POMC neurons [14]. Electrophysiological evidence indicates that leptin's ability to activate

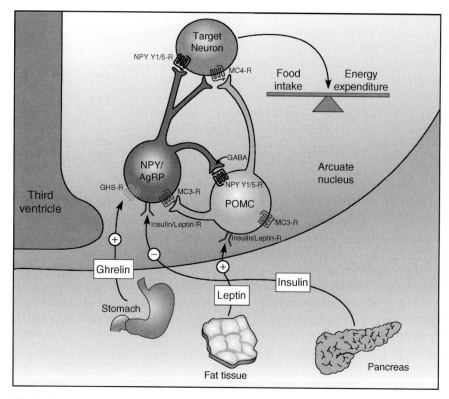

Fig. 1. Actions of leptin, insulin and ghrelin on distinct neuronal populations in the arcuate nucleus of the hypothalamus. Leptin and insulin inhibit activity of agouti-related peptide/ neuropeptide Y (AgRP/ NPY) neurons while stimulating activity of pro-opiomelanocortin (POMC) neurons. Ghrelin stimulates activity of AgRP/NPY neurons, and this results in inhibition of POMC neurons. NPY and AgRP (a melanocortin receptor antagonist) can increase food intake potently and result in accumulation of increased stored calories. POMC is a precursor for several biologically active peptides, including alpha-melanocyte stimulating hormone (α-MSH). α-MSH acts as a melanocortin receptor agonist. Through these disparate actions on distinct cell types in the arcuate nucleus, peripheral signals can influence the amount of NPY and melanocortin signaling in downstream target neurons.
Abbreviations: Insulin/leptin-R, insulin/leptin receptor; MC-R, melanocortin receptor; NPY Y-R, NPY receptor; GHS-R, growth hormone secretagogue receptor. (*Adapted from* Barsh GS, Schwartz MW. Nat Rev Genet 2002;3:589–600.)

POMC neurons is caused by direct actions of leptin on POMC neurons but also because of disinhibiting of the GABA tone as leptin inhibits the AgRP/ NPY neurons [14].

Serotonin

The regulation of energy balance depends critically on the interaction of peripheral signals with a network of neurons in which the arcuate nucleus plays a critical role. It has long been known, however, that other neurotransmitter and hormonal systems implicated in psychiatric disorders can have dramatic impacts on food intake and body weight. One of these is serotonin. Serotonin (5-HT) is a widespread neurotransmitter synthesized in the raphe nucleus and in the peripheral nervous system [68]. At least 14 distinct 5-HT receptors have been identified and are widely localized within the CNS, including in hypothalamic nuclei implicated in the control of energy balance [69]. Experiments in rodents and people have demonstrated that several serotonin agonists or reuptake inhibitors are anorexigenics [70,71] and stimulate energy expenditure [72]. Compounds reducing 5-HT neurotransmission have the opposite effects; they are orexigenics, and they inhibit energy expenditure [73].

Although an association between the serotonin system and feeding was postulated several decades ago (Tecott) [68], the mechanisms underlying 5-HT-induced anorexia have just started to be unraveled. Although multiple receptor subtypes are likely involved in 5-HT's effect on appetite, recent evidence suggests an important role for $5-HT_{2C}$ receptor in particular [74]. Genetic deletion of $5-HT_{2C}$ induces hyperphagia and obesity in mice [75–77]. The opposite effect is observed with administration of relatively selective $5-HT_{2C}$ agonists. As an example, dexfenfluramine (d-fenfluramine), an agonist of the $5-HT_{2A/2C}$ receptors, has been reported to cause hypophagia and weight loss in obese individuals [78]. Early studies suggested that d-fenfluramine-induced anorexia occurs at least partially through activation of $5-HT_{2C}$ in the hypothalamus. Site-specific injection of d-fenfluramine into various subregions of the hypothalamus causes anorexia [79], and d-fenfluramine is much less effective in mice with targeted genetic disruption of $5-HT_{2C}$ receptors [80]. The authors note that d-fenfluramine was removed from the market on Sept. 15, 1997, when it was found to be associated with valvular heart disease in people.

An important question is whether 5-HT's potent anorexic effects are mediated by the arcuate nucleus circuits that also integrate peripheral information about energy stores. A recent report makes a compelling argument that the arcuate nucleus melanocortin system is an important target of 5-HT action on food intake. $5-HT_{2C}$ receptors are found on POMC-producing neurons in the arcuate nucleus [81]. In vitro electrophysiological recordings demonstrate that d-fenfluramine activates POMC neurons [82]. Finally, similar to leptin and insulin, melanocortin receptor antagonists greatly diminish d-fenfluramine's effects to reduce food intake [82]. As a consequence, it would appear that this melanocortin system is a critical node that integrates multiple influences on food intake and body weight from peripheral and central sources.

Several drugs used to treat depression, schizophrenia, anxiety, hallucinations, dysthymia, and sleep disorders modulate $5-HT_{2C}$ [83]. Some of these medications have antagonistic properties for the $5-HT_{2C}$ [84,85]. Others can cause an atypical down-regulation of this receptor subtype [83]. It is therefore reasonable to hypothesize that a reduction of activity in the CNS melanocortin system may be a component of the weight gain experienced by patients treated with antidepressants and antipsychotics. Further, pharmacogenomic data indicate an association between polymorphism of the 5-HT_{2C} promoter and weight gain observed in first-episode schizophrenic patients treated with antipsychotics [86], and the authors would hypothesize that this may be the result of changes in melanocortin activity.

Glucocorticoids

Much literature has tried to link the secretion and actions of glucocorticoids to several psychiatric disorders [87,88]. Although it is beyond the scope of this article to synthesize that literature, it is clear that glucocorticoids have important peripheral and central effects to regulate energy balance [89,90]. Glucocorticoids are steroid hormones secreted by the zona fasciculata of the adrenal cortex that bind to two subtypes of intracellular receptors: the mineralocorticoid receptors (type I, MR) and the glucocorticoid receptors (type II, GR). Under basal conditions with low glucocorticoid secretion, the occupancy of MR is close to saturation. When glucocorticoid levels rise during stress or the peak of the circadian cycle, MR becomes fully occupied, and glucocorticoids start binding to GR [91]. Because rodents are nocturnally active, corticosterone peaks before the onset of the dark phase and decreases to attain its lowest concentration at the end of this [92]. In people, this pattern is reversed, so that peak concentrations of cortisol are reached early in the morning, before awakening [93]. The circadian rhythm of glucocorticoid secretion also is regulated by the timing of meal intake in rodents and in people [94,95]. Glucocorticoid levels rise before the consumption of a meal, and manipulations of the pattern of meals alter the pattern of glucocorticoid secretion [94,95]. Low energy stores rapidly stimulate ACTH and glucocorticoid secretion in situations of negative energy balance [96]. This effect is persistent, because glucocorticoid negative feedback efficacy on the hypothalamo-pituitary-adrenal (HPA) axis also is reduced in these conditions [96].

The critical role of glucocorticoids in regulating feeding behavior and body weight is illustrated best in conditions associated with hypersecretion or hyposecretion of glucocorticoids. Patients with glucocorticoid excess, of either endogenous (Cushing's syndrome) or exogenous (corticosteroids treatment) origin, report a marked elevation in appetite and accumulate additional abdominal fat [97,98]. On the other hand, patients with glucocorticoid deficiency (Addison's disease) report reduced appetite and weight loss [99]. Studies in animals lead to similar conclusions. Chronic administration of dexamethasone, a synthetic GR agonist, in the CNS markedly stimulates hyperphagia and obesity in normal rats [100]. Conversely, removal of glucocorticoids by adrenalectomy significantly reduces daily food intake and slows body weight gain in normal rats [101]. Similarly, adrenalectomy abolishes hyperphagia and reduces fat stores of diet- or genetically induced obese rats [99]. Absence of glucocorticoids is associated with a reduction in plasma leptin and insulin [102] levels and an elevation in plasma ghrelin levels [103]. All those characteristics dose-dependently reappear upon corticosterone supplementation, demonstrating that they specifically are caused by the absence of glucocorticoids [104].

Glucocorticoids appear to have important effects on the CNS melanocortin system. Animals with reduced glucocorticoids have increased anorexia in response to leptin and insulin [99,105,106]. Moreover, reduced glucocorticoids have a potent effect to alter the ability of arcuate nucleus-derived peptides to increase or decrease food intake. Low glucocorticoids result in increased sensitivity to the anorexic effects of the synthetic MC4-R agonist MTII and decreased orexigenic effects of NPY and AgRP [105]. The conclusion is that at least part of the impact of glucocorticoids on food intake and body weight appears to be the result of potent effects to alter the arcuate nucleus circuits. This opens up the possibility that the psychiatric disorders associated with both alterations in glucocorticoid levels and body weight may owe part of that effect to alterations in activity of these critical hypothalamic circuits.

Summary

This article highlighted some of the growing understanding of how body weight is regulated over time. The pace of scientific progress in this area continues to accelerate. That increased understanding provides hope that safe and effective therapeutic strategies to curb the rising tide of obesity will result. This new understanding also provides an opportunity to reveal the common neural substrates that account for the strong relationship between some psychiatric conditions and obesity. In particular, both 5-HT and glucocorticoids have been associated with the pathophysiology of several psychiatric conditions. Both of these systems have potent actions on the hypothalamic circuits that transduce peripheral signals about the status of energy stores into changes in food intake and energy expenditure that maintain energy balance. Thus, alterations in the actions of 5-HT and glucocorticoids could result in increased risk of psychiatric disorders and obesity. Future research advances on the neural underpinnings of psychiatric conditions and obesity will increase the understanding of the overlap between them and increase the ability to treat both.

References

[1] Malhotra S, McElroy SL. Medical management of obesity associated with mental disorders. J Clin Psychiatry 2002;63(Suppl 4):24–32.
[2] Specker S, de Zwaan M, Raymond N, et al. Psychopathology in subgroups of obese women with and without binge eating disorder. Compr Psychiatry 1994;35(3):185–90.

[3] de Zwaan M, Mitchell JE, Raymond NC, et al. Binge eating disorder: clinical features and treatment of a new diagnosis. Harv Rev Psychiatry 1994;1(6):310–25.

[4] Woods SC, Seeley RJ. Adiposity signals and the control of energy homeostasis. Nutrition 2000;16(10):894–902.

[5] Halaas JL, Gajiwala KS, Maffel M, et al. Weight-reducing effects of the plasma protein encoded by the obese gene. Science 1995;269:543–6.

[6] Zhang Y, Proenca R, Maffie M, et al. Positional cloning of the mouse obese gene and its human homologue. Nature 1994;372:425–32.

[7] Considine RV, Sinha MK, Heiman ML, et al. Serum immunoreactive-leptin concentrations in normal-weight and obese humans. N Engl J Med 1996;334(5):292–5.

[8] Caro JF, Kolaczynski JW, Nyce MR, et al. Decreased cerebrospinal-fluid/serum leptin ratio in obesity: a possible mechanism for leptin resistance. Lancet 1996;348:159–61.

[9] Farooqi IS, Jebb SA, Langmack G, et al. Effects of recombinant leptin therapy in a child with congenital leptin deficiency. N Engl J Med 1999;341:913–5.

[10] Heymsfield SB, Greenberg AS, Fujioka K, et al. Recombinant leptin for weight loss in obese and lean adults: a randomized, controlled, dose-escalation trial. JAMA 1999;282(16):1568–75.

[11] Schwartz MW, Seeley RJ, Campfield LA, et al. Identification of hypothalamic targets of leptin action. J Clin Invest 1996;98:1101–6.

[12] Seeley RJ, van Dijk G, Campfield LA, et al. The effect of intraventricular administration of leptin on food intake and body weight in the rat. Horm Metab Res 1996;28:664–8.

[13] Cohen P, Zhao C, Cai X, et al. Selective deletion of leptin receptor in neurons leads to obesity. J Clin Inves 2001;108:1113–21.

[14] Cowley MA, Smart JL, Rubinstein M, et al. Leptin activates anorexigenic POMC neurons through a neural network in the arcuate nucleus. Nature 2001;411(6836):480–4.

[15] Polonsky KS, Given BD, Hirsch L, et al. Quantitative study of insulin secretion and clearance in normal and obese subjects. J Clin Invest 1988;81:435–41.

[16] Polonsky KS, Given E, Carter V. Twenty-four-hour profiles and pulsatile patterns of insulin secretion in normal and obese subjects. J Clin Invest 1988;81:442–8.

[17] Baskin DG, Sipols AJ, Schwartz MW, White MF. Insulin receptor substrate-1 (IRS-1) expression in rat brain. Endocrinology 1994;134:1952–5.

[18] Woods SC, Lotter EC, McKay LD, et al. Chronic intracerebroventricular infusion of insulin reduces food intake and body weight of baboons. Nature 1979;282:503–5.

[19] Air EL, Benoit SC, Blake Smith KA, et al. Acute third ventricular administration of insulin decreases food intake in two paradigms. Pharmacol Biochem Behav 2002;72:423–9.

[20] Chavez M, Kaiyala K, Madden LJ, et al. Intraventricular insulin and the level of maintained body weight in rats. Behav Neurosci 1995;109:528–31.

[21] Brüning JC, Gautam D, Burks DJ, et al. Role of brain insulin receptor in control of body weight and reproduction. Science 2000;289:2122–5.

[22] Woods SC, Seeley RJ. Insulin as an adiposity signal. Int J Obes Relat Metab Disord 2001;25(Suppl 5):S35–8.

[23] Zhang B, Salituro G, Szalkowski D, et al. Discovery of a small molecule insulin mimetic with antidiabetic activity in mice. Science 1999;284:974–7.

[24] Air EL, Strowski MZ, Benoit SC, et al. Small molecule insulin mimetics reduce food intake and body weight and prevent development of obesity. Nat Med 2002;8(2):179–83.

[25] Cummings DE, Schwartz MW. Genetics and pathophysiology of human obesity. Annu Rev Med 2003;54:453–71.

[26] Tschöp M, Smiley DL, Heiman ML. Ghrelin induces adiposity in rodents. Nature 2000;407(6806):908–13.

[27] Nakazato M, Murakami N, Date Y, et al. A role for ghrelin in the central regulation of feeding. Nature 2001;409(6817):194–8.

[28] Inui A. Ghrelin: an orexigenic and somatotrophic signal from the stomach. Nat Rev Neurosci 2001;2:551–60.

[29] Nagaya N, Uematsu M, Kojima M, et al. Elevated circulating level of ghrelin in cachexia associated with chronic heart failure: relationships between ghrelin and anabolic/catabolic factors. Circulation 2001;104(17):2034–8.

[30] Wisse BE, Frayo RS, Schwartz MW, et al. Reversal of cancer anorexia by blockade of central melanocortin receptors in rats. Endocrinology 2001;142(8):3292–301.

[31] Wisse BE, Campfield LA, Marliss EB, et al. Effect of prolonged moderate and severe energy restriction and refeeding on plasma leptin concentrations in obese women. Am J Clin Nutr 1999;70:321–30.

[32] Kojima M, Hosoda H, Kangawa K. Purification and distribution of ghrelin: the natural endogenous ligand for the growth hormone secretagogue receptor. Horm Res 2001; 56(Suppl 1):93–7.

[33] Kojima M, Hosoda H, Date Y, et al. Ghrelin is a growth-hormone-releasing acylated peptide from stomach. Nature 1999;402(6762):656–60.

[34] Wren AM, Small CJ, Ward HL, et al. The novel hypothalamic peptide ghrelin stimulates food intake and growth hormone secretion. Endocrinology 2000;141(11): 4325–8.

[35] Asakawa A, Inui A, Kaga T, et al. Ghrelin is an appetite-stimulatory signal from stomach with structural resemblance to motilin. Gastroenterology 2001;120(2):337–45.

[36] Guan XM, Yu H, Palyha OC, et al. Distribution of mRNA encoding the growth hormone secretagogue receptor in brain and peripheral tissues. Brain Res Mol Brain Res 1997;48(1): 23–9.

[37] Cowley MA, Smith RG, Diano S, et al. The distribution and mechanism of action of ghrelin in the CNS demonstrates a novel hypothalamic circuit regulating energy homeostasis. Neuron 2003;37(4):649–61.

[38] Date Y, Murakami N, Toshinai K, et al. The role of the gastric afferent vagal nerve in ghrelin-induced feeding and growth hormone secretion in rats. Gastroenterology 2002;123: 1120–8.

[39] Gantz I, Fong TM. The melanocortin system. Am J Physiol Endocrinol Metab 2003;284(3):E468–74.

[40] Fan W, Boston B, Kesterson R, et al. Role of melanocortinergic neurons in feeding and the agouti obesity syndrome. Nature 1997;385:165–8.

[41] Thiele T, van DG, Yagaloff K, et al. Central infusion of melanocortin agonist MTII in rats: assessment of c-Fos expression and taste aversion. Am J Physiol 1998;274: R248–54.

[42] Tsujii S, Bray GA. Acetylation alters the feeding response to MSH and beta-endorphin. Brain Res Bull 1989;23:165–9.

[43] Huszar D, Lynch CA, Fairchild-Huntress V, et al. Targeted disruption of the melanocortin-4 receptor results in obesity in mice. Cell 1997;88(1):131–41.

[44] Butler AA, Kesterson RA, Khong K, et al. A unique metabolic syndrome causes obesity in the melanocortin-3 receptor-deficient mouse. Endocrinology 2000;141(9):3518–21.

[45] Yasuda T, Masaki T, Kakuma T, et al. Hypothalamic melanocortin system regulates sympathetic nerve activity in brown adipose tissue. Exp Biol Med (Maywood) 2004;229(3):235–9.

[46] Hahn TM, Breininger JF, Baskin DG, et al. Coexpression of Agrp and NPY in fasting-activated hypothalamic neurons. Insulin activates ATP-sensitive K + channels in hypothalamic neurons of lean, but not obese rats. 1998;1:271–2.

[47] Chen P, Li C, Haskell-Luevano C, et al. Altered expression of agouti-related protein and its colocalization with neuropeptide Y in the arcuate nucleus of the hypothalamus during lactation. Endocrinology 1999;140(6):2645–50.

[48] Nijenhuis WA, Oosterom J, Adan RA. AgRP(83–132) acts as an inverse agonist on the human-melanocortin-4 receptor. Mol Endocrinol 2001;15(1):164–71.

[49] Ollmann M, Wilson B, Yang Y, et al. Antagonism of central melanocortin receptors in vitro and in vivo by agouti-related protein. Science 1997;278:135–8.

[50] Rossi M, Kim M, Morgan D, et al. A C-terminal fragment of Agouti-related protein increases feeding and antagonizes the effect of alpha-melanocyte stimulating hormone in vivo. Endocrinology 1998;139:4428–31.

[51] Hagan MM, Rushing PA, Pritchard LM, et al. Long-term orexigenic effects of AgRP-(83–132) involve mechanisms other than melanocortin receptor blockade. Am J Physiol 2000; 279:R47–52.

[52] Billington CJ, Levine AS. Hypothalamic neuropeptide Y regulation of feeding and energy metabolism. Curr Opin Neurobiol 1992;2(6):847–51.

[53] Blomqvist AG, Herzog H. Y-receptor subtypes–how many more? Trends in Neurosci 1997;20:294–8.

[54] Xu B, Li B-H, Rowland NE, Kalra SP. Neuropeptide Y injection into the fourth cerebroventricle stimulates c-Fos expression in the paraventricular nucleus and other nuclei in the forebrain: effect of food consumption. Brain Res 1995;698:227–31.

[55] Stanley BG, Magdalin W, Seirafi A, et al. Evidence for neuropeptide Y mediation of eating produced by food deprivation and for a variant of the Y_1 receptor mediating this peptide's effect. Peptides 1992;13:581–7.

[56] Mizuno T, Kleopoulos S, Bergen H, et al. Hypothalamic proopiomelanocortin mRNA is reduced by fasting and in ob/ob and db/db mice, but is stimulated by leptin. Diabetes 1998; 47:294–7.

[57] Cheung CC, Clifton DK, Steiner RA. Proopiomelanocortin neurons are direct targets for leptin in the hypothalamus. Endocrinology 1997;138:4489–92.

[58] Schwartz MW, Seeley RJ, Weigle DS, et al. Leptin increases hypothalamic proopiomelanocortin (POMC) mRNA expression in the rostral arcuate nucleus. Diabetes 1997;46: 2119–23.

[59] Satoh N, Ogawa Y, Katsuura G, et al. Satiety effect and sympathetic activation of leptin are mediated by hypothalamic melanocortin system. Neurosci Lett 1998;249:107–10.

[60] Seeley R, Yagaloff K, Fisher S, et al. Melanocortin receptors in leptin effects. Nature 1997; 390:349.

[61] Benoit SC, Air EL, Coolen LM, et al. The catabolic action of insulin in the brain is mediated by melanocortins. J Neurosci 2002;22(20):9048–52.

[62] Cusin I, Dryden S, Wang Q, et al. Effect of sustained physiologic hyperinsulinemia on hypothalamic neuropeptide Y and NPY mRNA levels in the rat. J Neuroendocrinol 1995;7: 193–7.

[63] McMinn JE, Seeley RJ, Wilkinson CW, et al. NPY-induced overfeeding suppresses hypothalamic NPY mRNA expression: potential roles of plasma insulin and leptin. Regul Pept 1998;75–76:425–31.

[64] Wang Q, Bing C, Al-Barazanji K, et al. Interactions between leptin and hypothalamic neuropeptide Y neurons in the control of food intake and energy homeostasis in the rat. Diabetes 1997;46(3):335–41.

[65] Schwartz MW, Baskin DG, Bukowski TR, et al. Specificity of leptin action on elevated blood glucose levels and hypothalamic neuropeptide Y gene expression in ob/ob mice. Diabetes 1996;45:531–5.

[66] Shintani M, Ogawa Y, Ebihara K, et al. Ghrelin, an endogenous growth hormone secretagogue, is a novel orexigenic peptide that antagonizes leptin action through the activation of hypothalamic neuropeptide Y/Y1 receptor pathway. Diabetes 2001;50(2):227–32.

[67] Chen HY, Trumbauer ME, Chen AS, et al. Orexigenic action of peripheral ghrelin is mediated by neuropeptide Y (NPY) and agouti-related protein (AgRP). Endocrinology 2004;145(6):2607–12.

[68] Blundell JE. Serotonin and appetite. Neuropharmacology 1984;23:1537–51.

[69] Peroutka SJ. Molecular biology of serotonin (5-HT) receptors. Synapse 1994;18(3):241–60.

[70] Heal DJ, Cheetham SC, Prow MR, et al. A comparison of the effects on central 5-HT function of sibutramine hydrochloride and other weight-modifying agents. Br J Pharmacol 1998;125(2):301–8.

[71] Jackson HC, Bearham MC, Hutchins LJ, et al. Investigation of the mechanisms underlying the hypophagic effects of the 5-HT and noradrenaline reuptake inhibitor, sibutramine, in the rat. Br J Pharmacol 1997;121(8):1613–8.

[72] Stock MJ. Sibutramine: a review of the pharmacology of a novel anti-obesity agent. Int J Obes Relat Metab Disord 1997;21(Suppl 1):S25–9.

[73] Simansky KJ. Serotonergic control of the organization of feeding and satiety. Behav Brain Res 1996;73:37–42.

[74] Giorgetti M, Hotsenpiller G, Froestl W, et al. In vivo modulation of ventral tegmental area dopamine and glutamate efflux by local GABA(B) receptors is altered after repeated amphetamine treatment. Neuroscience 2002;109(3):585–95.

[75] Tecott LH, Sun LM, Akana SF, et al. Eating disorder and epilepsy in mice lacking 5–HT2c serotonin receptors. Nature 1995;374(6522):542–6.

[76] Nonogaki K, Strack AM, Dallman MF, et al. Leptin-independent hyperphagia and type 2 diabetes in mice with a mutated serotonin 5–HT2C receptor gene. Nat Med 1998;4(10): 1152–6.

[77] Heisler LK, Chu HM, Tecott LH. Epilepsy and obesity in serotonin 5–HT2C receptor mutant mice. Ann N Y Acad Sci 1998;861:74–8.

[78] Rowland NE, Carlton J. Neurobiology of an anorectic drug: fenfluramine. Prog Neurobiol 1986;27(1):13–62.

[79] Shor-Posner G, Grinker JA, Marinescu C, et al. Hypothalamic serotonin in the control of meal patterns and macronutrient selection. Brain Res Bull 1986;17(5):663–71.

[80] Vickers SP, Clifton PG, Dourish CT, et al. Reduced satiating effect of d-fenfluramine in serotonin 5-HT(2C) receptor mutant mice. Psychopharmacology (Berl) 1999;143(3): 309–14.

[81] Wright DE, Seroogy KB, Lundgren KH, et al. Comparative localization of serotonin1A, 1C, and 2 receptor subtype mRNAs in rat brain. J Comp Neurol 1995;351(3): 357–373.

[82] Heisler LK, Cowley MA, Tecott LH, et al. Activation of central melanocortin pathways by fenfluramine. Science 2002;297(5581):609–11.

[83] Van Oekelen D, Luyten WH, Leysen JE. 5–HT2A and 5–HT2C receptors and their atypical regulation properties. Life Sci 2003;72(22):2429–49.

[84] Giorgetti M, Tecott LH. Contributions of 5-HT(2C) receptors to multiple actions of central serotonin systems. Eur J Pharmacol 2004;488:1–9.

[85] Ni YG, Miledi R. Blockage of 5HT2C serotonin receptors by fluoxetine (Prozac). Proc Natl Acad Sci USA 1997;94(5):2036–40.

[86] Reynolds GP, Zhang ZJ, Zhang XB. Association of antipsychotic drug-induced weight gain with a 5–HT2C receptor gene polymorphism. Lancet 2002;359(9323):2086–7.

[87] Young AH. Glucocorticoids, serotonin and mood. Br J Psychiatry 1994;165(2):271–2.

[88] Hanley NR, Van de Kar LD. Serotonin and the neuroendocrine regulation of the hypothalamic–pituitary-adrenal axis in health and disease. Vitam Horm 2003;66: 189–255.

[89] Dallman MF, La Fleur SE, Pecoraro NC, et al. Glucocorticoids: food intake, abdominal obesity wealthy nations in 2004. Endocrinology 2004;145(6):2633–8.

[90] Dallman MF, Strack AM, Akana SF, et al. Feast and famine: critical role of glucocorticoids with insulin in daily energy flow. Front Neuroendocrinol 1993;14(4):303–47.

[91] Reul JM, de Kloet ER. Two receptor systems for corticosterone in rat brain: microdistribution and differential occupation. Endocrinology 1985;117(6):2505–11.

[92] La Fleur SE, Kalsbeek A, Wortel J, et al. A suprachiasmatic nucleus generated rhythm in basal glucose concentrations. J Neuroendocrinol 1999;11(8):643–52.

[93] Krieger DT. Central nervous system disease. Clin Endocrinol Metab 1979;8(3): 467–85.

[94] Honma KI, Honma S, Hiroshige T. Critical role of food amount for prefeeding corticosterone peak in rats. Am J Physiol 1983;245(3):R339–44.

[95] Bogdan A, Bouchareb B, Touitou Y. Ramadan fasting alters endocrine and neuroendo-crine circadian patterns. Meal-time as a synchronizer in humans? Life Sci 2001;68(14): 1607–15.

[96] Dallman MF, Akana SF, Bhatnagar S, et al. Starvation: early signals, sensors, and sequelae. Endocrinology 1999;140(9):4015–23.

[97] Cavagnini F, Croci M, Putignano P, et al. Glucocorticoids and neuroendocrine function. Int J Obes Relat Metab Disord 2000;24(Suppl 2):S77–9.

[98] Tataranni PA, Larson DE, Snitker S, et al. Effects of glucocorticoids on energy metabolism and food intake in humans. Am J Physiol 1996;271:E317–25.

[99] Zakrzewska KE, Cusin I, Sainsbury A, et al. Glucocorticoids as counter-regulatory hormones of leptin. Diabetes 1997;46:717–9.

[100] Zakrzewska KE, Cusin I, Stricker-Krongrad A, et al. Induction of obesity and hyperleptinemia by central glucocorticoid infusion in the rat. Diabetes 1999;48(2):365–70.

[101] Green PK, Wilkinson CW, Woods SC. Intraventricular corticosterone increases the rate of body weight gain in underweight adrenalectomized rats. Endocrinology 1992;130:269–75.

[102] Sainsbury A, Cusin I, Rohner-Jeanrenaud F, et al. Adrenalectomy prevents the obesity syndrome produced by chronic central neuropeptide Y infusion in normal rats. Diabetes 1997;46:209–14.

[103] Proulx K, Vahl TP, Drazen DL, et al. The orexigenic effect of ghrelin is enhanced in the absence of glucocorticoids. J Neuroendocrinol (in revision).

[104] Jeanrenaud B, Rohner-Jeanrenaud F. CNS-periphery relationships and body weight homeostasis: influence of the glucocorticoid status. Int J Obes Relat Metab Disord 2000; 24(Suppl 2):S74–6.

[105] Drazen DL, Wortman MD, Schwartz MW, et al. Adrenalectomy alters the sensitivity of the central nervous system melanocortin system. Diabetes 2003;52(12):2928–34.

[106] Chavez M, Seeley RJ, Green PK, et al. Adrenalectomy increases sensitivity to central insulin. Physiol and Behav 1997;62:631–4.

ELSEVIER
SAUNDERS

PSYCHIATRIC
CLINICS
OF NORTH AMERICA

Psychiatr Clin N Am 28 (2005) 39–54

Obesity, Psychiatric Status, and Psychiatric Medications

Robert I. Berkowitz, MD*,
Anthony N. Fabricatore, PhD

*Weight and Eating Disorders Program, Department of Psychiatry,
University of Pennsylvania School of Medicine, 3535 Market Street,
Philadelphia, PA 19104, USA*

The medical complications of overweight and obesity are known well. These include type 2 diabetes, hypercholesterolemia, osteoarthritis, and increased risk of all-cause mortality [1,2]. The psychological correlates of carrying excess weight, however, are documented less well. Clinicians and laypersons frequently assume that obesity is either a cause or a consequence of emotional disturbance or psychiatric disorder. This article examines the relationship between psychopathology and obesity. In addition, the association of psychiatric medications with changes in weight is examined.

Early theoretical papers conceptualized obesity as the manifestation of underlying psychopathology and suboptimal development [3]. To the authors' knowledge, no empirical studies have lent support to such ideas. Instead, studies have yielded inconsistent findings. Some comparisons of overweight and average-weight individuals showed that the former experienced greater psychological distress [4]. Others showed lower rates of psychiatric disorder at higher body weights [5]. Studies conducted over the past 10 to 15 years have become increasingly representative of the general population and methodologically sophisticated [6–8]. The primary question being examined has shifted from, "Is obesity related to psychopathology?" to, "Which obese individuals are at greatest risk for psychiatric disturbance [9,10]?" A few studies also have sought to determine the temporal relationship between obesity and psychopathology (specifically depression) when they co-occur [11,12]. This evolution in the literature has enhanced understanding of the psychosocial correlates of obesity and has created a database from which to judge common stereotypes and assumptions.

---

* Corresponding author.
E-mail address: rberk@mail.med.upenn.edu (R.I. Berkowitz).

0193-953X/05/$ - see front matter © 2005 Elsevier Inc. All rights reserved.
doi:10.1016/j.psc.2004.10.005   *psych.theclinics.com*

This section reviews the literature regarding the comorbidity of obesity and psychopathology. Most extant studies have focused on depression. Recently, however, the links between obesity and more severe mental illnesses such as bipolar disorder have begun to be investigated. Before the comorbidity literature is presented, however, the authors briefly discuss the problems of prejudice and discrimination against obese individuals.

Sobal and Stunkard [13] have called bias toward obese persons "the last socially acceptable form of prejudice." Negative attitudes toward significantly overweight people have persisted even as the prevalence of obesity has doubled from 15% of the adult population in 1980 to 31% in 2002 [14].

Biases toward obesity are developed early in life, remain active throughout adulthood, and are present in several contexts. Nearly 40 years ago, Staffieri [15] found that 6-year-old children assumed silhouettes of an overweight child to be "lazy," "dirty," "stupid," and "ugly." More recently, children as young as 3 years old were found to rate drawings of overweight children more negatively than otherwise equivalent lean or average-weight children [16]. Researchers have uncovered bias against obese individuals not only in social situations, but also in educational and occupational settings [17]. There is even evidence of "stigma by association," as demonstrated by Hebl and Mannix [18]. Male job applicants received more negative evaluations if they were depicted seated next to an obese versus a lean woman. The negative evaluation was independent of the rater's own sex and whether the rater thought the woman was the applicant's romantic partner or a stranger.

Health care professionals also have been found to hold negative attitudes toward obese persons [19]. Even clinicians and researchers who specialize in obesity appear to hold antifat biases [20]. Their responses to a test of implicit attitudes (which measures difficulty in pairing target constructs with specific attributes) revealed stereotypes relating obesity to laziness, stupidity, and worthlessness. These findings are tempered somewhat by additional analyses that indicated that these health care professionals held much weaker stereotypes than members of the general population and that their implicit negative attitudes do not manifest invariably in explicit bias or discriminatory behavior toward their obese patients. Collectively, these investigations imply that no one is immune to antifat biases. Health care professionals must be particularly alert to their own attitudes to ensure that they treat patients on the basis of their clinical presentations, rather than on their own implicitly held stereotypes or biases.

Obesity and psychopathology

Depression

On the basis of three large studies that included representative samples of the US population, two conclusions can be drawn about the relationship between obesity and depression [6–8]. First, the relationship differs between the sexes, such that obese men are at no greater risk of depression than nonobese men, but obese women are significantly more likely to be depressed than their average-weight counterparts. Second, extremely obese individuals (ie, body mass index (BMI) of at least 40 kg/m^2) are at particular risk of clinically significant mood disturbance. These findings have been supported by studies of nonrepresentative samples (ie, clinical studies of individuals seeking weight loss therapy) also [21]. Other epidemiological studies have provided preliminary evidence to suggest that the onset of obesity precedes the onset of depression in adults, and that the opposite is true in children and adolescents [11,12].

The obesity-depression relationship differs between sexes

This conclusion is derived from studies by Istvan et al, Carpenter et al, and Onyike et al [6–8]. Istvan et al [6] analyzed data from the First National Health and Nutrition Examination Survey (NHANES I), which was conducted from 1971 to 1975. They examined the relationship between BMI and depression, as indicated by a score of at least 16 on the Center for Epidemiological Studies Depression scale (CES-D), for men and women. Men in the highest BMI quintile (greater than 28.65 kg/m^2) were no more likely to score in the depressed range on the CES-D than men in the lower four quintiles (odds ratio of 0.97, 95% confidence interval [CI]: 0.48, 1.47). For women, however, the relationship was quite different. The risk of depression was 38% greater for women in the highest BMI quintile (greater than 28.96 kg/m^2) than for those in the lower four quintiles (95% CI: 1.07, 1.69).

Carpenter et al [7] examined the relationship between obesity and depression–diagnosed according to *Diagnostic and Statistical Manual of Mental Disorders, Fourth Edition (DSM-IV)* criteria and related variables in a nationally representative sample of more than 40,000 individuals. In their sample, obesity appeared to have a protective effect for men. Obese men (BMI of at least 30 kg/m^2) were 37% less likely to report a history of major depression (95% CI: 0.60, 0.67) or suicide attempts (95% CI: 0.48, 0.83) in the past year than average-weight or overweight men (BMI of 20.8 to 29.9 kg/m^2). Underweight men (BMI less than 20.8 kg/m^2), by contrast, had a 25% increased risk of depression (95% CI 1.18, 1.32), 81% increased risk of suicidal ideation (95% CI: 1.71, 1.89), and 77% increased risk of suicide attempts (95% CI: 1.34, 2.33), compared with average-weight men. Similar to Istvan et al, Carpenter et al found that obesity was related to poorer mental health among women. The 1-year prevalence of major depression was 37% (95% CI: 1.09, 1.73) higher among women with a BMI of at least 30 kg/m^2 than those with a BMI of 20.8 to 29.9 kg/m^2. Obese women also were 20% more likely to report suicidal ideation (95% CI: 0.96, 1.50) and 23% more likely to have made a suicide attempt (95% CI: 0.74, 2.03) in the past year, but these increases were not statistically significant. These findings are depicted in Fig. 1.

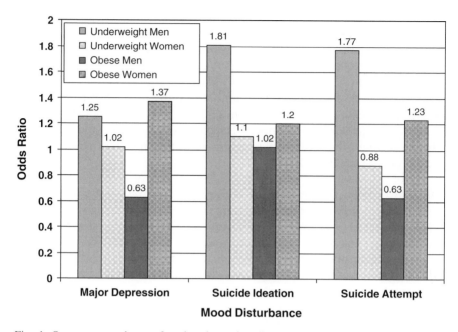

Fig. 1. One-year prevalence of major depressive disorder, suicidal ideation, and suicide attempts by weight status and gender. The reference group (BMI = 20.8–29.9 kg/m^2) has an odds ratio of 1 and is a normal-weight control group. *Data from* Carpenter KM, Hasin DS, Allison DB, et al. Relationships between obesity and DSM-IV major depressive disorder, suicide ideation, and suicide attempts: Results from a general population study. Am J Public Health 2000;90:251–7.

Onyike et al [8] updated the study by Istvan et al [6]. These researchers analyzed data from the Third National Health and Nutrition Examination Survey (NHANES-III), which were collected from 1988 to 1994. This study used standard definitions of normal weight (BMI of 18.5 to 24.9 kg/m^2), obesity (BMI of at least 30 kg/m^2), and depression (diagnosed with the Diagnostic Interview Schedule according to *Diagnostic and Statistical Manual of Mental Disorders, Third Edition [DSM-III]* criteria). Like the Istvan [6] and Carpenter [7] studies, the Onyike examination [8] found no significant increase in the risk of depression in obese men (odds ratio = 1.73, 95% CI: 0.56, 5.37) versus normal-weight men. The association between obesity and depression in women (odds ratio of 1.82, 95% CI: 1.01, 3.3) was significant and stronger than it was in the two previous epidemiological investigations.

Extremely obese persons are at greatest risk of depression

Onyike et al re-examined the relationship between obesity and depression after stratifying their sample according to obesity severity [8]. Obese individuals were separated into class I (BMI of 30 to 34.9 kg/m^2), class II

(BMI of 35 to 39.9 kg/m^2), and class III obesity (BMI of at least 40 kg/m^2). Logistic regression analyses revealed that neither class I nor class II obesity was associated with an increased risk of past-month depression in women or men. Class III (or extreme) obesity, however, significantly increased the likelihood of past-month depression in both sexes. Extremely obese women were nearly four times more likely to meet criteria than were normal-weight women (odds ratio of 3.78, 95% CI: 1.64, 8.68). The risk was almost eight times greater for extremely obese versus normal-weight men (odds ratio of 7.68, 95% CI: 1.03, 57.26). When results were adjusted for age, education, marital status, physician-rated health, substance use, and use of psychiatric medication, the increase in risk remained high (odds ratio of 4.63, 95% CI: 2.06, 10.42). Fig. 2 shows the adjusted odds of past-month depression across BMI categories.

The fact that more severe obesity increases the risk of depression is not surprising; however, the mechanisms accounting for this finding are not understood well. Researchers have suggested that more extremely obese individuals experience greater prejudice and discrimination than do less obese persons, and that the increase in experienced bias may account for the higher risk of depression [21]. To the authors' knowledge, however, these hypotheses have not been tested empirically.

Another mechanism that may help to explain the increased risk of depression among extremely obese persons is health-related quality of life

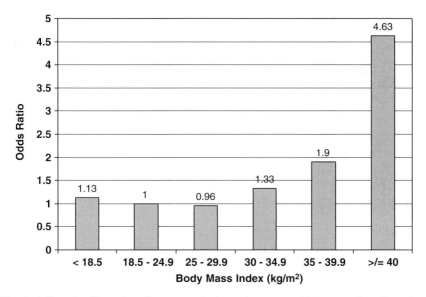

Fig. 2. Adjusted odds ratios of past-month depression across BMI categories. *Data from* Onyike CU, Crum RM, Lee HB, et al. Is obesity associated with major depression? Results from the Third National Health and Nutrition Examination Survey. Am J Epidemiol 2003;158:1139–47.

(HRQL). Several studies have shown that the extent to which physical health interferes with daily functioning is related positively to BMI and symptoms of depression [22–25].

Preliminary evidence suggests that impaired HRQL may account for poorer psychosocial outcomes among extremely obese individuals. Fabricatore et al examined whether the relationship between extreme obesity and depression is mediated by impairments in HRQL [26]. Their sample included 261 individuals who sought diet, exercise, and behavior therapy (with or without adjunctive pharmacotherapy) and 178 candidates who sought gastric bypass surgery. Patients' BMI ranged from 27.4 to 85.2 kg/m^2, with a mean ($\pm$ standard deviation [SD]) of 41.8 $\pm$ 10.5 kg/m^2. As expected, BMI was related to greater symptoms of depression (assessed with the Beck Depression Inventory [BDI]-II) and poorer HRQL in the domains of bodily pain, role limitations due to physical health, and physical functioning (assessed with the SF-36). When controlling for these aspects of HRQL, however, the association between BMI and symptoms of depression became nonsignificant (Fig. 3). Thus, these findings suggest that poorer HRQL mediates (ie, accounts for) the relationship between increasing obesity severity and symptoms of depression.

The temporal relationship between obesity and depression

The study by Fabricatore et al was limited by its cross-sectional nature [26]. Longitudinal data are necessary to conclude that increasing BMI leads to greater impairments in HRQL, which in turn lead to greater severity of

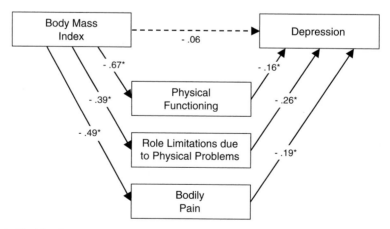

Fig. 3. Health-related quality of life mediates the relationship between increasing BMI and depression. Dotted line represents the correlation between BMI and depressive symptoms when controlling for quality-of-life variables. Values reflect correlation coefficients. * = p < 0.05. *Data from* Fabricatore AN, Wadden TA, Sarwer DB. Depressive symptoms as a function of body mass index and health-related quality of life in treatment-seeking obese adults. Obes Res 2003;11:A10.

mood disturbance. Although they did not focus on any particular mechanisms that would account for the comorbidity of obesity and depression, at least two studies have investigated the temporal sequence of the onset of these disorders.

Goodman and Whittaker [12] followed a nationally representative sample of over 9000 US adolescents, grades 7 through 12. Height and weight were self-reported, and depression was assessed by questionnaire at baseline and after 1 year. No relationship was found between obesity and depression at baseline, and baseline obesity did not increase the risk of depression at follow-up. Depression at baseline, however, was associated with a twofold risk of becoming obese in the next year.

Roberts et al explored the temporal relationship between obesity and depression among 2123 US adults aged 50 and up [11]. Height, weight, and depressive symptoms were assessed by interview at baseline and 5 years later. Those who were depressed (but not obese) at baseline were no more likely to have become obese by the end of the 5-year study when controlling for age, gender, education, and marital status (odds ratio of 1.27, 95% CI: 0.62, 2.62). The risk of depression at follow-up, controlling for the same variables, was twice as high (odds ratio of 2.06, 95% CI: 1.26, 3.37) for individuals who were obese (but not depressed) at baseline than it was for those who were not obese at baseline. When financial strain, life events, social variables, health, and functional limitations were controlled, the increased risk of incident depression remained significant (odds ratio of 1.79, 95% CI: 1.06, 3.02) for those who were obese versus not obese at baseline.

Together, these longitudinal studies suggest that depression precedes obesity in adolescents and that obesity precedes depression in older adults [11,12]. These findings, however, must be viewed as preliminary. More research is needed to replicate these findings, to examine temporal relationships among younger and middle-aged adults, and to discover the mechanisms that mediate the association between depression and obesity.

Depression and weight gain

Although the studies did not compare the rate of weight gain among depressed and nondepressed adults, at least one longitudinal study has addressed this issue. DiPietro et al analyzed data from NHANES-I and the National Health Epidemiologic Follow-up Study; this analysis included 1794 US adults [27]. They divided their sample according to sex and age (younger than 55 years old versus those 55 years old and older) and found that younger men who were depressed at baseline gained significantly more weight over 7 to 10 years than their counterparts who were free of depression (4.2 kg versus 1.2 kg, respectively). Younger women, however, gained significantly less weight if they were depressed versus not depressed at baseline (1.4 kg versus 3.1 kg, respectively). The direction of weight change and the relationship to depression were different for individuals over 55 years of age. Older adults lost more weight if they were depressed at baseline than if they were not depressed (1.6 kg versus 1.2 kg for men, 3.1 kg versus 1.6 kg for women).

Loss of appetite and unintentional weight loss are symptomatic of classic unipolar depression [28]. Individuals with atypical presentations of depression, however, may display an increase in appetite and weight during depressive episodes [29]. Although the direction and magnitude of weight change varies between depressed adults, a study by Stunkard et al suggests that these characteristics remain consistent across episodes of depression in the same individual [30]. In a small sample of 53 patients with recurrent depression, 45 (85%) experienced the same direction of weight change across two episodes. Nearly 38% of those patients reported gaining weight during their episodes, compared with 51% who reported losing weight, and 11% who reported no change.

Obesity and bipolar disorder

Two studies by Fagiolini et al concluded that overweight and obesity are much more prevalent in individuals with bipolar disorder (36% and 32%, respectively) than in the general population [31,32]. These investigators referenced an obesity prevalence rate of 19.8% in the general population, which was obtained from self-reported heights and weights. The latest data from NHANES-III, however, indicated that the prevalence of overweight and obesity are 35% and 31%, respectively, based on measured height and weight [14]. In comparison to these figures, individuals with bipolar disorder may exhibit modestly greater rates of overweight and obesity than the US population at large.

A comparison of obese and nonobese patients with bipolar disorder revealed that obese patients had significantly more manic episodes (9.6 plus or minus 13.3 versus 7.0 plus or minus 11.7), depressive episodes (15.0 plus or minus 15.5 versus 10.5 plus or minus 14.6), and greater severity of depressive symptoms on the 25-item Hamilton Depression Rating Scale (22.3 plus or minus 9.5 versus 18.2 plus or minus 9.8) than did patients who were not obese [32]. Obese patients also had poorer treatment outcomes than nonobese patients, as evidenced by a greater percentage of recurrence (54.3% versus 35.4%, respectively), and a shorter time to recurrence of depressive episodes. There were no differences, however, with respect to recurrence of manic or mixed episodes.

Obesity and schizophrenia

Individuals with schizophrenia have been reported to have greater odds of being overweight or obese than the population without the disorder [33,34]. Allison et al used a BMI of 27 or higher to define obesity and found that 42% of people with schizophrenia and 27% of the general population were obese. A major factor describing these differences was the very high percentage of women with schizophrenia with obesity, in particular for young women. It was not possible to determine to what degree this weight gain related to the use of antipsychotic medications. Schizophrenia is associated with a 20% shorter life expectancy [35,36] and a greater frequency for several illnesses including obesity, diabetes, coronary heart disease, hypertension, and emphysema.

Obesity and psychiatric medications

Until recently, there was little information from pharmaceutical companies about the risk of weight gain with psychotropic medications. Several of these drugs are now known to be associated with weight gain, and these include the atypical antipsychotic medications, antidepressant medications (selective serotonin reuptake inhibitors [SSRIs], tricyclic antidepressants, and mirtazapine), and mood stabilizers (including lithium and some anticonvulsants) [37].

Antipsychotic medications

The antipsychotic medications used in the treatment of schizophrenia, bipolar disorder, and other psychotic conditions have been associated with clinically significant weight gain. A consensus statement (2004) was developed by four medical associations to alert health care professionals to assess patients receiving atypical antipsychotic medications for rapid weight gain and for metabolic effects, including the development of diabetes and dyslipidemia [38]. The consensus statement, published simultaneously in the February 2004 issues of *Diabetes Care* and *Journal of Clinical Psychiatry*, was written by a panel representing the American Association of Clinical Endocrinologists, the American Diabetes Association, American Psychiatric Association, and the North American Association for the Study of Obesity.

The consensus statement reported that antipsychotic medications have been an important therapy for psychotic conditions and other serious psychiatric disorders. The first-generation antipsychotics (FGAs) treated the positive symptoms of psychosis (hallucinations and delusions) but have been less effective in the treatment of the negative symptoms of psychotic disorders such as withdrawal, apathy, and affective disorder. The FGAs were more likely to be associated with movement disorders, including dystonic reactions, akathisia, drug-induced parkinsonism, and the potentially irreversible serious effect of tardive dyskinesia.

The atypical antipsychotic medications, also referred to as second-generation antipsychotics (SGA), were developed with the aims of improving efficacy and minimizing adverse effects [38]. The SGAs indeed had fewer extrapyramidal and other movement disorders associated with them. In addition to treating the positive symptoms of psychosis, SGAs were significantly more helpful in treating the negative symptoms. The consensus statement reported that except for clozapine, the other SGAs have become used widely in recent years as the primary treatment modality for psychotic disorders and other severe psychiatric syndromes. In addition to clozapine, these medications include risperidone, olanzapine, ziprasidone, quetiapine, and aripiprazole. Several SGAs, however, have been associated with weight gain and metabolic abnormalities.

Allison et al [39] reported in a meta-analysis that FGAs and SGAs cause varying degrees of weight gain within the first 10 weeks of treatment. Placebo treatment resulted in a mean weight reduction of 0.74 kg. Of the FGAs, a 3.19 kg weight gain was reported with thioridazine. Among the SGAs (atypical antipsychotic medications), mean increases were 4.45 kg for clozapine, 4.15 kg for olanzapine, 2.92 kg for sertindole, 2.10 kg for risperidone, and 0.04 kg for ziprasidone. Little data were available to evaluate quetiapine at 10 weeks [39], and aripiprazole was not available. Table 1 contains a summary of the consensus report of weight gain [38].

The consensus statement suggested that although the precise neurobiology describing how the SGAs are associated with weight gain is not understood, both hunger and satiety may be affected by these medications. It hypothesized that the SGAs most likely work by their activities at the receptor sites for dopamine, serotonin, norepinephrine, and histamine-H1, which also are related to mechanisms involved in weight regulation. Thus, the mechanisms involved in the therapeutic value of these medications also may be involved directly in the development of increased food intake and excess weight gain.

A note of caution must be made, however. The risks of developing obesity and other complications (such as diabetes and dyslipidemia) ought to be considered along with the patient's diagnosis and response to treatment with a specific medication. For example, it is not clear whether a patient who is treated successfully for a severe psychiatric condition on

Table 1
Second-generation antipsychotics and metabolic abnormalities

Drug	Weight gain	Risk for diabetes	Worsening lipid profile
Clozapine	+++	+	+
Olanzapine	+++	+	+
Risperidone	++	D	D
Quetiapine	++	D	D
Arpiprazole*	+/−	−	−
Ziprasidone*	+/−	−	−

+, increase effect; −, no effect; D, discrepant results.
* Newer drugs with limited long-term data.
Adapted from Consensus Development Conference on Antipsychotic Drugs and Obesity and Diabetes. Diabetes Care 2004;27(2):596–601; with permission.

one antipsychotic will do as well when switched to another medication. Clozapine, for example, may be associated with improved therapeutic gains for the patient with treatment-resistant schizophrenia or suicidal risk. At the same time, it may be associated with higher risk for the development of weight gain and metabolic abnormalities. Consideration of the potential for development of obesity, diabetes, and dyslipidemia, however, ought to be considered when a psychotropic medication is chosen for a specific condition, such as for the treatment of schizophrenia.

Type 2 diabetes mellitus and dyslipidemia

As noted earlier, people suffering from schizophrenia have a greater likelihood of developing obesity and diabetes. Some of the antipsychotic medications, however, have a greater likelihood of being associated with the development of obesity and type 2 diabetes mellitus and lipid disorders. Although there have been some limitations in the studies, the consensus report found that there was evidence [40–43] for increased risk for diabetes with clozapine and olanzapine (see Table 1). Henderson et al [44] evaluated patients taking clozapine for 5 years and reported that 36.6% had a diagnosis of type 2 diabetes mellitus. Increased insulin resistance secondary to weight gain has been suggested as one possible mechanism for this association with antipsychotic medication usage.

Lipids disorders also are associated with the weight gain found with use of the SGAs. As noted in Table 1, the greatest increases in low-density lipoprotein (LDL) cholesterol and triglycerides and reductions in high-density lipoprotein (HDL) are found with the most weight gain, especially in those treated with clozapine and olanzapine. Aripiprazole and ziprasidone appear to have minimal weight gain and dyslipidemia associated with their use.

Monitoring

The consensus panel advised that there be monitoring at baseline and during treatment with antipsychotic medications (Table 2). Panel members suggested that history of obesity, diabetes, dyslipidemia, hypertension, or cardiovascular disease (including family history) be obtained. Similarly, height and weight should be obtained (to calculate BMI) and waist circumference. In addition, they suggested that blood pressure and fasting glucose and lipid profile be obtained initially. When obesity, hypertension, metabolic disorders, or dyslipidemia are diagnosed, treatment should be initiated, including referral to the appropriate health care professionals. Although it may be clinically challenging when the patient is acutely psychiatrically ill, both nutritional and physical activity counseling should be initiated when treatment is begun, because of the propensity that an SGA may be related to significant weight gain.

The consensus panel also recommended that health care professionals, patients, and family members be educated to the signs and symptoms of

Table 2
Monitoring protocol for patients on second-generation antipsychotics*

	Baseline	4 weeks	8 weeks	12 weeks	Quarterly	Annually	Every 5 years
Personal/family history	X					X	
Weight (BMI)	X	X	X	X	X		
Waist circumference	X					X	
Blood pressure	X			X		X	
Fasting plasma glucose	X			X		X	
Fasting lipid profile	X			X			X

* More frequent assessments may be warranted based on clinical status.

Adapted from Consensus Development Conference on Antipsychotic Drugs and Obesity and Diabetes. Diabetes Care 2004;27(2):596–601; with permission.

diabetes and to the development of diabetic ketoacidosis (DKA), a potentially fatal condition. The recommendations state that DKA may present uncommonly, but rapidly, and include the following symptoms: polyuria, polydipsia, weight loss, nausea, vomiting, dehydration, rapid respiration, and delirium or coma. In addition, it advised that drugs be chosen that minimize the risk of weight gain for patients at higher risk for diabetes who require antipsychotic (or mood stabilizing) drugs.

The panel recommended that once SGA treatment is started, the weight of the patient be taken at 4, 8, and 12 weeks. If the patient has gained more than 5% of initial weight, consideration of switching to another SGA should be made; such a switch should be made in a gradual manner. It is important to assess the psychiatric status of the patient and the potential benefit, however, of the SGA, before discontinuing. Fasting lipid and glucose along with blood pressure measures ought to be made also at 12 weeks. These may be made quarterly, and appropriate referral to other health care providers for management of hypertension, dyslipidemia, hyperglycemia, or symptoms of diabetes or DKA should be made as clinically indicated. The choice of SGA may reduce the frequency of the onset of diabetes or cardiovascular disease. There is some initial short-term evidence that adding a dietary and physical activity intervention may minimize weight gain with the SGAs, and more research is needed to evaluate the effectiveness of this strategy.

Antidepressant medications

Some antidepressant medications also have been associated with significant weight gain [37]. Initially, this was observed with the use of the tricyclic antidepressants (TCAs), such as amitriptyline. Since the arrival of SSRIs, the TCAs are used uncommonly for the treatment of depression. There was significant weight gain associated with the use of both imipramine and amitriptyline, however. One study [45] compared imipramine with the atypical antidepressant nefazodone and found that a greater number of patients gained weight (at least 7%) during the first 2 months (4.9% versus 0.9%) and during longer-term treatment (24.5% versus 9.5%) respectively.

Fava et al [46] assessed changes in weight during a randomized study of the treatment of major depressive disorder with the SSRIs fluoxetine, sertraline, and paroxetine (n = 284). They reported that 25.5% of paroxetine-treated patients had weight gains of at least 7% compared with those treated with fluoxetine (6.8%) and sertraline (4.2%). Bupropion and nefazodone are less likely to be associated with increases in weight than are the SSRIs, although further controlled trials are needed [47]. Bupropion has been assessed as a potential treatment for weight loss in obese patients who also have depressive symptoms [48]. These patients were obese, had depressive symptoms, but did not meet criteria for major depressive disorder. They were treated with a 2100 kJ per day deficit diet and either bupropion SR or placebo. The bupropion SR group lost an average of 4.4 kg (4.6% of baseline weight) versus 1.7 kg (1.8% of baseline weight) among those on placebo ($P < 0.001$). Depressive symptoms improved more in the bupropion SR group than with placebo in subjects with a history of major depressive disorder. This study serves as an important model for future studies evaluating the pharmacological treatment of obese patients in whom depression is co-occurring.

As with the antipsychotic medications, treatment with the antidepressants requires attention not only to response to treatment for depression but also attention to increases in weight and BMI. It is recommended that weight and BMI be monitored with antidepressants, and use of antidepressants that are associated with minimal weight gain, especially in those at risk or already obese, should be considered. Switching to another antidepressant when weight gain occurs will require particular attention and caution with regard to the depressed patient's psychiatric status and clinical response. For example, if a patient is being treated successfully with an antidepressant but beginning to gain weight, initiating changes in diet with a nutritionally balanced deficit diet of 2100 to 4200 kJ per day reduction and an increase in physical activity may be helpful to help maintain a lower BMI.

Mood stabilizers

Mood stabilizers are an important treatment modality for bipolar disorder. Several of these medications also can be associated with weight gain, however. In addition to the antipsychotic medications reviewed earlier, certain mood stabilizers have been associated with weight gain, including valproic acid, carbamazepine, and lithium [37].

Lithium treatment has been associated with weight gain, with mean changes of 10 kg when used from 6 to 10 years [49]. A concern is that patients receiving mood stabilizers may discontinue treatment, with serious consequences for their mood disorder. Chengappa et al [50] completed an open-label, nonrandomized chart review (n = 214) study to assess change in weight in patients receiving topiramate, lithium, or valproate. Patients treated with lithium gained a mean (SD) of 6.3 (9.0) kg; those with valproate gained 6.4 (9.0) kg, while those receiving topiramate were found to have a reduction in body weight of 1.2 (6.3) kg. The weight gains with lithium and valproate were significantly greater than when topiramate was used ($P <$ 0.001). It is not clear, however, whether topiramate is effective in the treatment of bipolar disorder, and controlled studies are needed to better assess its use for psychiatric disorders. Patients with bipolar disorder are at greater risk for overweight and obesity, and weight gain may be associated with use of mood stabilizing medications [51]. Lamotrigine increasingly is being used as a mood stabilizer, and it has not been associated with weight gain. More research is needed to help prevent weight gain when mood stabilizers are used. Prevention and treatment programs for patients with bipolar disorder might include behavioral interventions for weight management and use of combination pharmacotherapy with medications that may induce weight loss [51]. Again, mood stabilizers are important for managing bipolar disorder, and the psychiatric status of patients with this disorder needs to be considered before switching medications because of weight gain to minimize the risk of destabilizing the patient's psychiatric condition.

Summary

Obesity has been associated with psychiatric disorders. There appears to be an association with depression and overweight, particularly in women. However, the picture is mixed during the course of depression, with some depressed patients gaining or losing weight during an episode. Obesity is also associated with bipolar disorder and schizophrenia. A number of psychiatric medications are associated with significant weight gain. Several second generation antipsychotic medications are associated not only with increases in weight but also with increased risk for type 2 diabetes mellitus and lipid disorders. It is important to monitor patients treated with the SGAs for weight gain and increases in metabolic and lipid measures. In addition, certain antidepressants and mood stabilizing drugs are associated with weight gain. Prevention and treatment programs need further research to better understand how to manage more effectively the weight gain and consequent increased risk for diabetes, hypertension, and lipid disorders in patients with serious psychiatric disorders.

References

[1] National Institutes of Health/National Heart, Lung, and Blood Institute. Clinical guidelines on the identification, evaluation, and treatment of overweight and obesity in adults: the evidence report. Obes Res 1998;6:51S–210S.

[2] Calle EE, Thun MJ, Petrelli JM, et al. Body mass index and mortality in a prospective cohort of US adults. N Engl J Med 1999;341:1097–105.

[3] Bychowski G. On neurotic obesity. Psychoanal Rev 1950;37:301–19.

[4] Moore ME, Stunkard AJ, Srole L. Obesity, social class and mental illness. JAMA 1962;181: 962–6.

[5] Stewart AL, Brook RH. Effects of being overweight. Am J Public Health 1983;73:171–8.

[6] Istvan J, Zavela K, Weidner G. Body weight and psychological distress in NHANES I. Int J Obes 1992;16:999–1003.

[7] Carpenter KM, Hasin DS, Allison DB, et al. Relationships between obesity and DSM-IV major depressive disorder, suicide ideation, and suicide attempts: results from a general population study. Am J Public Health 2000;90:251–7.

[8] Onyike CU, Crum RM, Lee HB, et al. Is obesity associated with major depression? Results from the third National Health and Nutrition Examination Survey. Am J Epidemiol 2003; 158:1139–47.

[9] Friedman MA, Brownell KD. Psychological correlates of obesity: moving to the next research generation. Psychol Bull 1995;117:3–20.

[10] Fabricatore AN, Wadden TA. Psychological aspects of obesity. Clin Dermatol, in press.

[11] Roberts RE, Deleger S, Strawbridge WJ, et al. Prospective association between obesity and depression: evidence from the Alameda County Study. Int J Obes 2003;27:514–21.

[12] Goodman E, Whitaker RC. A prospective study of the role of depression in the development and persistence of adolescent obesity. Pediatrics 2002;110:497–504.

[13] Sobal J, Stunkard AJ. Socioeconomic status and obesity: a review of the literature. Psychol Bull 1989;105:260–75.

[14] Hedley AA, Ogden CL, Johnson CL, et al. Prevalence of overweight and obesity among US children, adolescents, and adults, 1999–2002. JAMA 2004;291:2847–50.

[15] Staffieri JR. A study of social stereotype of body image in children. J Pers Soc Psychol 1967;7: 101–4.

[16] Cramer P, Steinwert T. Thin is good, fat is bad: how early does it begin? J Appl Dev Psychol 1998;19:429–51.

[17] Puhl R, Brownell KD. Bias, discrimination, and obesity. Obes Res 2001;9:788–805.

[18] Hebl MR, Mannix LM. The weight of obesity in evaluating others: a mere proximity effect. J Pers Soc Psychol Bull 2003;29:28–38.

[19] Harris JE, Hamaday V, Mochan E. Osteopathic family physicians' attitudes, knowledge, and self-reported practices regarding obesity. J Am Osteopath Assoc 1999;99:358–65.

[20] Schwartz MB, Chambliss HO, Brownell KD, et al. Weight bias among health professionals specializing in obesity. Obes Res 2003;11:1033–9.

[21] Wadden TA, Womble LG, Stunkard AJ, et al. Psychosocial consequences of obesity and weight loss. In: Wadden TA, Stunkard AJ, editors. Handbook of obesity treatment. New York: Guilford Press; 2002. p. 144–69.

[22] Doll HA, Petersen SEK, Stewart-Brown SL. Obesity and physical and emotional well-being: associations between body mass index, chronic illness, and the physical and mental components of the SF-36 questionnaire. Obes Res 2000;8:160–70.

[23] Fontaine KR, Cheskin LJ, Barofsky I. Health-related quality of life in obese persons seeking treatment. J Fam Pract 1996;43:265–70.

[24] Kolotkin RL, Crosby RD, Williams GR. Health-related quality of life varies among obese subgroups. Obes Res 2002;10:748–56.

[25] Dixon JB, Dixon ME, O'Brien PE. Depression in association with severe obesity: changes with weight loss. Arch Intern Med 2003;163:2058–65.

[26] Fabricatore AN, Wadden TA, Sarwer DB. Depressive symptoms as a function of body mass index and health-related quality of life in treatment-seeking obese adults. Obes Res 2003;11: A10.

[27] DiPietro L, Anda RF, Williamson DF, et al. Depressive symptoms and weight change in a national cohort of adults. Obes Res 1992;16:745–53.

[28] American Psychiatric Association. Diagnostic and statistical manual of mental disorders. 4th edition. Washington (DC): American Psychiatric Association; 1994.

[29] Matza LS, Revicki DA, Davidson JR, et al. Depression with atypical features in the national comorbidity survey. Arch Gen Psychiatry 2003;60:817–26.

[30] Stunkard AJ, Fernstrom MH, Price RA, et al. Direction of weight change in recurrent depression. Arch Gen Psychiatry 1990;47:857–60.

[31] Fagiolini A, Frank E, Houck PR, et al. Prevalence of obesity and weight change during treatment in patients with bipolar 1 disorder. J Clin Psychiatry 2002;63:528–33.

[32] Fagiolini A, Kupfer DJ, Houck PR, et al. Obesity as a correlate of outcome in patients with bipolar 1 disorder. Am J Psychiatry 2003;160:112–7.

[33] Allison DB, Fontaine KR, Heo M, et al. The distribution of body mass index among individuals with and without schizophrenia. J Clin Psychiatry 1999;60:215–20.

[34] Homel P, Casey D, Allison DB. Changes in body mass index for individuals with and without schizophrenia, 1987–1996. Schizophr Res 2002;55:277–84.

[35] Newman SC, Bland RC. Mortality in a cohort of patients with schizophrenia: a record linkage study. Can J Psychiatry 1991;36:239–45.

[36] Marder ST, Essock SM, Buchanan RW, et al. Physical health monitoring of patients with schizophrenia. Am J Psychiatry 2004;161:1334–49.

[37] Aronne LJ, Bray GA, Pi-Sunyer FX, et al, editors. Management of drug-induced weight gain: a continuing education monograph for physicians. The University of Wisconsin School of Medicine and Boron LePore Group Companies, Madison, WI; 2002.

[38] Consensus Development Conference on Antipsychotic Drugs and Obesity and Diabetes. Diabetes Care 2004;27(2):596–601.

[39] Allison DB, Mentore JL, Heo M, et al. Antipsychotic-induced weight gain: a comprehensive research synthesis. Am J Psychiatry 1999;156:1686–96.

[40] Gianfrancesco FD, Grogg AL, Mahmoud RA, et al. Differential effects of risperidone, olanzapine, clozapine, and conventional antipsychotics on type 2 diabetes: findings from a large health plan database. J Clin Psychopharmacol 2003;23:328–35.

[41] Genuth S, Alberti KG, Bennett P, et al. Expert committee on the diagnosis and classification of diabetes mellitus: follow-up report on the diagnosis of diabetes mellitus. Diabetes Care 2003;26:3160–7.

[42] Koller EA, Doraiswamy PM. Olanzapine-associated diabetes mellitus. Pharmacotherapy 2002;22:841–52.

[43] Newcomer JW, Haupt DW, Fucetola R, et al. Abnormalities in glucose regulation during antipsychotic treatment of schizophrenia. Arch Gen Psychiatry 2002;59:337–45.

[44] Henderson DC, Cagliero E, Gray C, et al. Clozapine, diabetes mellitus, weight gain, and lipid abnormalities: a five-year naturalistic study. Am J Psychiatry 2000;157:975–81.

[45] Sussman N, Ginsberg DL, Bikoff J. Effects of nefazodone on body weight: a pooled analysis of selective serotonin reuptake inhibitors and imipramine controlled trials. J Clin Psychiatry 2004;62(4):256–60.

[46] Fava M, Judge R, Hoog SL, et al. Fluoxetine versus sertraline and paroxetine in major depressive disorder: changes in weight with long-term treatment. J Clin Psychiatry 2000; 61(11):863–7.

[47] Fava M. Weight gain and antidepressants. J Clin Psychiatry 2000;61(11):37–41.

[48] Jain AK, Kaplan RA, Gadde KM, et al. Bupropion SR vs. placebo for weight loss in obese patients with depressive symptoms. Obes Res 2002;10(10):1049–56.

[49] Garland EJ, Remick RA, Zis AP. Weight gain: a side-effect with antidepressants and lithium. J Clin Psychopharmacol 1988;8:323–30.

[50] Chengappa KN, Chalasani L, Brar JS, et al. Changes in body weight and body mass index among psychiatric patients receiving lithium, valproate, or topiramate: an open label, nonrandomized chart review. Clin Ther 2002;24(10):1576–84.

[51] Keck PE, McElroy SL. Bipolar disorder, obesity, and pharmacotherapy-associated weight gain. J Clin Psychiatry 2003;64(12):1426–35.

ELSEVIER
SAUNDERS

PSYCHIATRIC
CLINICS
OF NORTH AMERICA

Psychiatr Clin N Am 28 (2005) 55–67

Obesity and Eating Disorders

Kelly C. Allison, PhD*, Albert J. Stunkard, MD

*Weight and Eating Disorders Program, University of Pennsylvania School of Medicine,
3535 Market Street, 3rd Floor, Philadelphia, PA 19104-3309, USA*

Understanding of the relationship between obesity and eating disorders has evolved over the past century. Obesity itself was considered by many to be an eating disorder until the middle of the last century. It has emerged, however, that most overweight and obese individuals do not overeat in any distinctive pattern. For a minority, however, two clear patterns have been identified: binge eating disorder (BED) and night eating syndrome (NES). Both disorders are more prevalent among overweight and obese persons than among those of normal weight. Their clinical features and treatments follow.

Binge eating disorder

Binge eating was described as far back as the times of Hippocrates, who called it bulimia (ox hunger) and viewed it as a sick form of hunger [1]. The first proposal of this type of disordered eating as a syndrome came in 1959 when Stunkard described binge eating syndrome. Since then, formal diagnostic criteria have been proposed and appear in the *Diagnostic and Statistical Manual of Mental Disorders, Fourth Edition, Text Revision (DSM-IV-TR)* as a provisional diagnosis. Criteria are based on two large studies (of 1984 and 1785 subjects, respectively) conducted at 12 eating disorder programs [2,3]. Two core features and several associated features were identified.

Diagnostic features

The first core feature of the diagnosis is "eating, in a discrete period of time...., an amount that is definitely larger than most individuals would eat

---

* Corresponding author.

E-mail address: kca@mail.med.upenn.edu (K.C. Allison).

under similar circumstances" [4]. The second core feature is experiencing
a loss of control over eating during this period of time, as if one cannot
either stop eating or limit the quantity that one eats. BED is to be
distinguished from bulimia nervosa by the absence of compensatory
behaviors such as vomiting, laxative abuse, or compulsive exercising. There
is also a sense of shame and disgust with oneself associated with the binge
eating episode that causes significant distress.

Compared with control groups of obese persons, people with BED suffer
from more severe obesity; earlier onset of overweight; earlier onset of, and
more frequent, dieting; and greater psychopathology.

Prevalence

Prevalence figures for BED range widely, depending on the assessment
methods used (eg, survey versus interview) and the definition of a binge. In
two community studies, the prevalence rate was as low as 1.8% [5] and 2%
[2]. In one study of 1450 persons who had identified themselves as binge
eaters on a phone screen following a television show, only 50 subjects (3.4%)
met interview-based criteria for BED [6]. Interview-based studies of
treatment-seeking obese persons found rates of 8.9% [7] and 18.8% [8].
BED is more common the more severe the obesity, as manifested by rates
for persons undergoing bariatric surgery of 27% [9], 38% [10], and 47%
[11]. Equal numbers of white men and women are affected with BED, while
black men report the disorder less frequently than black women [12–14].

Psychiatric comorbidity

Two risk factors for BED have been documented: psychiatric disorders
and obesity. Psychopathology, especially depression, has been reported
consistently among people with BED [15–24]. Axis II disorders, particularly
clusters B (dramatic-emotional) and C (anxious-fearful), [16,18,20] also
occur frequently in binge eaters (Table 1). In a community study, binge
eaters showed several vulnerabilities compared with healthy control
subjects, including frequent parental depression; greater susceptibility to
obesity; more exposure to negative comments about shape, weight, and
eating; morbid perfectionism; and negative self-evaluation [25]. Compared
with subjects with other psychiatric disorders, binge eaters were distinctive
only by more frequent reports of childhood obesity and awareness of
negative comments about shape, weight, and eating. Persons with BED
reported less exposure to risk factors for general psychopathology than
those with bulimia nervosa [25].

Risk factors

The influence of genetics on BED is unclear. A latent class analysis of
a large number of twins [27] revealed that one of the generated classes

Table 1
Percentage of binge eating disorder patents with lifetime comorbidity of Diagnostic and Statistical Manual of Mental Disorders diagnoses, as assessed by Structured Clinical Interview for DSM-IV Axis I Disorders

Study	Major depression	Any substance abuse or dependence	Any anxiety disorder	Any axis I disorder	Personality disorder
Yanovski et al, 1993	51	12		60	35
Specker et al, 1994	47	72	11.6	72.1	33
Mussel et al, 1996	47	23	18.8	70	
Telch and Stice, 1998	49	9		59	20
Wilfley et al, 2002				63	31

Data from ref. [26]. Stunkard AJ, Allison KC. Binge eating disorder: disorder or marker? Int J Eat Disord 2003;34:S107–16.

approximated the features of BED, and that monozygotic twin pairs more often fell into the same class than did dizygotic pairs. On the other hand, Lee et al [28] did not find a familial tendency for BED, or a familial relationship between BED and other eating disorders.

A once popular theory of development of BED has been put to rest in recent years, the theory that dieting causes BED. Spitzer et al [2,3] reported that dieting occurred after the onset of binge eating, and this finding was confirmed by five subsequent studies [29–34]. The National Task Force on the Prevention and Treatment of Obesity concluded that empirical studies do not support the belief that dieting induces binge eating in obese adults [35].

Treatment

Three treatment options for BED are: psychotherapy developed specifically for BED, medication, and behavioral weight loss programs. Although the first two options seem obvious, the last, behavioral weight loss programs, is surprising.

Psychotherapy
Both cognitive–behavioral therapy (CBT) and interpersonal psychotherapy (IPT), usually administered in a group format, are effective in decreasing the number of binge episodes, with reductions ranging from 48% to 96% [36–43]. Only one of the studies showed weight loss and a decrease in body mass index (BMI), and that changed only from 37.4 ± 5.1 kg/m^2 to 36.3 ± 5.4 kg/m^2 [43]. Similar results have been reported when CBT treatments were administered through self-help methods [37,39,44]. IPT also reduces binging, but again, with no clinically meaningful weight loss [41–43]. These results question the overall health benefits of these BED-specific treatments.

Psychopharmacology
Most controlled medication trials have used antidepressants [45]. Four of five placebo-controlled trials with selective serotonin reuptake inhibitors

(SSRIs), including citalopram [46], fluoxetine [47], fluvoxamine [48], and sertraline [49], significantly decreased binge frequency. Table 2 shows the percentage of patients achieving cessation of binging. All four successful trials produced significant decreases in weight over placebo, ranging from 1.2 kg [48] to 5.6 kg [49]. One trial of fluoxetine did not show significant benefit over placebo [50].

Two small (n = 23 in each) controlled trials that used tricyclic anti-depressants failed to produce significant weight loss; one decreased binges [51], and one did not [52].

One controlled medication trial for BED with an appetite suppressant (d-fenfluramine) reduced binges significantly without weight loss [6], while another (sibutramine) reduced binges with weight loss (7.4 kg) [53]. Finally, one controlled study of the anticonvulsant topiramate significantly de-creased binge frequency (from 3.4 to 0.3 episodes per week) and weight, with a loss of 5.9 kg [54].

Placebo responsiveness

Although medication trials reduced the number of binges, they also reported strong placebo responses. Alger et al [52] found that reductions in binging of 88% with imipramine and 79% with naltrexone did not differ significantly from the reduction induced by placebo treatment (68%). Trials with SSRIs produced high placebo remission rates (Table 2) and also high response rates (50% reduction in binges per week) in placebo versus medication: 49% *vs.* 62% with fluvoxamine [48]; 42% *vs.* 74% with citalopram [46]; 64% *vs.* 86% with sertraline [49]; and 57% *vs.* 76% with fluoxetine [47]. The trials with the appetite suppressants d-fenfluramine and sibutramine employed placebo run-in periods before randomizing participants; 44% [6]

Table 2
Remission rates of binge eating disorders with pharmacotherapy and placebos

Study	Active medication	Medication: % remission of binges	Placebo: % remission of binges
McElroy et al, 2003 [46]	Citalopram	47	21
Arnold et al, 2002 [47]	Fluoxetine	45	24
Hudson et al, 1998 [48]	Fluvoxamine	38	26
McElroy et al, 2000 [49]	Sertraline	47	14
Grilo et al, 2002 [50]	Fluoxetine	29	30
Stunkard et al, 1996 [6]	d-Fenfluramine	67	33
Appolinario et al, 2003 [53]	Sibutramine	52	32
McElroy et al, 2003 [54]	Topiramate	64	30
McCann, Agras, 1990 [51]	Desipramine	60	15

Data from Carter WP, Hudson JI, Lalonde JK, et al. Pharmacologic treatment of binge eating disorder. Int J Eat Disord 2003;34:S74–88; Stunkard AJ, Allison KC. Two forms of disordered eating in obesity: binge eating and night eating. Int J Obes Relat Metab Disord 2003;27:1–12.

and 24% [53] of the participants no longer met criteria for BED after the run-in and were not randomized. Even the impressive 94% reduction in binges on topiramate was accompanied by a decrease in bingeing of 46% on placebo [54]. Thus, the average placebo responses to BED come close to achieving responder status. The modest weight losses attained with medication together with placebo responsiveness raise questions as to the value of pharmacotherapy for binge eating [26,55].

Behavioral weight loss programs

Traditional behavioral weight loss programs that do not pay special attention to BED have been surprisingly effective in reducing binges. Marcus et al [59] found an 83% reduction in binges with a traditional behavioral weight loss program, while Agras et al [60] found that CBT alone reduced binging slightly more and weight slightly less than a combination of behavioral therapy and pharmacotherapy. Data from a community behavioral weight loss program (Trevose Weight Loss Program, Trevose, PA) showed that BED status was not related to weight loss, which averaged 18.7 (7.9) kg over 12 months [61]. Overweight and obese persons with BED also lost comparable amounts of weight in two additional studies [38,62]. One study has even shown that people with BED lost more weight than people without BED, while also significantly lowering their levels of depression [63]. BED status before treatment with very low calorie diets did not affect weight loss outcomes [22,56–58]. Behavioral weight loss programs appear to be as effective in reducing binging as treatments that specifically address binge eating behaviors. In addition, they are even more successful than CBT, IPT and most pharmacologic interventions in producing weight loss.

Variability

A recent study of BED among morbidly obese persons awaiting bariatric surgery indicated that BED was so variable that it was necessary to include a subthreshold group because of the small number of patients who consistently binged twice per week, for a period of 6 months, as per *DSM-IV-TR* provisional criteria [64]. Latner and Wilson [65] also found notable symptom fluctuation in BED; dietary self-monitoring alone reduced binge episodes by 45%. Nine of 18 patients with BED no longer met the full diagnostic criteria, and 28% were abstinent from binge eating at the end of a 1-week trial of self-monitoring. In contrast, of the 12 patients with bulimia nervosa in the same study, only 16% no longer met full diagnostic criteria, and none was abstinent [65].

Binge eating disorder appears to be a reactive disorder that waxes and wanes with clinical attention, or no attention at all. BED has a high placebo response rate in controlled trials. Binge episodes are reduced dramatically during placebo run-in trials, and BED responds well to nonspecific self-monitoring behavioral techniques. This variability severely limits the value of the diagnosis of BED in choosing treatments. The most distinctive aspect of the diagnosis of BED is its extensive psychiatric comorbidity. The extensive comorbidity with which it is associated suggests that BED may serve better as a marker for psychopathology [26].

Night eating syndrome

The night eating syndrome (NES) is an eating disorder characterized by a phase delay in the circadian pattern of eating, manifested by (1) evening hyperphagia, (2) awakenings accompanied by nocturnal ingestions, or (3) both. NES was originally described in 1955 based on a single patient and on the subsequent treatment of 25 obese persons referred to a special study clinic because of difficulties in the management of their obesity [66]. The features noted in this original study were the consumption of 25% of caloric intake after the evening meal, initial insomnia at least half of the time, and morning anorexia. A major revision of the criteria occurred in the course of a study by Birketvedt et al [67] that revealed nighttime awakenings, which were very often the occasion for the consumption of food. Consequently, provisional criteria for NES included morning anorexia, evening hyperphagia, and awakenings accompanied by frequent nocturnal ingestions [67].

More recently, an Item Response Theory (IRT) analysis, using data from 1479 Night Eating Questionnaires [68], examined the symptoms of NES described above (Allison et al, unpublished data, 2004). IRT revealed that *evening hyperphagia*, defined by eating 25% or more of the daily caloric intake after the evening meal, and/or the presence of *nocturnal ingestions*, more than half of the time upon awakening, were the most predictive symptoms of a diagnosis of NES. Morning anorexia and delayed ingestion of the first meal did not add enough information to be considered essential in diagnosing NES.

Prevalence

Night eating syndrome is uncommon in the general population (1.5%) [69]. As in the case of BED, prevalence of NES increases with increasing weight, from 8.9% [70] to 15% [71] in obesity clinics and from 10% [72] to 27% [69] and 42% [10] among obese persons undergoing assessment for bariatric surgery.

A recent discovery has been the occurrence of NES in persons of normal weight. This fact came to light through responses to the NES Web site, which provided the Night Eating Questionnaire (NEQ) [68]. The results showed one major difference between the responses of 40 obese night eaters and 40 nonobese night eaters. The normal weight night eaters were 7 years younger (33.1 plus or minus 10.7 years compared with 40.0 plus or minus 14.3 years for the obese night eaters). The younger age of the nonobese subjects suggests that NES may contribute to the development of their obesity. This suggestion is supported by the fact that more than half of obese night eaters reported that their night eating began before their obesity.

Features of night eating syndrome

Five studies have confirmed aspects of the NES. Gluck et al [71] reported that NES subjects consumed more of their food intake than did controls during the latter part of the day, and that a test meal at this time was larger in night eaters than in controls. This study also found elevated levels of depression in NES subjects. Aronoff et al [73] reported that 70% of the 24-hour food intake of night eaters was consumed after 7 p.m. Allison et al [74] found that NES subjects awakened 1.7 times per night, and 73% of these awakenings were associated with nocturnal snacks. Manni et al [75] found NES, as confirmed by polysomnography, in 7 of 120 sleep clinic patients. Patients ate compulsively shortly after awakening, and ingestions were limited to small snacks. Spaggiari et al [76] noted frequent awakenings, also confirmed by polysomnography, in 10 patients who ate during half of these occasions.

Stress plays a strong role in the development and maintenance of NES. In the authors' experience, approximately 75% of NES sufferers linked the onset of their disorder to a specific stress-related event. Those who reported a stress-related onset were nearly 15 years older at age of onset than the 25% of respondents who did not experience such an event (34.2 years versus 19.6 years; t (36) = 5.1, $P = 0.001$) suggesting a particular vulnerability among night eaters with younger age of onset (Allison et al, unpublished data, 2004). Additional evidence of the role of stress is provided by measures of cortisol. Birketvedt et al [67] reported elevated serum cortisol over a 24-hour period in the controlled environment of a general clinical research center, and daytime salivary cortisol also is elevated among night eaters (Allison et al, unpublished data, 2004).

As in the case with BED, psychiatric comorbidity is common among people with NES [26,55]. Over 75% of NES participants in one study had a lifetime history of an axis I disorder [55]. Specifically, night eaters met DSM-IV criteria significantly more often than controls for a history of major depressive disorder (47%), any anxiety disorder (37%), and any substance abuse or dependence (24%). Beck Depression Inventory scores are moderately elevated among people with NES [77]. Napolitano et al [78] also reported even higher levels of state and trait anxiety and disinhibition of food intake among obesity clinic patients with NES than among those with BED or with no disordered eating.

There is a strong familial link in NES. A study in progress by the authors has found that 36% of NES participants reported at least one first-degree relative with night eating behaviors compared with significantly fewer (16%) matched controls ($\chi^2(1) = 4.6$, $P = 0.03$). This comparison is biased in favor of the night eaters, since they are far more likely to be aware of family members with the disorder than are persons without NES.

Eating versus sleep disorder

The disturbed sleep with frequent awakenings had led to the view that NES is a combined eating and sleeping disorder. The recent study by O'Reardon et al [79], however, revealed no significant differences between night eaters and controls for sleep onset (23:31 ± 1:40 versus 23:32 ± 1:06) and sleep offset (07:24 ± 1:07 versus 06:59 ± 1:12). This finding suggests that, among night eaters, it is the eating pattern that is disturbed and not the sleeping pattern. NES thus appears to be a disorder of biological rhythm, characterized by a phase delay onset of eating (Fig. 1). This view encompasses the continuation of overeating into the night and the delay in onset of appetite in the morning.

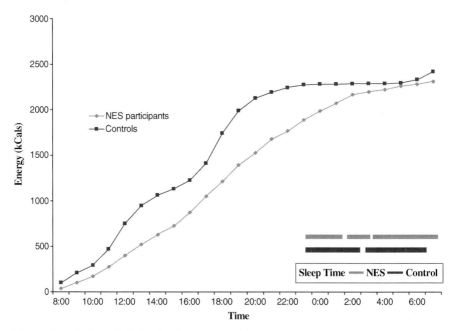

Fig. 1. Cumulative caloric intake for persons with night-eating syndrome shows a delayed circadian shift relative to matched control participants, while the timing of the sleep period for both groups does not differ. Persons with night-eating syndrome have more frequent awakenings than controls, and they occur earlier in the sleep period [79].

Treatment

A history of dramatic response of NES to fenfluramine by two small groups suggested that an SSRI might be effective in its treatment [75,78]. An open-label trial of the SSRI sertraline with 17 patients strongly supported this suggestion [78]. Sertraline was administered in a dose that averaged 188 mg per day over a period of 12 weeks. Analyses revealed highly significant improvements in all four primary outcome measures: number of nocturnal awakenings, number of nocturnal ingestions, total daily caloric intake after the evening meal, and an overall rating change on the Clinical Global Impression of Improvement scale (CGI-I). Although five subjects dropped out of treatment for various reasons, five others achieved full remission of symptoms (CGI-I score of 1) and, in addition, lost a significant amount of weight (4.8 ± 2.6 kg, $p < 0.05$). Two others reduced their NES by at least 50%, and five had only minimal improvement. The weight loss found among remitters suggests that successful treatment of NES might contribute to control of the associated obesity. A double-blind, placebo-controlled trial of sertraline, now underway, is finding results as promising as those of the earlier open-label trial (O'Reardon et al, unpublished data, 2004).

Another treatment modality has been effective in the treatment of NES. Pawlow et al [77] reported that abbreviated progressive muscle relaxation therapy delivered for a period of 1 week, resulted in significantly better outcome for 20 night eaters compared with 20 untreated night eaters. Significant reductions were noted in stress and anxiety and levels of hunger that were significantly lower at nighttime and higher in the morning.

Summary

In conclusion, two subtypes of disordered eating affect a segment of the overweight and obese population. BED and NES represent opportunities to recognize, treat, and prevent these disorders that, at the least, maintain, and at the worst, promote, overweight and obesity.

The constellation of symptoms that comprise BED is recognized readily, while the stability of the diagnosis is low, with very high placebo responsiveness. Psychotherapeutic efforts reduce the number of binges without affecting body weight. SSRIs are modestly effective in decreasing binges and facilitating weight loss. Traditional behavioral weight loss programs, however, may be the most effective. The marked psychopathology with which BED is associated suggests that the disorder may serve best as a marker for psychopathology.

Night eating syndrome is an eating disorder characterized by a delayed shift in the circadian pattern of eating. By contrast, circadian sleep rhythms are intact, although sleep is disturbed and subject to awakenings to eat. Stress plays a major part in the onset and maintenance of NES, and psychiatric comorbidity is high. NES may be a pathway to obesity.

Treatment with sertraline and muscle relaxation has shown considerable promise.

References

[1] Stunkard AJ. A history of binge eating. In: Fairburn CG, Wilson GT, editors. Binge eating: nature, assessment and treatment. New York: Guilford; 1993. p. 15–34.

[2] Spitzer RL, Devlin M, Walsh BT, et al. Binge eating disorder: a multisite field trial of the diagnostic criteria. Int J Eat Disord 1992;11:191–203.

[3] Spitzer RL, Yanovski S, Wadden TA, et al. Binge-eating disorder: its further validation in a multi-site study. Int J Eat Disord 1993;13:137–50.

[4] American Psychiatric Association. Diagnostic and statistical manual of mental disorders, Fourth edition, text revision. Washington, DC: American Psychiatric Association; 2000. p. 787.

[5] Bruce B, Agras WS. Binge eating in females: a population-based investigation. Int J Eat Disord 1992;12:365–73.

[6] Stunkard AJ, Berkowitz R, Tanrikut C, et al. d-fenfluramine treatment of binge eating disorder. Am J Psychiatry 1996;153:1455–9.

[7] Stunkard AJ, Berkowitz R, Wadden T, et al. Binge eating disorder and the night eating syndrome. Int J Obes Relat Metab Disord 1996;20:1–6.

[8] Brody ML, Walsh BT, Devlin MJ. Binge eating disorder: reliability and validity of a new diagnostic category. J Consult Clin Psychol 1994;62:381–6.

[9] Wadden TA, Sarwer DB, Womble LG, et al. Psychosocial aspects of obesity and obesity surgery. Surg Clin North Am 2001;81:1001–24.

[10] Hsu LKG, Betancourt S, Sullivan SP. Eating disturbances before and after vertical banded gastroplasty: a pilot study. Int J Eat Disord 1996;19:23–34.

[11] Adami GF, Bandolfo P, Bauer B, et al. Binge eating in massively obese patients undergoing bariatric surgery. Int J Eat Disord 1995;17:45–50.

[12] le Grange D, Telch CF, Agras WS. Eating and general psychopathology in a sample of Caucasian and ethnic minority subjects. Int J Eat Disord 1997;21:285–93.

[13] Pike KM, Dohm FA, Striegel-Moore RH, et al. A comparison of black and white women with binge eating disorder. Am J Psychiatry 2001;158:1455–60.

[14] Smith DE, Marcus MD, Lewis CE, et al. Prevalence of binge eating disorder, obesity, and depression in a biracial cohort of young adults. Ann Behav Med 1998;20:227–32.

[15] Marcus MD, Wing RR, Hopkin J. Obese binge eaters: affect, cognitions and response to behavioral weight control. J Consult Clin Psychol 1988;56:433–9.

[16] Marcus MD, Wing RR, Ewing L, et al. Psychiatric disorders among obese binge eaters. Int J Eat Disord 1996;9:69–77.

[17] Yanovski SZ, Nelson JE, Dubbert BK, et al. Association of binge eating disorder and psychiatric comorbidity in obese subjects. Am J Psychiatry 1993;150:1472–9.

[18] Mitchell JE, Mussell MP. Comorbidity and binge eating disorder. Addict Behav 1995;20: 725–32.

[19] Antony MM, Johnson WG, Carr-Nangle RE, et al. Psychopathology correlates of binge eating and binge eating disorder. Compr Psychiatry 1994;35:386–92.

[20] Specker S, De Zwaan M, Raymond N, Mitchell J. Psychopathology in subgroups of obese women with and without binge eating disorder. Compr Psychiatry 1994;35:185–90.

[21] Telch C, Stice E. Psychiatric comorbidity in a nonclinical sample of women with binge eating disorder. J Consult Clin Psychol 1998;66:768–76.

[22] Wadden TA, Foster GD, Letizia KA. One-year behavioral treatment of obesity: comparison of moderate and severe caloric restriction and the effects of weight maintenance therapy. J Consult Clin Psychol 1994;62:165–71.

[23] Kuehnel RH, Wadden TA. Binge eating disorder, weight cycling, and psychopathology. Int J Eat Disord 1994;15:321–9.

[24] Mussell MP, Mitchell JE, de Zwaan M, et al. Clinical characteristics associated with binge eating in obese females: a descriptive study. Int J Obes Relat Metab Disord 1996;20:324–31.

[25] Fairburn CG, Doll HA, Welch SL, et al. Risk factors for binge eating disorder - a community based, case-control study. Arch Gen Psychiatry 1998;55:425–32.

[26] Stunkard AJ, Allison KC. Binge eating disorder: disorder or marker? Int J Eat Disord 2003; 34:S107–16.

[27] Bulik CM, Sullivan PF, Kendler KS. An empirical study of the classification of eating disorders. Am J Psychiatry 2000;157:851–3.

[28] Lee YH, Abbott DW, Seim H, et al. Eating disorders and psychiatric disorders in the first-degree relatives of obese probands with binge eating disorder and obese nonbinge eating disorder controls. Int J Eat Disord 1999;26:322–32.

[29] Wilson GT, Nonas CA, Rosenblum GD. Assessment of binge eating in obese patients. Int J Eat Disord 1993;150:1472–9.

[30] Berkowitz R, Stunkard AJ, Stallings VA. Binge eating disorder in obese adolescent girls. Annual New York Academy of Medicine 1993;699:200–96.

[31] Spurrell EM, Wilfley DE, Tanofsky MB, et al. Age of onset for binge eating disorder: are there different pathways to binge eating? Int J Eat Disord 1997;21:55–65.

[32] Grilo CM, Masheb RM. Onset of dieting vs. binge eating in outpatients with binge eating disorder. Int J Obes Relat Metab Disord 2000;24:404–9.

[33] Abbott DW, de Zwaan M, Mussell MP, et al. Onset of binge eating and dieting in overweight women: implications for etiology, associated features and treatment. J Psychosom Res 1998; 44:367–74.

[34] Mussell MP, Mitchell JE, Fenna CJ, et al. A comparison of onset of binge eating versus dieting in the development of bulimia nervosa. Int J Eat Disord 1997;12:353–60.

[35] National Task Force on the Prevention and Treatment of Obesity. Dieting and the development of eating disorders in overweight and obese adults. Arch Intern Med 2000;160: 2581–9.

[36] Agras WS, Telch CF, Arnow B, et al. One-year follow-up of cognitive behavioral therapy for obese individuals with binge eating disorder. J Consult Clin Psychol 1997;65:343–7.

[37] Carter JC, Fairburn CG. Cognitive behavioral self-help for binge eating disorder: a controlled effectiveness study. J Consult Clin Psychol 1998;66:616–23.

[38] Nauta H, Hospers H, Kok G, et al. A comparison between a cognitive and a behavioral treatment for obese binge eaters and obese nonbinge-eaters. Behav Ther 2000;31:441–61.

[39] Peterson CB, Mitchell JE, Engbloom S, et al. Group cognitive-behavioral treatment of binge eating disorder: a comparison of therapist-led versus self-help formats. Int J Eat Disord 1998;24:125–36.

[40] Smith DE, Marcus MD, Kaye W. Cognitive–behavioral treatment of obese binge eaters. Int J Eat Disord 1992;12:257–62.

[41] Wilfley DE, Cohen LR. Psychological treatment of bulimia nervosa and binge eating disorder. Psychopharmacol Bull 1997;33:437–54.

[42] Wilfley DE, Agras WS, Telch CF, et al. Group cognitive–behavioral therapy and group interpersonal psychotherapy for the nonpurging bulimic individual: a controlled comparison. J Consult Clin Psychol 1993;61:296–305.

[43] Wilfley DE, Welch RR, Stein RI, et al. A randomized comparison of group cognitive–behavioral therapy and group interpersonal psychotherapy for the treatment of overweight individuals with binge eating disorder. Arch Gen Psychiatry 2002;59:713–21.

[44] Fairburn CG. Overcoming binge eating. New York: Guilford Press; 1995.

[45] Carter WP, Hudson JI, Lalonde JK, et al. Pharmacologic treatment of binge eating disorder. Int J Eat Disord 2003;34:S74–88.

[46] McElroy SL, Hudson JI, Malhotra S, et al. Citalopram in the treatment of binge eating disorder: a placebo-controlled trial. J Clin Psychiatry 2003;64:807–13.

[47] Arnold LM, McElroy SL, Hudson JI, et al. A placebo-controlled randomized trial of fluoxetine in the treatment of binge eating disorder. J Clin Psychiatry 2002;63:1028–33.

[48] Hudson JI, McElroy SL, Raymond NC, et al. Fluvoxamine in the treatment of binge eating disorder: a multi-center placebo-controlled, double-blind trial. Am J Psychiatry 1998;155: 1756–62.

[49] McElroy SL, Casuto L, Nelson E, et al. Placebo-controlled trial of sertraline in the treatment of binge eating disorder: a randomized trial. Am J Psychiatry 2000;157:1004–6.

[50] Grilo CM, Masheb RM, Heniger G. Controlled comparison of cognitive behavioral therapy and fluoxetine for binge eating disorder. Presented at 2002 Annual Meeting of the Academy of Eating Disorders. Boston, April 28, 2002.

[51] McCann UD, Agras WS. Successful treatment of nonpurging bulimia nervosa with desipramine: a double-blind, placebo-controlled study. Am J Psychiatry 1990;147:1509–13.

[52] Alger SA, Schwalberg MD, Bigaoutte JM, et al. Effect of a tricyclic antidepressant and opiate antagonist on binge eating behavior: a double-blind, placebo-controlled study. Am J Clin Nutr 1991;53:865–71.

[53] Appolinario JC, Bacaltchuk J, Sichieri R, et al. A randomized, double-blind, placebo-controlled study of sibutramine in the treatment of binge-eating disorder. Arch Gen Psychiatry 2003;60:1109–16.

[54] McElroy SL, Arnol LM, Shapira NA, et al. Topiramate in the treatment of binge eating disorder associated with obesity: a randomized placebo-controlled trial. Am J Psychiatry 2003;160:255–61.

[55] Stunkard AJ, Allison KC. Two forms of disordered eating in obesity: binge eating and night eating. Int J Obes Relat Metab Disord 2003;27:1–12.

[56] LaPorte DJ. Treatment response in obese binge eaters: preliminary results using a very low calorie diet (VLCD) and behavior therapy. Addict Behav 1992;17:247–57.

[57] Telch CF, Agras WS. The effects of a very low calorie diet on binge eating. Behav Ther 1993; 24:177–93.

[58] Wadden TA, Foster GD, Letizia KA. Response of obese binge eaters to treatment by behavior therapy combined with very low calorie diet. J Consult Clin Psychol 1992;60: 808–11.

[59] Marcus MD, Wing RR, Fairburn CG. Cognitive behavioral treatment of binge eating vs. behavioral weight control on the treatment of binge eating disorder. Ann Behav Med 1995; 17:S090.

[60] Agras WS, Telch CF, Arnow B, et al. Weight loss, cognitive, behavioral and desipramine treatments in binge eating disorder: an additive design. Behav Ther 1994;25:225–38.

[61] Latner JD, Delinsky SS, Wilson GT. Binge eating and weight loss in a self-help behavioral treatment program for obesity. Presented at the Australasian Society for Psychiatric Research. Christchurch, New Zealand, December 2, 2003.

[62] Ho KSI, Nichaman MZ, Taylor WC, et al. Binge eating disorder, retention and drop-out rate in an adult obesity program. Int J Eat Disord 1995;18:291–4.

[63] Gladis MM, Wadden TA, Vogt R, et al. Behavioral treatment of obese binge eaters: do they need different care? J Psychosom Res 1998;44:375–84.

[64] Hsu LKG, Mulliken B, McDonagh B, et al. Binge eating disorder in extreme obesity. Int J Obes 2002;26:1398–403.

[65] Latner JD, Wilson GT. Self-monitoring and the assessment of binge eating. Behav Ther 2002;33:465–77.

[66] Stunkard AJ, Grace WJ, Wolff HG. The night-eating syndrome: a pattern of food intake among certain obese patients. Am J Med 1955;19:78–86.

[67] Birketvedt G, Florholmen J, Sundsfjord J, et al. Behavioral and neuroendocrine characteristics of the night eating syndrome. JAMA 1999;282:657–63.

[68] Marshall HM, Allison KC, O'Reardon JO, et al. The night eating syndrome among nonobese persons. Int J Eat Disord 2004;35:217–22.

[69] Rand CSW, Macgregor MD, Stunkard AJ. The night eating syndrome in the general population and among post-operative obesity surgery patients. Int J Eat Disord 1997;22: 65–9.

[70] Stunkard AJ. Eating patterns and obesity. Psychiatr Q 1959;33:284–94.

[71] Gluck ME, Geliebter A, Satov T. Night eating syndrome is associated with depression, low self-esteem, reduced daytime hunger, and less weight loss in obese outpatients. Obes Res 2001;9:264–7.

[72] Powers PS, Perez A, Boyd F, Rosemurgy A. Eating pathology before and after bariatric surgery: a prospective study. Int J Eat Disord 1999;25:293–300.

[73] Aronoff NJ, Geliebter A, Zammit G. Gender and body mass index as related to the night eating syndrome in obese outpatients. J Am Diet Assoc 2001;101:102–4.

[74] Allison KC, O'Reardon J, Stunkard AJ, et al. Characterizing the night eating syndrome. Obes Res 2001;9:93S.

[75] Manni R, Ratti MT, Tartara A. Nocturnal eating: prevalence and features in 120 insomniac referrals. Sleep 1997;20:734–8.

[76] Spaggiari MC, Granella F, Parrino L, et al. Nocturnal eating syndrome in adults. Sleep 1994; 17:339–44.

[77] O'Reardon JO, Stunkard AJ, Allison KC. A clinical trial of sertraline in the treatment of the night eating syndrome. Int J Eat Disord 2004;35:16–26.

[78] Napolitano MA, Head S, Babyak MA, et al. Binge eating disorder and night eating syndrome: psychological and behavioral characteristics. Int J Eat Disord 2001;30:193–203.

[79] O'Reardon JO, Ringel BL, Dinges DF, et al. Circadian eating and sleeping patterns in the night eating syndrome. Obes Res 2004;12:1789–96.

PSYCHIATRIC
CLINICS
OF NORTH AMERICA

Psychiatr Clin N Am 28 (2005) 69–87

Body Image and Obesity in Adulthood

David B. Sarwer, PhD[a],*, J. Kevin Thompson, PhD[b],
Thomas F. Cash, PhD[c]

[a]Departments of Psychiatry and Surgery, The Edwin and Fannie Gray Hall
Center for Human Appearance, University of Pennsylvania School of Medicine,
3535 Market Street, Suite 3108, Philadelphia, PA 19104, USA
[b]Department of Psychology, University of South Florida,
4202 Fowler Avenue, Tampa, FL 33620-8200, USA
[c]Department of Psychology, Old Dominion University, Norfolk 23529, VA, USA

The body image concerns of obese individuals first were described in the late 1960s [1]. Initially, body image disturbance was thought to be limited to persons who experienced a prepubescent onset of obesity, those who received negative appearance evaluations from parents and siblings, and those with the presence of an emotional disturbance. After 25 years of relatively little discussion, the last decade has witnessed a dramatic growth in empirical attention to the relationship between body image and obesity [2,3]. This research has focused on the prevalence and nature of body image dissatisfaction and its clinical significance.

Prevalence of body image dissatisfaction

Dissatisfaction with physical appearance appears to be more the rule than the exception. Based on the results of the 1996 survey published in *Psychology Today* [4], most women (56%) and almost half (43%) of men are dissatisfied with their overall appearance. Two-thirds of women and more than half of men report dissatisfaction with their body weight. Features likely to be affected negatively by excess body weight, such as the abdomen, hips, and thighs, generate greater dissatisfaction among women.

The validity of findings from surveys like this frequently is called into question [5]. Magazine surveys are often subject to sample biases; it is

This paper was supported, in part, by funding from the National Institute of Diabetes and Digestive and Kidney Diseases (Grant No. K23 DK60023-03) (D.B. Sarwer).
* Corresponding author.
E-mail address: dsarwer@mail.med.upenn.edu (D.B. Sarwer).

unknown how representative the readers of *Psychology Today* magazine who responded to this survey are of the general population. Studies that have used sampling strategies to ensure a more representative sample of the American population [6] have found lower levels of body image dissatisfaction relative to the *Psychology Today* surveys from 1985 [7] and 1996 [5]. Still, a substantial percentage of women reported being discontented with various aspects of their body—especially their midtorso (51%), lower torso (47%), and weight (46%).

As the prevalence of overweight and obesity has increased [8], it is logical to expect that rates of body image dissatisfaction would rise similarly. No evidence of a recent worsening of body image, however, exists. Prospective and cross-sectional studies suggest a recent modest improvement of college women's body satisfaction despite their heavier weights [9–11]. Perhaps the threshold for weight-related body dissatisfaction has shifted upwards as the population has become heavier. This hypothesis, however, awaits further study.

Body image dissatisfaction is common but varies across different groups. Women, who have been the focus of most of the research, typically are far more dissatisfied with their body image than men [12,13]. Differences also exist across ethnic groups. African American women, as compared with Caucasian women, typically report less body image dissatisfaction [14]. Among other ethnic groups, body image dissatisfaction appears to be related to the degree of acculturation. As Asian and Hispanic American individuals acculturate to American customs, body image dissatisfaction appears to increase and mirror that of Caucasian Americans [15].

The nature of body image dissatisfaction

Overweight and obese women report greater body image dissatisfaction than normal weight women [16]. In a society that puts such premium on thinness for women, this observation is not surprising. Counter to intuition, several studies [17–21], but not all [22], have found no relationship between body image dissatisfaction and body mass index (BMI) in overweight and obese women. This finding is consistent with theories of body image, which have suggested that there may be little relationship between what one thinks about the body and the objective reality of one's appearance [23,24]. It may be that some overweight or obese individuals experience a threshold effect with regard to body image dissatisfaction [25,26]. As individuals become overweight or obese, they experience an increase in body image dissatisfaction. Similarly, if they lose weight, they experience an improvement in body image. If they continue to gain or lose weight beyond the threshold, however, their body dissatisfaction may remain stable. This interpretation, however, must be made cautiously. Each of the studies cited used truncated distributions of overweight and obese individuals, typically excluding those with extreme obesity. Studies investigating large samples of individuals with a wide range of BMIs are need to clarify the relationship between body mass and body image dissatisfaction.

Certain characteristics and experiences of obese individuals appear to be associated with increased body image dissatisfaction [15,16]. Childhood onset of obesity and experience of weight-related teasing are related to increased body image dissatisfaction in adulthood [27,28]. Adults with binge eating disorder, a history of weight cycling, and those who reported being stigmatized secondary to their obesity also report greater body image dissatisfaction [21,29–31].

For many women, the degree of dissatisfaction is profound and adversely affects behavior. More than 80% of overweight women who sought body image therapy scored greater than one standard deviation above the norms of the Body Dysmorphic Disorder Examination and the Body Shape Questionnaire [32]. A significantly greater percentage of obese women than nonobese women reported, on more than half of the days of the month, camouflaging their bodies with clothing, changing their posture or body movements, avoiding looking at their bodies, and becoming upset when thinking about their appearance [20]. Similarly, a greater percentage of obese women also reported moderate-to-extreme embarrassment in social situations, such as work or parties, because of their weight [20].

Perhaps the degree of distress associated with excess body weight is illustrated best by the extremely obese. Men and women who underwent bariatric surgery were asked if they would prefer to return to their previous level of obesity or be of a normal weight and have one of the following disabilities: deafness, severe acne, heart disease, dyslexia, diabetes, blindness, or losing a leg [33]. Typically, most persons presented with this forced-choice question will select their own worst-handicap (in this case, obesity) rather than a new disability. No patient elected a return to extreme obesity over being deaf, dyslexic, or diabetic, or over having severe acne or heart disease. Five patients selected obesity over blindness, and four patients selected obesity over losing a leg. Although this study did not specify the reasons why persons almost exclusively chose another disability over obesity, the fact that 100% of the participants reported improvements in body image following surgery suggests that the body image dissatisfaction experienced preoperatively may have contributed to this decision.

Clinical significance of body image dissatisfaction

Several studies have found a relationship between increased body image dissatisfaction, increased depressive symptoms, and decreased self-esteem among obese women who sought weight loss treatment [18,20,27]. These relationships appear to occur independently from the degree of obesity. Sarwer et al [20] found that while obese women and nonobese women differed in body image dissatisfaction, they did not differ on self-reported depressive symptoms or self-esteem. In a nonclinical sample, Annis et al [29] also found no differences among currently, formerly, and never-overweight women on depressive symptoms or social anxiety. Compared with their nonobese counterparts, obese adolescent girls reported greater dissatisfaction with their weight and figure, but not greater symptoms of depression [34]. In contrast, Cash et al [35] recently found that increasing BMI levels were related to a poorer body image quality of life among women. This finding underscores the need for additional study of the relationships between body weight, body image dissatisfaction, and psychological symptoms.

A small minority of obese women, however, appears to experience extreme body image dissatisfaction. Eight percent of obese women reported a degree of body image dissatisfaction consistent with the diagnosis of body dysmorphic disorder (BDD) [20]. BDD is defined as a preoccupation with an imagined or slight defect in appearance that causes clinically significant distress or impairment in social, occupational, or other important areas of functioning [36]. Five of the six women were concerned with their appearance as it related to their obesity. As a result, the formal diagnosis could not be applied, as it requires that the preoccupation and distress be focused on a slight defect in appearance. The *Diagnostic and Statistical Manual of Mental Disorders, Fourth Edition, Text Revised (DSM-IV-TR)* does not have a diagnostic category for patients with marked distress about medical conditions that affect physical appearance. These women also reported significantly more depressive symptoms compared with other obese women. Thus, a subset of obese women experiences body image dissatisfaction to an extent that entails clinically significant psychological impairment.

Motivation for weight loss and body image dissatisfaction

Regardless of the relationship of body image dissatisfaction and psychological symptoms, body image dissatisfaction has been hypothesized to play a significant role in motivating people to lose weight. Heinberg et al [37] have suggested that individuals with a moderate degree of dissatisfaction might be motivated to lose weight or improve health status by changing their diet and physical activity. In contrast, those with a low level of dissatisfaction might not be inclined to change these behaviors. Of importance here is the possibility that highly body-dissatisfied obese individuals, because of their perceived inability to lose weight, might actually give up and not attempt healthy eating and exercise behaviors.

For many overweight and obese adults, weight reduction may be the most popular form of body image therapy [38]. Although some individuals may be motivated to lose weight to improve their health, most people do so to improve physical appearance [39]. Even among the extremely obese who seek bariatric surgery (who often present with serious obesity-related comorbid health problems such as hypertension, diabetes, and osteoarthritis), improving appearance, and not health, is the primary motivator for weight loss [40,41].

Assessment of body image in obese adults

Body image is considered a multi-dimensional construct [15,42–44]. The assessment of body image dissatisfaction is also multi-dimensional and includes the measurement of subjective (dis)satisfaction, cognitive distortions, affective reactions, behavioral avoidance, and perceptual inaccuracy [43]. The number of assessment tools for such aspects of body image has increased substantially over the past 20 years, producing a wide variety of measures [45–48]. The following discussion will focus rather selectively on those instruments most relevant for the particular appearance concerns of obese individuals (ie, body weight and shape).

One of the first considerations in the assessment of body image is to ensure that the measure under consideration actually indexes the particular dimension of body image of interest [42]. Just because a measure has body image, body dissatisfaction, or some similar body-related word or phrase in its title does not mean that the measure assesses the same aspect of body image as a different scale with a similar name. The authors suggest that investigators and clinicians scan the items of a measure to ensure that the name of the measure adequately captures the content of the instrument.

Additionally, it is important to realize that subscales of a particular measure may capture different components of body image. For instance, the widely used Multi-dimensional Body Self-Relations Questionnaire (MBSRQ) [45,49] has two subscales (Appearance Evaluation [AE] and Appearance Orientation [AO]) that index orthogonal aspects of body image. The AE scale captures a general subjective satisfaction with appearance, whereas the AO scale assesses one's investment in appearance. In a study that readily demonstrates the distinction between the two dimensions, Smith et al [50] found that Caucasian men and women had higher levels of appearance evaluation than African American men and women, whereas African Americans had higher levels of appearance orientation. In terms of the practical application to research and clinical endeavors, this example illustrates that care should be taken in the selection of a body image measure and the interpretation of the results.

Measures of weight satisfaction

Table 1 describes some of the more commonly used measures that index weight (dis)satisfaction. These measures include scales such as the Eating Disorder Inventory—Body Dissatisfaction scale and the Body Shape

Table 1
Measures of body satisfaction and related concepts

Name of instrument	Author(s)	Description	Author address
Figure Rating Scale	Stunkard et al (1983)	Select self and ideal percepts from nine figures varying from underweight to overweight	Albert J. Stunkard, MD, University of Pennsylvania, 3535 Market Street, Philadelphia, PA 19104-2648
Contour Rating Scale	Thompson and Gray (1995)	Select self and ideal percepts from nine male and nine female schematic figures ranging from underweight to overweight	James J. Gray, PhD, Department of Psychology, Asbury Building, American University, Washington, DC 20016-8062
None given	Collins (1991)	Select self and ideal from seven boy and seven girl figures that vary in size	M.E. Collins, HSD, MPH, Centers for Disease Control and Prevention, 4770 Buford Highway, NE, Mailstop K26, Atlanta, GA 30341-3724
Body Image Assessment Procedure	Williamson et al (1989)	Select self and ideal from nine figures of various sizes	Donald A. Williamson, PhD, Department of Psychology, Louisiana State University, Baton Rouge, LA 70803-5501
Somatomorphic Matrix	Gruber et al (1999)	Computer program allows selection of self and ideal bodies from 100 male and 100 female schematic figures, ranging on muscularity and fatness	Amanda J. Gruber, McLean Hospital, 115 Mill Street, Belmont, MA 02478
Eating Disorder Inventory, Body Dissatisfaction subscale	Garner et al (1983)	Rate degree of agreement with statements about body parts being large (seven items)	David M. Garner, PhD, c/o Psychological Assessments Resources, Inc., P.O. Box 998, Odessa, FL 33556

Multidimensional Body-Self Relations Questionnaire, Appearance Evaluation (AE) subscale and Body Areas Satisfaction Scale (BASS)	Cash (2000)	AE: seven-item scale that measures overall appearance evaluation; BASS: assesses satisfaction with nine body areas/attributes	Thomas F. Cash, PhD*, Department of Psychology, Old Dominion University, Norfolk, VA 23529
Body Satisfaction Scale	Slade et al (1990)	Indicate degree of satisfaction with 16 parts (three subscales: general, head, body)	P.D. Slade, PhD, Department of Psychiatry and Department of Movement Science, Liverpool University Medical School, P.O. Box 147, Liverpool L69 3BX, England
Body-Esteem Scale-Revised	Mendelson et al (1998)	23-item scale with three subscales: appearance, attribution, and weight	Beverly K. Mendelson, PhD, Department of Psychology, Concordia University, 7141 Sherbrooke Street, Montreal, Quebec, H4B 1R6, Canada
Body Image Ideals Questionnaire	Szymanski & Cash (1995)	Assesses extent of discrepancy from ideals for 11 physical characteristics weighted by each ideal's importance	Thomas F. Cash, PhD*, Department of Psychology, Old Dominion University, Norfolk, VA 23529
Body Shape Questionnaire	Cooper et al (1987)	34 Items on concerns with one's body shape	Peter Cooper, PhD, Department of Psychiatry, University of Cambridge Addenbrooke's Hospital, Hills Road, Cambridge CB2 2QQ, England
Self-Image Questionnaire for Young Adolescents, Body Image subscale	Peterson et al (1984)	Designed for 10 to 15-year-olds; 11-item body image subscale assesses positive feelings toward the body	Anne C. Peterson, PhD, College of Health and Human Development, Pennsylvania State University, 101 Henderson Building, University Park, PA 16802

(continued on next page)

Table 1 (*continued*)

Name of instrument	Author(s)	Description	Author address
Body Image States Scale	Cash et al (2002)	Six items assess momentary evaluative/affective body image states	Thomas F. Cash, PhD* Department of Psychology, Old Dominion University, Norfolk, VA 23529
Physical Appearance State and Trait Anxiety Scale	Reed et al (1991)	Rate anxiety associated with 16 body parts (eight weight-relevant; eight non weight-relevant); trait and state versions available	J. Kevin Thompson, PhD, Department of Psychology, University of South Florida, 4202 Fowler Avenue, Tampa, FL 33620-8200
Physical Appearance Behavioral Avoidance Test	Thompson et al (1994)	Approach own body image in a mirror, from a distance of 20 ft; subjective units of distress ratings and approach distance are dependent measures	J. Kevin Thompson, PhD, Department of Psychology, University of South Florida, 4202 Fowler Avenue, Tampa, FL 33620-8200
Situational Inventory of Body Image Dysphoria–Short Form	Cash (2002)	Rate how often one experiences negative body image emotions in 20 situations	Thomas F. Cash, PhD*, Department of Psychology, Old Dominion University, Norfolk, VA 23529
Appearance Schemas Inventory–Revised	Cash, Melnyk, and Hrabosky (2004)	20-Item assessment of one's psychological investment in one's appearance (two subscales)	Thomas F. Cash, PhD*, Department of Psychology, Old Dominion University, Norfolk, VA 23529
Body Image Quality of Life Inventory	Cash and Fleming (2002)	19 Items that measure negative-to-positive effects of one's body image on one's life	Thomas F. Cash, PhD*, Department of Psychology, Old Dominion University, Norfolk, VA 23529

Drive for Muscularity Scale	McCreary and Sasse (2000)	15 Items assessing attitudes and behaviors related to the pursuit of a muscular appearance	Dr. Don McCreary, PhD, Stress & Coping Group, Defense R&D, Canada—Toronto 1133 Sheppard Avenue West, P.O. Box 2000, Toronto, Ontario Canada M3M 3B9
Muscle Appearance Satisfaction Scale (MASS)	Mayville et al (2002)	Rate symptoms of muscle dysmorphia on 19-items with five subscales	Donald A. Williamson, PhD, Department of Psychology, Louisiana State University, Baton Rouge, LA 70803-5501

* Available at www.body-images.com for a nominal fee.

Questionnaire. These scales appear to be ideal for use with obese samples, because the focus is on the subjective rating of weight-related aspects of the body.

Another method to assess body image dissatisfaction involves the use of schematic figure rating methodologies. These consist of a range of figures varying in size from thin/underweight to obese. Generally, individuals rate the figures using an instructional protocol designed to determine their ideal body size and their current or actual body size. The discrepancy between the two ratings is used as the index of dissatisfaction, which has been shown to be correlated highly with questionnaire measures of satisfaction [48]. These measures include the Figure Rating Scale, the Contour Rating Scale, and the Body Image Assessment Procedure. Unfortunately, most of these assessments have limited gradation in the depiction of obesity and other psychometric limitations [47,51].

Measures of appearance satisfaction

The broader notion of body image dissatisfaction can be assessed by measures of overall appearance satisfaction. These measures may focus on nonweight-related features, such as discrete body parts or muscularity, or include items that attempt to assess an individual's conception of how he or she looks in clothes or appears to other people. The MBSRQ AE scale is likely the most widely used measure of more general appearance satisfaction. This scale and other measures may be particularly useful, as they provide information regarding the generality or specificity of the obese individual's appearance concerns. For instance, it might be clinically useful to determine if satisfaction is specific to certain body areas (for example, using the Body Areas Satisfaction Scale of the MBSRQ or the Body Image Ideals Questionnaire) [45,49] or generalized to other aspects of appearance. Similarly, it might be relevant to examine the extent to which people experience negative body image emotions in specific day-to-day-life contexts with the Situational Inventory of Body Image Dysphoria [45,52]. Moreover, it may be especially useful to measure how individuals' psychosocial functioning is influenced by his or her body image using the Body Image Quality of Life Inventory [35,45,53].

Measures of body image investment

Equating people's body image experiences purely with their level of satisfaction or dissatisfaction with appearance has a limited perspective. Cash et al [54,55] have maintained that one also should take into account the extent to which people are invested in their appearance psychologically. The AO subscale of the MBSRQ provides a general assessment of appearance investment. Recent investigation has suggested that this dimension may consist of two cognitive–behavioral facets, as measured by the Appearance Schemas Inventory-Revised [45,55]. One facet is termed "motivational salience" and refers to the extent to which people value appearance management (ie, pay attention to their looks and engage in grooming behaviors). The second facet, called "self-evaluative salience," reflects how much one's physical appearance defines self-worth. The latter seems to be a more pivotal determinant of psychological functioning and body image quality of life. Most research on body image and obesity has focused on body image satisfaction and has ignored body image investment.

Measures of size perception

No discussion of body image assessment is complete without some reference to perceptual aspects of body image. This is perhaps the most controversial area in body image assessment. Many of the early studies of people with eating disorders noted a tendency of anorexics to actually overestimate the size of their bodies. As a result, the field of body image was somewhat dominated by interest in this phenomenon until the late 1980s [56]. Recent work has questioned the specificity of overestimation to any diagnostic group (eating disordered or obese) and has demonstrated that perceptual ratings are affected by attitudinal and affective factors [44]. Many of the perceptual assessment methods are costly and logistically impractical, making the inclusion of such a strategy difficult for many clinicians. Finally, these measures do not appear to be associated strongly with body image satisfaction. [43,51].

General considerations

A measure of weight or shape satisfaction may be the most appropriate initial screening instrument for an obese individual. Results from a weight satisfaction measure should provide a general picture of the body image of an obese person. Based on the analysis of these data, overall appearance scales, cognitive measures, or behavioral indices of body image could be included to provide more detailed information. In addition, a useful adjunctive strategy might involve the addition of a self-monitoring form, such as the Body Image Diary [57], designed to allow for daily self-monitoring of body image experiences. Finally, the aforementioned Body Image Quality of Life Inventory is valuable in assessing how and to what extent the person's body image affects his or her life and psychosocial functioning.

Gender and ethnicity should be considered when choosing a body image assessment tool (or any psychological test), as the instrument may have been developed and validated on a sample with different characteristics. This may be particularly true for the assessment of body size. Many of the measures listed in Table 1 were developed, normed, and validated on college students. Certainly, these samples contained some proportion of overweight or obese individuals; however, studies often have failed to provide information on the body mass of the respondents or to evaluate the psychometric characteristics of the scales that assessed body weight. Similarly, the psychometric qualities of a scale developed on nonpatient samples may not generalize to patient samples. For these reasons, the authors recommend contacting the authors of specific scales and requesting any normative and psychometric data for obese samples, by gender and ethnicity.

Treatment of body image dissatisfaction in obese adults

The treatment of body image concerns of obese people is still in the developmental stages. Through 1990, no study in the obesity treatment literature had addressed body image specifically [58,59]. Since that time, several studies have investigated the efficacy of psychotherapeutic interventions to improve body image. Perhaps as a result, many comprehensive behavior modification weight loss interventions now address body image concerns [26].

Nevertheless, the specific role of body image treatment in behavioral weight control programs has not been determined fully. Studies have shown that improvements in the body image of obese people occur with weight loss. Other studies have shown that body image improvements can occur without weight reduction. The importance of body image in satisfaction with weight loss treatment and long-term weight maintenance is unknown.

Improvements in body image accompanying weight loss

Several studies have assessed changes in body image in obese people during weight loss. Cash [60] reported significant improvements in the body image of obese women who achieved an average weight loss of 22 kg. Foster et al [18] assessed changes in body image in women following 48 weeks of weight loss. At the midpoint of treatment, women had lost an average of 19 kg and reported significant improvements in body image. A weight regain of approximately 3 kg from weeks 24 to 48 was associated with a slight but significant worsening in body image. Nevertheless, at the end of treatment, patients reported significant improvements in body image as compared with baseline. These improvements were related only modestly to the amount of weight lost.

Another approach to understanding body image in relation to obesity and weight loss involves a cross-sectional comparison of overweight/obese, formerly overweight/obese, and never overweight/obese cohorts, in which the latter two groups are of equal average weight [61]. This methodology examines the proposition that the body image experiences associated with obesity may not be lost fully when the weight is lost, a phenomenon termed "phantom fat" or "vestigial body image." Annis et al [29] found that relative to never overweight women, currently overweight women reported more body dissatisfaction/distress, overweight preoccupation, and dysfunctional appearance investment, in addition to greater binge eating pathology, poorer social self-esteem, and less satisfaction with life. Consistent with a phantom fat interpretation, formerly overweight women were comparable to currently overweight women but worse than never overweight women on overweight preoccupation and dysfunctional appearance investment. On the other hand, formerly and never overweight women did not differ on body satisfaction.

Several studies have suggested that extremely obese patients who undergo bariatric surgery experience improvements in body image [62–65]. Two cross-sectional investigations have documented improvements in body image using the AE subscale of the MBSRQ [64,65]. Anecdotal reports, however, suggest that some bariatric surgery patients report dissatisfaction with their bodies following the massive weight loss. Some may experience phantom fat, reflecting vestigial body image concerns. Others may be experiencing a different type of body image dissatisfaction, perhaps related to body frame size or other nonweight-related concerns, such as the development of loose or sagging skin at different areas of the body [66,67].

Improvements in body image without weight loss

Several studies have investigated the efficacy of improving body image in overweight and obese people without weight loss. Roughan et al [68] reported significant improvements in body image, self-esteem, and depressive symptoms following a program designed to promote weight acceptance and decrease overeating and dietary restraint. Obese women enrolled in a similar "Undieting" program reported improvements in self-esteem and depression, but did not find improvements in body image [69]. One possible explanation for the difference in body image findings may be that Roughan et al's participants lost 3 kg, while Polivy et al's participants gained approximately 6 kg.

Based in large part on the work of Cash et al [57,70,71], Rosen et al developed an extensive cognitive–behavioral body image therapy program specifically tailored for overweight and obese individuals [32]. Obese women treated by this approach reported marked improvements in body image and self-esteem compared with the nontreatment condition [32]. They did not, however, experience weight loss. At the end of treatment, 70% of women in body image intervention demonstrated significant improvements on the body image measures, with scores moving from the clinically severe range (at pretreatment) to within the normal range. Subsequently, Strachan et al [72] examined the outcomes of a self-directed cognitive–behavioral body image improvement program in which one-third of the participants were obese. Participants did not lose weight, and obese and nonobese persons reported equivalently favorable body image improvements.

More recently, Ramirez et al [73] combined their body image therapy program with a 16-week behavioral weight control intervention to assess if the combined treatment, as compared with behavioral weight control alone, would be more effective in improving body image. Following treatment, both groups lost approximately 10% of their initial weight and reported significant improvement in body image, self-esteem, and eating concerns. During the 1-year follow-up period, the two groups did not differ on weight maintenance or body image. Thus, it appears that weight reduction alone is as effective in improving body image as a combined weight loss/body image treatment.

Cooper et al [74] and Sarwer et al [26] have suggested that the treatment of body image concerns may be most useful during the maintenance phase of treatment. As such, it may improve long-term weight maintenance. Several studies of the efficacy of body image therapy to improve weight maintenance are in progress.

In summary, a growing number of interventions exist to help people improve their body image with or without losing weight. The utility of these inventions for people with a variety of more general body image concerns is unquestioned. Their ultimate usefulness for obese individuals, however, remains undetermined. Many obese people have significant medical comorbidities that are made worse by their excess body weight. For these individuals, weight reduction is clearly more than an aesthetic issue. Enhancing the body image of these people may be a less critical issue compared with improving their overall health through weight reduction.

Summary

Research on the relationship between body image and obesity is relatively new. Several areas await additional investigation. Many obese individuals have body image concerns, but these concerns are not universal. Furthermore, there appears to be little relationship between the degree of obesity and the intensity of the dissatisfaction. The nature of the obesity and its effect on body size and shape may moderate the relationship with the degree of body image dissatisfaction. Similarly, obesity-related comorbidities, such as osteoarthritis, may contribute to body image dissatisfaction further.

The clinical significance of body image dissatisfaction also warrants additional study. Among obese women, body image dissatisfaction appears to be related to lower self-esteem and increased symptoms of depression. For most people, it does not appear to be related to clinically significant depression. Furthermore, such body image dissatisfaction cannot be equated with body image disturbance necessarily, which entails dissatisfaction that also produces significant distress and psychosocial impairment [5]. A small minority of obese persons, however, reports body image disturbance consistent with that of body dysmorphic disorder. Major depression and extreme body image dissatisfaction, and significant social anxiety, may not only prevent individuals from seeking weight loss but also may compromise the potential effectiveness of certain treatment approaches.

Most body image studies have relied heavily on paper-and-pencil measures of general body image dissatisfaction. As a result, the perceptual component of body image has been neglected somewhat. Recently developed computer programs that allow for the morphing of body features may provide interesting opportunities to assess body image in obese persons. This technology potentially could be used to assess patients' expectations about changes in body size and shape following weight loss. Future studies also should incorporate other important body image dimensions, such as body image investment (or schematicity) and body image quality of life. Investigators should strive to include a wider range of subgroups of obese individuals, including those with binge eating disorder and the rapidly increasing number of extremely obese individuals who pursue bariatric surgery. Most research in this area has focused on obese women. There has been some research on obese children and adolescents [75,76], but comparatively little study of men [77].

Treatment for body image dissatisfaction in obese people has drawn heavily from cognitive–behavioral models of psychotherapy. Most studies support their effectiveness; however, there has been little study of the components of treatment that are most critical to success. It is unclear if the behaviorally based strategies, such as exposure to avoided situations and behavioral changes to promote body acceptance, or if the cognitive elements of treatment, such as cognitive restructuring or coping skills training, play a more central role in treatment outcome. Ultimately, studies of the differential effectiveness of these strategies may provide important information on the treatment of body image dissatisfaction.

Presently, it appears that two separate camps of research on the relationship between obesity and body image are developing. The first group is looking primarily at changes in body image that accompany weight loss. These investigators are focusing more on how changes to the physical body influence the body image. The second group is looking more specifically at changes in body image, through the use of psychotherapy, often independent of weight loss. The focus of this group is changing the body image without changing the body. Although both areas have evidence to support their effectiveness, it may turn out that the combination of both approaches—changing the body and the body image simultaneously—may lead to the most successful outcomes. Alternatively, ongoing research ultimately may suggest that body image interventions play their most important role during weight maintenance. Regardless, the relationship between obesity and body image likely will continue to generate much research and clinical interest.

Acknowledgments

The authors would like to thank Lauren M. Gibbons for her editorial assistance during the preparation of the paper.

References

[1] Stunkard AJ, Mendelson M. Obesity and body image: I. Characteristics of disturbances in the body image of some obese persons. Am J Psychiatry 1967;123:1296–300.
[2] Thompson JK, editor. Body image, eating disorders, and obesity: an integrative guide for assessment and treatment. Washington (DC): American Psychological Association; 1996.
[3] Thompson JK, editor. Handbook of eating disorders and obesity. Hoboken (NJ): John Wiley & Sons; 2004.
[4] Garner DM. The 1997 body image survey results. Psychol Today 1997;31:30.
[5] Cash TF. A negative body image: evaluating epidemiological evidence. In: Cash TF, Pruzinsky T, editors. Body image: a handbook of theory, research, and clinical practice. New York: Guilford Press; 2002. p. 269–76.
[6] Cash TF, Henry P. Women's body images: the results of a national survey in the USA. Sex Roles 1995;33:19–28.
[7] Cash TF, Winstead BA, Janda LH. The great American shape-up: body image survey report. Psychol Today 1986;20:30–7.
[8] Flegal KM, Carroll MD, Ogden CL, et al. Prevalence and trends in obesity among US adults, 1999–2000. JAMA 2002;288:1723–7.
[9] Cash TF, Morrow JA, Hrabosky JI, et al. How has body image changed? A cross-sectional study of college women and men from 1983 to 2001. J Consult Clin Psychol, in press.
[10] Heatherton TF, Nichols P, Mahamedi F, et al. Body weight, dieting, and eating disorder symptoms among college students, 1982 to 1992. Am J Psychiatry 1995;152:1623–9.
[11] Heatherton TF, Mahamedi F, Striepe M, et al. A 10-year longitudinal study of body weight, dieting, and eating disorder symptoms. J Abnorm Psychol 1997;106:117–25.
[12] Cash TF. Women's body images. In: Wingood G, DiClemente R, editors. Handbook of women's sexual and reproductive health. New York: Plenum, 2002. p. 175–94.
[13] Feingold A, Mazzella R. Gender differences in body image are increasing. Psychol Sci 1998; 9:190–5.
[14] Celio AA, Zabinski MF, Wilfley DE. African American body images. In: Cash TF, Pruzinsky T, editors. Body image: a handbook of theory, research, and clinical practice. New York: Guilford Press; 2002. p. 234–42.
[15] Cash TF, Pruzinsky T, editors. Body image: a handbook of theory, research, and clinical practice. New York: Guilford Press; 2002.
[16] Schwartz MB, Brownell KD. Obesity and body image. Body Image: An International Journal of Research 2004;1:43–56.
[17] Eldrige KL, Agras WS. Weight and shape overconcern and emotional eating in binge eating disorder. Int J Eat Disord 1996;19:73–82.
[18] Foster GD, Wadden TA, Vogt RA. Body image before, during, and after weight loss treatment. Health Psychol 1997;16:226–9.
[19] Matz PE, Foster GD, Faith MS, et al. Correlates of body image dissatisfaction among overweight women seeking weight loss. J Consult Clin Psychol 2002;70:1040–4.
[20] Sarwer DB, Wadden TA, Foster GD. Assessment of body image dissatisfaction in obese women: specificity, severity and clinical significance. J Consult Clin Psychol 1998;66(4): 651–4.
[21] Wilfley DE, Schwartz MB, Spurrell EB, et al. Using the eating disorder examination to identify the specific psychopathology of binge eating disorder. Int J Eat Disord 2000;27: 259–69.

[22] Hill AJ, Williams J. Psychological heath in a nonclinical sample of obese women. Int J Obes 1998;22:578–83.

[23] Cash TF. The psychology of physical appearance: aesthetics, attributes, and images. In: Cash TF, Pruzinsky T, editors. Body images: development, deviance and change. New York: Guilford Press; 1990. p. 51–79.

[24] Sarwer DB, Wadden TA, Pertschuk MJ, et al. The psychology of cosmetic surgery: a review and reconceptualization. Clin Psychol Rev 1998;18(1):1–22.

[25] Foster GD, Matz PE. Weight loss and changes in body image. In: Cash TF, Pruzinsky T, editors. Body image: a handbook of theory, research, and clinical practice. New York: Guilford Press; 2003. p. 405–13.

[26] Sarwer DB, Thompson JK. Obesity and body image disturbance. In: Wadden TA Stunkard AJ, editors. Handbook of obesity treatment. New York: Guilford Press; 2002. p. 447–64.

[27] Grilo CM, Wilfley DE, Brownell KD, et al. Teasing, body image, and self-esteem in a clinical sample of obese women. Addict Behav 1994;19:443–50.

[28] Jackson TD, Grilo CM, Masheb RM. Teasing history, onset of obesity, current eating disorder psychopathology, body dissatisfaction, and psychological functioning in binge eating disorder. Obes Res 2000;8:451–8.

[29] Annis NM, Cash TF, Hrabosky JI. Body image and psychosocial differences among stable average-weight, currently overweight, and formerly overweight women: the role of stigmatizing experiences. Body Image: An International Journal of Research 2004;1: 155–67.

[30] Friedman MA, Schwartz MB, Brownell KD. Differential relation of psychological functioning with the history and experience of weight cycling: psychological correlates of weight cycling. J Consult Clin Psychol 1998;66:646–50.

[31] Myers A, Rosen JC. Obesity stigmatization and coping: Relation to mental health symptoms, body image, and self-esteem. Int J Obes 1999;23:221–30.

[32] Rosen JC, Orosan P, Reiter J. Cognitive–behavior therapy for negative body image in obese women. Behav Ther 1995;26:42.

[33] Rand CSW, Macgregor AMC. Successful weight loss following obesity surgery and the perceived liability of morbid obesity. Int J Obes 1991;15:577–9.

[34] Wadden TA, Foster GD, Stunkard AJ, et al. Dissatisfaction with weight and figure in obese girls: discontent but not depression. Int J Obes 1989;13:89–97.

[35] Cash TF, Jakatdar TA, Williams EF. The Body Image Quality of Life Inventory: further validation with college men and women. Body Image: An International Journal of Research 2004;1:279–87.

[36] American Psychiatric Association. Diagnostic and statistical manual of mental disorders. 4th edition, text revised. Washington (DC): American Psychiatric Association; 2000.

[37] Heinberg LJ, Thompson JK, Matzon JL. Body image dissatisfaction as a motivator for healthy lifestyle change: is some distress beneficial? In: Stiegel-Moore RH, Smolak L, editors. Eating disorders: innovative directions in research and practice. Washington (DC): American Psychological Association; 2001.

[38] Sarwer DB, Grossbart TA, Didie ER. Beauty and society. In: Kaminer MS, Dover JS, Arndt KA, editors. Atlas of cutaneous aesthetic surgery. Philadelphia: WB Saunders; 2001.

[39] Levy AS, Heaton AW. Weight control practices of US adults trying to lose weight. Ann Intern Med 1993;119:661–6.

[40] Krall JG. Surgical treatment of obesity. In: Wadden TA, VanItallie TB, editors. Treatment of the seriously obese patient. New York: Guilford Press; 1992. p. 496–506.

[41] Wadden TA, Sarwer DB, Arnold ME, et al. Psychosocial status of severely obese patients before and after bariatric surgery. Problems in General Surgery 2000;17:13–22.

[42] Thompson JK. The (mis)measurement of body image: ten strategies to improve assessment for applied and research purposes. Body Image: An International Journal of Research 2004; 1:7–14.

[43] Thompson JK, Heinberg LJ, Altabe M, et al. Exacting beauty: theory, assessment, and treatment of body image disturbance. Washington (DC): American Psychological Association; 1999.

[44] Thompson JK, Smolak L, editors. Body image, eating disorders, and obesity in youth: assessment, prevention, and treatment. Washington (DC): American Psychological Association; 2001.

[45] Cash TF. Questionnaires and manuals to assess body image 2004. Available at: www.body-images.com. Accessed October 15, 2004.

[46] Stewart TM, Williamson DA. Assessment of body image disturbances. In: Thompson JK, editor. Handbook of eating disorders and obesity. New York: Wiley; 2004. p. 495–514.

[47] Thompson JK, van den Berg P. Measuring body image attitudes among adolescents and adults. In: Cash TF, Pruzinsky T, editors. Body image: a handbook of theory, research, and clinical practice. New York: Guilford; 2002. p. 142–54.

[48] Thompson JK. Assessing body image disturbance: measures, methodology and implementation. In: Thompson JK, editor. Body image, eating disorders, and obesity: an integrative guide for assessment and treatment. Washington (DC): American Psychological Association; 1996. p. 49–81.

[49] Brown TA, Cash TF, Mikulka PJ. Attitudinal body image assessment: factor analysis of the Body-Self Relations Questionnaire. J Pers Assess 1990;55:135–44.

[50] Smith DE, Thompson JK, Raczynski JM, et al. Body image among men and women in a biracial cohort: the CARDIA study. Int J Eat Disord 1999;25:83–8.

[51] Thompson JK, Gardner RM. Measuring perceptual body image among adolescents and adults. In: Cash TF, Pruzinsky T, editors. Body image: a handbook of theory research, and clinical practice. New York: Guilford Press; 2002. p. 135–41.

[52] Cash TF. The Situational Inventory of Body Image Dysphoria: psychometric evidence and development of a short form. Int J Eat Disord 2002;32:362–6.

[53] Cash TF, Fleming EC. The impact of body image experiences: development of the Body Image Quality of Life Inventory. Int J Eat Disord 2002;31:455–60.

[54] Cash TF. Cognitive–behavioral perspectives on body image. In: Cash TF, Pruzinsky T, editors. Body image: a handbook of theory, research, and clinical practice. New York: Guilford Press; 2002. p. 38–46.

[55] Cash TF, Melnyk SE, Hrabosky JI. The assessment of body-image investment: an extensive revision of the Appearance Schemas Inventory. Int J Eat Disord 2004;35:305–16.

[56] Thompson JK. Body image disturbance: assessment and treatment. Elmsford (NY): Pergamon Press; 1990.

[57] Cash TF. The body image workbook: an 8-step program for learning to like your looks. Oakland (CA): New Harbinger Publications; 1997.

[58] Brownell KD, Wadden TA. Behavioral therapy for obesity: modern approaches and better results. In: Brownell KD, Foreyt JP, editors. Handbook of eating disorders: physiology, psychology, and treatment of obesity, anorexia, and bulimia. New York: Basic Books; 1986. p. 180–99.

[59] Rosen JC. Improving body image in obesity. In: Thompson JK, editor. Body image, eating disorders, and obesity: an integrative guide for assessment and treatment. Washington (DC): American Psychological Association; 1996. p. 425–40.

[60] Cash TF. Body image and weight changes in a multisite comprehensive very-low calorie diet program. Behav Ther 1994;25(2):239–54.

[61] Cash TF, Counts B, Huffine CE. Current and vestigial effects of overweight among women: fear of fat, attitudinal body image, and eating behaviors. J Psychopathol Behav Assess 1990; 12:157–67.

[62] Adami GF, Gandolfo P, Campostano A, et al. Body image and body weight in obese patients. Int J Eat Disord 1998;24:299–306.

[63] Camps MA, Zervos E, Goode S, et al. Impact of bariatric surgery on body image perception and sexuality in morbidly obese patients and their partners. Obes Surg 1996;6:356–60.

[64] Dixon JB, Dixon ME, O'Brien PE. Body image: appearance orientation and evaluation in the severely obese. Obes Surg 2002;12:65–71.

[65] Neven K, Dymek M, leGrange D, et al. The effects of Roux-en-Y gastric bypass surgery on body image. Obes Surg 2002;12:265–9.

[66] Bailey SM, Goldberg JP, Swap WC, et al. Relationships between body dissatisfaction and physical measurements. Int J Eat Disord 1990;9:457–61.

[67] Davis C, Durnin JVGA, Dionne M, et al. The influence of body fat content and bone diameter measurements on body dissatisfaction in adult women. Int J Eat Disord 1994;15:257–63.

[68] Roughan P, Seddon E, Vernon-Roberts J. Long-term effects of a psychologically based group programme for women preoccupied with body weight and eating behaviour. Int J Obes 1990;14:135–47.

[69] Polivy J, Herman CP. Undieting: a program to help people stop dieting. Int J Eat Disord 1992;11:261–8.

[70] Butters JW, Cash TF. Cognitive–behavioral treatment of women's body-image dissatisfaction. J Consult Clin Psychol 1987;55:889–97.

[71] Cash TF, Hrabosky JI. The treatment of body-image disturbances. In: Thompson JK, editor. Handbook of eating disorders and obesity. New York: Wiley; 2004. p. 515–41.

[72] Strachan MD, Cash TF. Self-help for a negative body image: a comparison of components of a cognitive–behavioral program. Behav Ther 2002;33:235–51.

[73] Ramirez EM, Rosen JC. A comparison of weight control and body image therapy for obese men and women. J Consult Clin Psychol 2001;69(3):440–6.

[74] Cooper Z, Fairburn CG. Cognitive behavioral treatment of obesity. In: Wadden TA, Stunkard AJ, editors. Obesity: theory and therapy. 3rd edition. New York: Guilford Press; 2002. p. 465–79.

[75] Ricciardelli LA, McCabe MP. Children's body image concerns and eating disturbance: a review of the literature. Clin Psychol Rev 2001;21(3):325–44.

[76] Smolak L. Body image in children and adolescents: where do we go from here? Body Image: An International Journal of Research 2004;1:15–28.

[77] McCabe MP, Ricciardelli LA. Weight and shape concerns of boys and men. In: Thompson JK, editor. Handbook of eating disorders and obesity. New York: Wiley; 2004. p. 606–34.

ELSEVIER
SAUNDERS

Psychiatr Clin N Am 28 (2005) 89–103

PSYCHIATRIC
CLINICS
OF NORTH AMERICA

Medical Evaluation of the Obese Individual

Robert F. Kushner, MD[a,b,*], Julie L. Roth, MD[a,b]

[a]*Northwestern University Feinberg School of Medicine, Galter Pavilion, Suite 3-150,*
251 East Huron Street, Chicago, IL 60611, USA
[b]*Wellness Institute, Northwestern Memorial Hospital, 150 East Huron Street,*
Suite 1100, Chicago, IL 60611, USA

Overweight and obesity are the most common medical problems seen in primary care practice, affecting over 60% of adults and 15% of adolescents [1]. Obesity affects at least nine organ systems, and it is linked to the most prevalent and costly medical problems seen in daily practice. Thus, treatment and control of obesity have the potential to have a significant impact on several chronic diseases. Yet despite the importance of screening and evaluating for obesity and the recommendation to do so from multiple organizations [2–8], detection and counseling rates among physicians remain low [9–11]. Several observational studies show that physicians are more likely to discuss weight problems with their patients only after they have developed moderate-to-severe obesity or associated comorbidities [12]. Reasons for this delayed action include lack of education and training in obesity management, time restraints, lack of reimbursement for obesity as a diagnostic code, and clinician attitudes of futility and lack of perceived benefit and reward. The ill fortune of this clinical inertia toward obesity care is that the most successful treatment is likely to be early intervention and prevention, before development of more severe obesity and comorbid conditions. According to Kristeller et al [13], three factors are necessary for physicians to intervene: adequate recognition of obesity as a medical problem, willingness to provide intervention, and adequate skills or resources to do so. For psychiatrists, the need to recognize obesity and the weight gain that occurs as a consequence of medications is important for several reasons. Patients are at risk of developing obesity-related silent

* Corresponding author.
E-mail address: rkushner@nmh.org (R.F. Kushner).

0193-953X/05/$ - see front matter © 2005 Elsevier Inc. All rights reserved.
doi:10.1016/j.psc.2004.09.004
psych.theclinics.com

conditions, such as prediabetes, diabetes, hypertension, and dyslipidemia, which typically do not present with symptoms [14]. Furthermore, even small gains in weight are associated with increased health risks [15,16]. Additionally, nonadherence to medications is more likely to occur if the patient perceives weight gain as an unacceptable adverse effect. This article reviews the current recommendations for medical evaluation of the obese adult patient.

Identification and evaluation of the obese patient

To provide guidance to physicians and associated health professionals and evidence for the effects of treatment, the National Heart, Lung, and Blood Institute (NHLBI) published the Clinical Guidelines on the Identification, Evaluation, and Treatment of Overweight and Obesity in Adults in 1998 [2]. This 228-page document containing over 750 references is an excellent resource on the research supporting the relationship between obesity and comorbid conditions and various treatment approaches. The Practical Guide to the Identification, Evaluation, and Treatment of Overweight and Obesity in Adults subsequently was developed cooperatively by the NHLBI and North American Association for the Study of Obesity (NAASO) and published in 2000 [17]. Both guidelines recommend proactive obesity care beginning with identification, classification, and categorization of risk. A treatment algorithm outlining this process can be found in both documents. Readers also are referred to the American Medical Association's Assessment and Management of Adult Obesity: A Primer for Physicians [18]. The Primer consists of 10 booklets covering the evaluation process, assessing readiness and making treatment decisions; setting up the office environment; communication and counseling strategies; using dietary, physical activity, pharmacological and surgical management; and suggested resources. Each booklet begins with a case presentation and is subdivided by targeted patient care-oriented questions that emphasize practical tips and expected outcomes.

Taking an obesity-focused history

The first step in providing obesity care is to take a comprehensive history that addresses issues and concerns specific to obesity treatment. This obesity-focused history allows the physician to develop tailored treatment recommendations that are more consistent with the needs and goals of the individual patient. Information from the history should address the following six questions:

1. What factors contribute to the patient's obesity?
2. How is obesity affecting the patient's health?

3. What is the patient's level of risk regarding obesity?
4. What are the patient's goals and expectations?
5. Is the patient motivated to enter a weight management program?
6. What kind of help does the patient need?

The following specific information is pertinent to an obesity focused history:

- Chronological history of weight gain. Age at onset, description of weight gain (and loss) and inciting events provide clues to potential factors contributing to the patient's obesity and how the patient views his or her problem. Asking the patient to graph his or her weight pattern over time is a useful reflective and oftentimes therapeutic activity. Common patterns include progressive weight gain, weight yo-yo cycling, and periods of weight stability followed by weight gain. Rapid cycling of weight often reflects mood instability or all-or-nothing thinking. For many patients, weight gain initially occurs or is accelerated coincident to smoking cessation, initiation of medication, or change in life events, such as marital status, occupation, or illness. A familial predisposition should be considered if at least one first-degree relative is also obese. At-risk times for women include pregnancy, child rearing years (25 to 34 years old), and menopause. Although most of overweight and obesity can be attributed to behavioral changes in diet and physical activity patterns, the patient's history may suggest several less common secondary causes that may warrant further evaluation. Endocrinological disorders causing obesity are exceedingly uncommon with the exception of polycystic ovarian syndrome (PCOS). Endocrinological etiologies include hypothyroidism, Cushing's syndrome, and hypothalamic tumors or damage to this part of the brain as a consequence of irradiation, infection, or trauma. PCOS should be considered in a woman who has hirsutism, irregular menstrual cycles, and obesity. Although not a diagnostic criteria, approximately 50% of women with PCOS are obese, and some have type 2 diabetes mellitus [19].
- Response to previous weight loss attempts. This is one of the most important and revealing areas of inquiry. The nature, duration, and response to past treatments should be discussed and documented. This information discloses patients' past commitment and adherence to treatment programs, perceptions of how their body functions, and what their needs are. Questions should focus on why they felt they were (or were not) successful, what elements of the programs were most useful or not helpful, and what led to eventual recidivism of behaviors. Exploration of the reasons for triggering entry into past weight loss attempts and what factors caused disengagement of the attempts are often quite revealing. A helpful empathetic question is, "What is hard about managing your weight?" Knowing whether the programs chosen were self-selected fads, commercial, or professionally supervised is also important. Many

patients selectively choose complementary and alternative medicine approaches to weight control based on self-beliefs and attitudes [20].

- Effect of excess body weight on health. It is important to elicit patients' own perceptions regarding how their overweight or obesity affects them physically, psychologically, and socially. According to the health belief behavior model, individuals are not likely to initiate behavior change unless they feel that their health is threatened and that the threat can be lessened by taking action. In many circumstances, the current or presenting complaint is linked to the burden of excess body weight. Targeted questions such as, "How does your body weight affect you?", and "Is there anything that you cannot do because of your weight?" are useful in obtaining this information. These triggers also serve as useful motivators that should be monitored during weight management. For patients who experience drug-induced weight gain, it is important to ask them whether and how it is impacting their health and well-being. Individuals with obesity uniformly perceive their general health as poorer than healthy weight individuals. Moreover, a continuum has been observed between mildly, moderately, and severely obese individuals and worsening perceived health status [21]. In large part, the poorer overall quality of life perceived in obesity is caused by worse physical functioning [22]. In sum, the quality of life for obese individuals worsens with increasing body weight and with the number of acquired comorbid illnesses.

- Expectations from a weight management program. Eliciting this information is vital before initiating any weight loss program. Unrealistic expectations will result in disappointment and frustration regardless of the outcome. Patient goals often are stated as achieving specific body weights, wearing certain clothes sizes, gaining a more attractive physical appearance, or improving their overall health status or an obesity-related medical problem.

Lifestyle history

A history of the patient's current diet and physical activity patterns along with existing or potential barriers to change is used to understand the contributing factors toward the development of obesity and target behaviors for treatment. A dietary and physical activity history can be obtained by having the patient fill out a short questionnaire while in the waiting room, or assessed as part of the patient interview. A useful and convenient technique is to ask the patient to describe a typical day. "I want to learn more about your diet. Can you take me through a typical day or an example of a day, starting first thing in the morning and continuing into the evening?" This open-ended and nonjudgmental approach allows patients to reveal their dietary pattern without guilt or embarrassment. The purpose is to obtain a description of the patient's habitual diet regarding meal and snack patterns, selection of types of foods and beverages, frequency of intake of food groups and portion sizes. Because weekday dietary patterns are often different from weekend patterns, a brief dietary recall of both may be useful. Dietary behaviors such as where food is eaten, what triggers eating, and whether there is binge eating is also important information. For some patients, their habitual diet may be managed well but episodically uncontrolled because of stress or mood. More detailed information can be obtained by asking the patient to keep a food and activity diary for several days to a week. This exercise serves to increase the patient's awareness of his or her dietary habits and forms the basis for targeted changes.

For physical activity information, the physician needs to establish how much activity is typically accumulated in an average day, and whether the patient engages in any routine physical exercise, including frequency, intensity, and duration. An informative open-ended question is, "What is the most physically active thing you do over the course of a week?" In today's society, walking to or from the car, train or bus often represents the extent of physical activity. Lastly, it is important to inquire about existing or potential barriers to lifestyle change, such as financial restraints, time limitations, lack of cooking skills, or dislike of certain food groups or activities. Many patients also may have medical conditions that limit higher levels of physical activity.

Social history

Any treatment plan for obesity must be implemented in the context of the patient's personal and social environment. This is consistent with the social learning theory of behavior change. Therefore, understanding the issues that are supportive of or interfere with a weight loss plan are important to identify during the interview. Descriptions of the home and work environment regarding pressures to eat, personal conflicts, flexibility in time and structure, and potential allies and saboteurs are particularly helpful.

Psychiatric/psychological history

Although there does not appear to be an increased association of severe psychopathology among obese patients, there are several psychological issues that should be looked for and explored if necessary. Many patients express emotional triggers for their eating, such as loneliness, boredom, or stress. Others express feelings of low self-esteem, social isolation, and depression. Associated eating disorders are discussed elsewhere in this issue.

Medication history

A thorough medication history should be taken to uncover possible drug-induced weight gain or medications interfering with weight loss. Box 1 provides a list of medications that are associated with body fat weight gain [23]. Other medications such as nonsteroidal anti-inflammatory drugs and calcium-channel blockers have been associated with peripheral edema rather than body fat weight gain. When possible, an alternative medication that is weight-neutral or weight-losing should be prescribed. The effect of psychotropic-induced weight gain is addressed in detail elsewhere in this issue [24].

Examination of the obese patient

According to the NHLBI guidelines, assessment of risk status caused by overweight or obesity is based on the patient's body mass index (BMI), waist circumference, and the existence of comorbid conditions. BMI is

---

Box 1. Medications associated with body fat weight gain

Psychiatric/neurological
- Antipsychotic agents: phenothiazines, olanzapine, clozapine, risperidone
- Mood stabilizers: lithium
- Antidepressants: tricyclics, MAOIs, SSRIs (paroxetine), mirtazapine
- Antiepileptic drugs: gabapentin, valproate, carbamazepine

Steroid hormones
- Corticosteroids
- Progestational steroids

Antidiabetic agents
- Insulin, sulfonylureas, thiazolidinediones

Antihypertensive agents
- Beta- and alpha-1 adrenergic receptor blockers

Antihistamines
- Cyproheptadine

HIV protease inhibitors: *lipodystrophy (central obesity)

Adapted from Aronne LJ, editor. A practical guide to drug-induced weight gain. Minneapolis (MN): Healthcare Information Programs, a Division of McGraw-Hill; 2002.

calculated as weight (kg)/height (m)^2, or as weight (pounds)/height (inches)^2 × 703. A BMI table is used for simple reference (Table 1). BMI is recommended, because it provides an estimate of body fat and is related to risk of disease. A desirable or healthy BMI is 18.5 to 24.9 kg/m^2; overweight is 25 to 29.9 kg/m^2, and obesity is at least 30 kg/m^2. Obesity is further subdefined into class I (30.0 to 34.9 kg/m^2), class II (35.0 to 39.9 kg/m^2), and class III (at least 40 kg/m^2) (Table 2). Although morbid obesity remains listed in the International Classification of Diseases, 9th Revision, Clinical Modification (ICD9 CM) for coding purposes, it is being replaced by other descriptive terms including class III obesity, extreme obesity, or clinically severe obesity. In practice, after obtaining the patient's measured height and weight, the BMI Table and Classification Table should be used to categorize overweight and obesity and to document this information in the medical record. Actual measurement of weight and height may not be a routine process of care in the psychiatric office. This is an important first step, however, for identifying at-risk individuals and during re-evaluation. Small amounts of weight gain likely will be missed if the patient is not weighed. To protect privacy, consideration should be given to placing the scale in a private area of the office to avoid unnecessary embarrassment.

In addition to BMI, the risk of overweight and obesity is associated independently with excess abdominal fat and fitness level. Population studies have shown that people with large waist circumferences have impaired health and increased cardiovascular risk compared with those with normal waist circumferences [25,26] within the healthy, overweight, and class I obesity BMI categories [27]. The threshold for excessive abdominal fat is defined as a waist circumference of at least 102 cm (40 in) in men and at least 88 cm (35 in) in women. According to the NHLBI/NAASO guide [17], "To measure waist circumference, locate the upper hip bone and the top of the right iliac crest. Place a measuring tape in a horizontal plane around the abdomen at the level of the iliac crest. Before reading the tape measure, ensure that the tape is snug, but does not compress the skin, and is parallel to the floor. The measurement is made at the end of a normal expiration." Measurement of abdominal girth is not a difficult procedure and only takes a few seconds. Overweight patients with waist circumferences exceeding these limits should be urged more strongly to pursue weight reduction, because a larger waist circumference categorically increases disease risk for each BMI class. The importance of measuring and documenting waist circumference in patients with a BMI less than 35 kg/m^2 is because of the independent contribution of abdominal fat to the development of comorbid diseases, particularly metabolic syndrome.

Determination of fitness level is another modifier to assessing risk associated with BMI. Ross et al [28] found that high cardiorespiratory fitness is associated with lower levels of total and abdominal obesity for a given BMI. Longitudinal studies from The Cooper Institute in Dallas, Texas, also have shown that cardiorespiratory fitness (as measured by

Table 1
Body mass index

BMI Height (inches)	19	20	21	22	23	24	25	26	27	28	29	30	31	32	33	34	35	36	37	38	39	40	41	42	43	44	45	46	47	48	49	50	51	52	53	54
	Body weight (pounds)																																			
58	91	96	100	105	110	115	119	124	129	134	138	143	148	153	158	162	167	172	177	181	186	191	196	201	205	210	215	220	224	229	234	239	244	248	253	258
59	94	99	104	109	114	118	124	128	133	138	143	148	153	158	163	168	173	178	183	188	193	198	203	208	212	217	222	227	232	237	242	247	252	257	262	267
60	97	102	107	112	118	123	128	133	138	143	148	153	158	163	168	174	179	184	189	194	199	204	209	215	220	225	230	235	240	245	250	255	261	266	271	276
61	100	106	111	116	122	127	132	137	143	148	153	158	164	169	174	180	185	190	195	201	206	211	217	222	227	232	238	243	248	254	259	264	269	275	280	285
62	104	109	115	120	126	131	136	142	147	153	158	164	169	175	180	186	191	196	202	207	213	218	224	229	235	240	246	251	256	262	267	273	278	284	289	295
63	107	113	118	124	130	135	141	146	152	158	163	169	175	180	186	191	197	203	208	214	220	225	231	237	242	248	254	259	265	270	278	282	287	293	299	304
64	110	116	122	128	134	140	145	151	157	163	169	174	180	186	192	197	204	209	215	221	227	232	238	244	250	256	262	267	273	279	285	291	296	302	308	314
65	114	120	126	132	138	144	150	156	162	168	174	180	186	192	198	204	210	216	222	228	234	240	246	252	258	264	270	276	282	288	294	300	306	312	318	324
66	118	124	130	136	142	148	155	161	167	173	179	186	192	198	204	210	216	223	229	235	241	247	253	260	266	272	278	284	291	297	303	309	315	322	328	334
67	121	127	134	140	146	153	159	166	172	178	185	191	198	204	211	217	223	230	236	242	249	255	261	268	274	280	287	293	299	306	312	319	325	331	338	344
68	125	131	138	144	151	158	164	171	177	184	190	197	203	210	216	223	230	236	243	249	256	262	269	276	282	289	295	302	308	315	322	328	335	341	348	354
69	128	135	142	149	155	162	169	176	182	189	196	203	209	216	223	230	236	243	250	257	263	270	277	284	291	297	304	311	318	324	331	338	345	351	358	365
70	132	139	146	153	160	167	174	181	188	195	202	209	216	222	229	236	243	250	257	264	271	278	285	292	299	306	313	320	327	334	341	348	355	362	369	376
71	136	143	150	157	165	172	179	186	193	200	208	215	222	229	236	243	250	257	265	272	279	286	293	301	308	315	322	329	338	343	351	358	365	372	379	386
72	140	147	154	162	169	177	184	191	199	206	213	221	228	235	242	250	258	265	272	279	287	294	302	309	316	324	331	338	346	353	361	368	375	383	390	397
73	144	151	159	166	174	182	189	197	204	212	219	227	235	242	250	257	265	272	280	288	295	302	310	318	325	333	340	348	355	363	371	378	386	393	401	408
74	148	155	163	171	179	186	194	202	210	218	225	233	241	249	256	264	272	280	287	295	303	311	319	326	334	342	350	358	365	373	381	389	396	404	412	420
75	152	160	168	176	184	192	200	208	216	224	232	240	248	256	264	272	279	287	295	303	311	319	327	335	343	351	359	367	375	383	391	399	407	415	423	431
76	156	164	172	180	189	197	205	213	221	230	238	246	254	263	271	279	287	295	304	312	320	328	336	344	353	361	369	377	385	394	402	410	418	426	435	443

Table 2
Classification of weight status and risk of disease (If patient is 18 years or older, use the body mass index (BMI) and waist circumference to estimate weight status and relative risk for diabetes, high blood pressure or heart disease.)

		Risk of disease (relative to having a healthy weight and waist size)	
		Waist circumference:* 35 inches or less (women) 40 inches or less (men)	Waist circumference:* More than 34 inches (women) More than 40 inches (men)
Underweight	BMI below 18.5		
Healthy weight	BMI 18.5–24.9		
Overweight	BMI 25.0–29.9	Increased	High
Obesity class I	BMI 30.0–34.9	High	Very High
Obesity class II	BMI 35.0–39.9	Very High	Very High
Obesity Class III (extreme obesity)	BMI 40 or more	Extremely High	Extremely High

* Measure waist circumference at the level of the iliac crest. An increased waist circumference may indicate increased disease risk even at a normal weight.

Adapted from National Institutes of Health, National Heart, Lung, and Blood Institute. Clinical guidelines on the identification, evaluation, and treatment of overweight and obesity in adults; 1998 US Department of Health and Human Services, Public Health Service, Bethesda, MD.

a maximal treadmill exercise test) is an important predictor of all-cause mortality independent of BMI and body composition. The authors observed that fit obese men had a lower risk of all-cause and cardiovascular disease mortality than did unfit, lean men [29]. Similarly among women, cardio-respiratory fitness was a more important predictor of all-cause mortality than was baseline BMI [30]. These observations highlight the importance of taking an exercise history during the assessment and emphasizing the incorporation of moderately vigorous physical activity as a treatment approach.

Identifying the high-risk obese patient

According to the NHLBI/NAASO guide, patients at very high absolute risk, in need of intense risk factor modification and management, include people with established coronary heart disease; patients with other atherosclerotic diseases such as peripheral arterial disease, abdominal aortic aneurysm, or symptomatic carotid artery disease; and people with type 2 diabetes or sleep apnea. Patients with metabolic syndrome and those most likely to be insulin-resistant also require urgent treatment [31]. The Third Report of the National Cholesterol Education Program Expert Panel on Detection, Evaluation, and Treatment of High Blood Cholesterol in Adults

Box 2. Obesity-related organ systems review

Cardiovascular
Hypertension
Congestive heart failure
Cor pulmonale
Varicose veins
Pulmonary embolism
Coronary artery disease

Respiratory
Dyspnea
Obstructive sleep apnea
Hypoventilation syndrome
Pickwickian syndrome
Asthma

Endocrine
Metabolic syndrome
Type 2 diabetes
Dyslipidemia
Polycystic ovarian syndrome (PCOS)/angrogenicity
Amenorrhea/infertility/menstrual disorders

Gastrointestinal
Gastroesophageal reflux disease (GERD)
Nonalcoholic fatty liver disease (NAFLD)
Cholelithiasis
Hernias
Colon cancer

Musculoskeletal
Hyperuricemia and gout
Immobility
Osteoarthritis (knees and hips)
Low back pain

Genitourinary
Urinary stress incontinence
Obesity-related glomerulopathy
Hypogonadism (male)
Breast and uterine cancer
Pregnancy complications

Psychological
Depression/low self esteem

Body image disturbance
Social stigmatization

Neurologic
Stroke
Idiopathic intracranial hypertension
Meralgia paresthetica

Integument
Striae distensae (stretch marks)
Stasis pigmentation of legs
Lymphedema
Cellulitis
Intertrigo, carbuncles
Acanthosis nigricans/skin tags

Adapted from Kushner RF, Roth JL. Assessment of the obese patient. Endocrinol Metab Clin N Am 2003;32(4):915–34.

(Adult Treatment Panel III) defines metabolic syndrome as presence of three or more of the following criteria:

1. Abdominal obesity
2. Hypertriglyceridemia (at least 150 mg/dL)
3. Low high-density lipoprotein (HDL) cholesterol (less than 40 mg/dL in men and less than 50 mg/dL in women)
4. High blood pressure (BP) (at least 130/85 mmHg)
5. High fasting glucose (at least 110 mg/dL) [32]

Other symptoms and diseases that are related to obesity directly or indirectly are listed in Box 2 [33]. Although individuals will vary, the number and severity of organ specific comorbid conditions usually rise with increasing levels of obesity [34]. Although many of these conditions may not be life threatening, they are often the chief concern and determine the quality of life for the patient and therefore should trigger active obesity treatment. Box 2 can be used as a checklist during the review of systems section of the history and when developing an obesity-related problem list.

There is no single laboratory test or diagnostic evaluation that is indicated for all patients with obesity. The specific evaluation performed should be based on presentation of symptoms, risk factors, and index of suspicion. Based on several other screening guideline recommendations, however, most if not all patients should have a fasting lipid panel (total, low-density lipoprotein (LDL) and HDL cholesterol and triglyceride levels) and blood glucose measured at presentation, along with BP determination. Checking the BP in the obese patient requires special consideration, however. A bladder cuff that is not the appropriate width for the patient's arm circumference will cause a systematic error in BP measurement; if the bladder is too narrow, the pressure will be overestimated and lead to a false diagnosis of hypertension. To avoid errors, the bladder width should be 40% to 50% of upper arm circumference. Therefore, a large adult cuff (15 cm wide) should be chosen for patients with mild-to-moderate obesity, while a thigh cuff (18 cm wide) will need to be used for patients whose arm circumferences are greater than 16 in [35].

Assessing patient's readiness to change behavior

Determining a patient's readiness for weight loss is the next essential part of the initial evaluation. Initiating change when the patient is not ready often leads to frustration and may hamper future efforts. Patients who are ready and have thought about the benefits and difficulties of weight management are more likely to succeed.

The NHLBI/NAASO guide for readiness recommends that physicians assess patient motivation and support, stressful life events, psychiatric status, time availability and constraints, and appropriateness of goals and expectations to help establish the likelihood of lifestyle change [17]. It is not enough to simply ask a patient, "Are you ready to lose weight?" Inquiring about readiness necessitates a more in-depth assessment of the patient and his or her environment. Readiness can be viewed as the balance of two opposing forces: motivation, or the patient's desire to change, and resistance, or the patient's resistance to change [36]. It is important to remember that most patients are ambivalent about changing long-standing lifestyle behaviors, fearing that it will be difficult, uncomfortable, or depriving. One helpful method to begin a readiness assessment is to anchor the patient's interest and confidence to change on a numerical scale. To measure this, simply ask the patient, "On a scale from 0 to 10, with 0 being not important and 10 being very important, how important is it for you to lose weight at this time?" "Also on a scale from 0 to 10, with 0 being not confident and 10 being very confident, how confident are you that you can lose weight at this time?" [37]. This is a very useful exercise to initiate further dialog such as, "What would it take to increase your confidence score from a 4 to a 7?"

The Transtheoretical or Stages of Change Model proposes that at any specific time, patients are in one of six discreet stages of change: precontemplation, contemplation, preparation, action, maintenance, and relapse. Assessing which stage of change the patient is in helps to tailor the advice and intensity of intervention [38]. For example, if the patient is in the precontemplation stage regarding weight control ("I'm not really interested in losing weight at this time"), the appropriate action would be to provide information about health risks and benefits of weight loss and encourage taking action when ready. In contrast, if the patient is in the preparation stage ("I have to lose weight, and I've already talked to my wife about supporting me"), a reasonable action would be to begin dietary and physical activity counseling.

There are known determinants of whether a patient is likely to institute behavioral changes. Whitlock et al [39] define certain change-predisposing attributes that typically lead to behaviors that promote weight loss. Assessing these qualities helps determine a ready candidate for lifestyle modification. Although it is unlikely that every patient will display all six qualities, they provide a useful benchmark for assessment. These patients:

- Strongly want and intend to change for clear, personal reasons
- Face a minimum of obstacles to change
- Have the requisite skills and self-confidence to make a change
- Feel positively about change and believe it will result in meaningful benefit
- Perceive the change as congruent with self-image and social group norms
- Receive encouragement and support to change from valued persons

Summary

Obesity may be the most significant medical problem that health care providers will face over the coming decades. Physicians must address this chronic disease aggressively, providing preventive and therapeutic care. Because this topic traditionally has not been taught in medical school or residency training, physicians will need to acquire the knowledge, skills, and attitudes necessary to be effective obesity care providers. Performing a detailed initial assessment, including an obesity-focused history, physical examination, and selected laboratory and diagnostic tests is fundamental to the process of care.

References

[1] Flegal KM, Carroll MD, Ogden CL, et al. Prevalence and trends in obesity among US adults, 1999–2000. JAMA 2002;288:1723–7.
[2] National Heart, Lung, and Blood Institute (NHLBI). Clinical guidelines on the identification, evaluation, and treatment of overweight and obesity in adults. The evidence report. Obes Res 1998;6(Suppl 2):51S–210S.
[3] US Preventive Services Task Force. Screening for obesity in adults: recommendations and rationale. Ann Intern Med 2003;139:930–2.
[4] American Association of Clinical Endocrinologists, American College of Endocrinology. AACE/ACE position statement on the prevention, diagnosis and treatment of obesity (1998 revision). Endocr Pract 1998;4:299–350.

[5] American Academy of Family Physicians. Recommendations for periodic health examination (RPHE) of the American Academy of Family Physicians. Leanwood (KS): American Academy of Family Physicians; 1997.

[6] Lyznicki JM, Young DC, Riggs JA, et al. Obesity: assessment and management in primary care. Am Fam Physician 2001;63(11):2185–96.

[7] Nawaz H, Katz DL. American College of Preventive Medicine Practice policy statement. Weight management counseling of overweight adults. Am J Prev Med 2001;21(1):73–8.

[8] Pearson TA, Blair SN, Daniels SR, et al. AHA guidelines for primary prevention of cardiovascular disease and stroke: 2002 update. Consensus panel guide to comprehensive risk reduction for adult patients without coronary or other atherosclerotic vascular diseases. Circulation 2002;106:388–91.

[9] Galuska DA, Will JC, Serdula MK, et al. Are health care professionals advising obese patients to lose weight? JAMA 1999;282(16):1576–8.

[10] Stafford RS, Farhat JH, Misra B, et al. National patterns of physician activities related to obesity management. Arch Fam Med 2000;9:631–8.

[11] Huang J, Yu H, Marin E, et al. Physicians' weight loss counseling in two public hospital primary care clinics. Acad Med 2004;79:156–61.

[12] Sciamanna CN, Tate DF, Lang W, et al. Who reports receiving advice to lose weight? Results from a multi-state survey. Arch Intern Med 2000;160:2334–9.

[13] Kristeller JL, Hoerr RA. Physician attitudes toward managing obesity: differences among six specialty groups. Prev Med 1997;26:542–9.

[14] American Diabetes Association. American Psychiatric Association, American Association of Clinical Endocrinologists, and North American Association for the Study of Obesity. Consensus development conference on antipsychotic drugs and obesity and diabetes. Obes Res 2004;12:362–8.

[15] Willett WC, Dietz WH, Colditz GA. Guidelines for healthy weight. N Engl J Med 1999;341: 427–34.

[16] Fontaine KR, Heo M, Harrigan EP, et al. Estimating the consequences of antipsychotic-induced weight gain on health and mortality rate. Psychiatry Research 2001;101:277–88.

[17] National Heart, Lung, and Blood Institute (NHLBI) and North American Association for the Study of Obesity (NAASO). Practical guide to on the identification, evaluation, and treatment of overweight and obesity in adults; 2000. Bethesda (MD), National Institutes of Health, NIH Publication # 00–4084.

[18] Kushner RF. Roadmaps for clinical practice: case studies in disease prevention and health promotion—assessment and management of adult obesity: a primer for physicians. Chicago: American Medical Association; 2003.

[19] Gambineri A, Vicennati V, Pagotto U, et al. Obesity and the polycystic syndrome. Int J Obes 2002;26:883–96.

[20] Blanck HM, Khan LK, Serdula MK. Use of nonprescription weight loss products: results from a multi-state survey. JAMA 2001;286:930–5.

[21] Kushner RF, Foster GD. Obesity and quality of life. Nutrition 2000;16:947–52.

[22] Doll HA, Peterson SEK, Stewart-Brown SL. Obesity and physical and emotional well being: association between body mass index, chronic illness, and the physical and mental components of the SF-36 questionnaire. Obes Res 2000;8:160–70.

[23] Aronne LJ, editor. A practical guide to drug-induced weight gain. Minneapolis (MN): Healthcare Information Programs, a Division of McGraw-Hill; 2002.

[24] Zimmermann U, Kraus T, Himmerich H, et al. Epidemiology, implications and mechanisms underlying drug-induced weight gain in psychiatric patients. Journal of Psychiatry Research 2003;37:193–220.

[25] Lean MEJ, Han TS, Seidell JC. Impairment of health and quality of life in people with large waist circumference. Lancet 1998;351(9106):853–6.

[26] Han TS, van Leer EM, Seidell JC, et al. Waist circumference action levels in the identification of cardiovascular risk factors: prevalence study in a random sample. BMJ 1995;311:1401–5.

[27] Janssen I, Katzmarzyk PT, Ross R. Body mass index, waist circumference, and health risk. Evidence in support of current national institutes of health guidelines. Arch Intern Med 2002;162:2074–9.

[28] Ross R, Katzmarzyk PT. Cardiorespiratory fitness is associated with diminished total and abdominal obesity independent of body mass index. Int J Obesity 2003;27:204–10.

[29] Lee CD, Blair SN, Jackson AS. Cardiorespiratory fitness, body composition, and all-cause and cardiovascular disease mortality in men. Am J Clin Nutr 1999;69:373–80.

[30] Farrell SW, Braun L, Barlow CE, et al. The relation of body mass index, cardiorespiratory fitness, and all-cause mortality in women. Obes Res 2002;10(6):417–23.

[31] Reaven GM. Importance of identifying the overweight patient who will benefit the most by losing weight. Ann Intern Med 2003;138(5):420–3.

[32] Expert Panel on Detection, Evaluation, and Treatment of High Blood Cholesterol in Adults Executive summary of the third reports of the National Cholesterol Education Program (NCEP) expert panel on detection, evaluation, and treatment of high blood cholesterol in adults (Adult Treatment Panel III). JAMA 2001;285:2486–97.

[33] Kushner RF, Roth JL. Assessment of the obese patient. Endocrinol Metab Clin North Am 2003;32(4):915–34.

[34] Must A, Spadano J, Coakley EH, et al. The disease burden associated with overweight and obesity. JAMA 1999;282(16):1523–9.

[35] Perloff D, Grimm C, Flack J, et al. Human blood pressure determination by sphygmomanometry. Circulation 1993;88:2460–70.

[36] Katz DL. Behavior modification in primary care: the pressure system model. Prev Med 2001; 32:66–72.

[37] Rollnick S, Mason P, Butler C. Health behavior change: a guide for practitioners. London: Churchill Livingstone; 1999.

[38] Prochaska JO, DiClemente CC. Toward a comprehensive model of change. In: Miller WR, editor. Treating addictive behaviors. New York: Plenum; 1986. p. 3–27.

[39] Whitlock EP, Orleans CT, Pender N, et al. Evaluating primary care behavioral counseling intervention: an evidence-based approach. Am J Prev Med 2002;22(4):267–84.

ELSEVIER
SAUNDERS

PSYCHIATRIC
CLINICS
OF NORTH AMERICA

Psychiatr Clin N Am 28 (2005) 105–116

Behavioral Assessment and Treatment Overview

James E. Mitchell, MD*, Tricia Cook Myers, PhD

Neuropsychiatric Research Institute and the Department of Neuroscience,
University of North Dakota School of Medicine and Health Sciences,
700 1st Avenue South, P.O. Box 1415, Fargo, ND 58107, USA

The behavioral assessment allows practitioners to gather information about weight history, previous weight loss attempts, environmental circumstances and social support, and any comorbid psychiatric disturbances that may complicate the course of weight loss treatment. Techniques for completing the assessment, however, may vary. In some instances, the clinician may conduct an intake interview with obesity identified as the presenting problem. In other circumstances, a provider may decide to broach the topic of weight loss after working with a patient for several weeks, months or even years. In both situations it is helpful to approach a discussion of weight in a supportive, nonjudgmental manner.

In the former situation, it can be beneficial to initiate the assessment with a discussion of neutral, demographic information such as marital status, current living situation, and occupation. This conversational tone can help establish rapport and may help the patient feel more at ease when disclosing information about this sensitive issue. It also can be helpful to orient the patient at the onset to the structure of the session, indicating that treatment recommendations will be reviewed at the close of the evaluation. Patients should be thanked for completing the self-report questionnaires, if used, and the interviewer should use this written information to guide the assessment. Although it is important to keep the patient on task and gather pertinent information, it is also worthwhile to allow patients the opportunity to freely discuss the impact their overweight status has had on their lives. Assessment tools such as the Impact of Weight on Quality of Life-Lite (IWQOL-Lite) can provide detailed information about this.

* Corresponding author.
E-mail address: mitchell@medicine.nodak.edu (J.E. Mitchell).

doi:10.1016/j.psc.2004.10.002

In the second scenario, a bit more delicacy may be needed. Patients may react with relief, surprise, defensiveness, or even anger; and the provider must be prepared for any of these. Often a verbal review of recent physical examination findings or laboratory results, if outside of the acceptable range and attributable to obesity, can open the door to this conversation in a manner that is meaningful to the patient and less likely to elicit strong negative emotional reactions. The practitioner may wonder aloud if the patient would like to consider a modest amount of weight loss, say 10 to 20 lbs, if this would bring the findings into healthier ranges. An alternative approach would be to ask an open-ended question about how the patient feels about his or her current weight, such as "I see that you were weighed this morning. What do you think about the number on the scale?" Generally, it is not helpful to take a scare tactic approach, as this may lead to defensiveness and damaged rapport.

Data-gathering strategies

The elements of an inclusive medical evaluation have been covered in the article by Kushner and Roth in this issue. One strategy to obtain detailed information about each patient's history is to use a patient self-report database, which the patient completes before the assessment visit. An example of such a database, the Eating Disorders Questionnaire (EDQ), is a comprehensive self-report inventory that provides detailed information about eating patterns, weight history, perceptions of shape and weight, as well as previous attempts at treatment. Another example is the Weight and Lifestyle Inventory (WALI) [1]. Such a database can be mailed to patients when they are scheduled for an evaluation, and they can be asked to return the completed form in advance or to bring it with them to the clinic visit. An alternative approach is to have patients come in 45 minutes to 1 hour early and complete the information on site. In addition, a review of these measures can provide the interviewer with appropriate suggestions for wording of queries during the clinical interview.

There are advantages to having the patient complete such a database at home, because they will have access there to other sources of information (dates, drug names and dosages) that they may not have at the time of their clinic visit. In the authors' experience, patients are willing to do this and appreciate the great attention to detail such an instrument provides. Clinicians find such database reports extremely useful. They can be examined by the evaluating clinician immediately before the interview. Also, if properly formatted, and if the software is available, they can be scanned and used to create a text narrative on the patient. Obtaining data in this way assures clinicians that they have the basic information on the patient, and allows them to focus the interview on points of particular interest or concern.

An important part of behavioral assessment includes obtaining a detailed history as to prior treatments and weight loss attempts and the patient's response to such interventions. Most individuals being seen for obesity have had numerous treatment episodes in the past and generally have found the outcome of most of their prior treatment exposures frustrating and disappointing. Such a careful review, however, will indicate what strategies are likely or unlikely to work, and also will allow one to gauge the degree of motivation and compliance of the patient when in treatment. It is important not to ask just about medically based interventions, but also self-help groups, various commercial programs, and prescription and nonprescription medications, particularly herbal preparations that increasingly are being used by patients in an attempt to lose weight, sometimes at great expense.

The database should include the assessment of mood, quality of life, and disordered eating behaviors and beliefs. Box 1 lists suggested self-report inventories that can be included in an assessment for weight loss treatment. If these are not to be presented to patients for them to complete, providers

---

Box 1. Suggested self-report inventories

Eating Disorders Questionnaire (EDQ; [Version 8.4] original version published by Mitchell et al) [2]. The EDQ provides demographic information and a detailed history of eating, weight, and previous treatment. It has recently been updated [Version 9.0] and can be obtained from the first author at the Neuropsychiatric Research Institute. The use of this instrument was discussed in the previous section.

Three Factor Eating Questionnaire (TFEQ) [3]. The TFEQ is a 51-item questionnaire with good reliability and validity, and three subscales: restraint, disinhibition and hunger.

Questionnaire on Eating and Weight Patterns–Revised (QEWP-R) [4]: The QEWP-R is a 28-item scale designed to assess binge eating and the presence of binge eating disorder (BED).

Social Function–36 (SF-36) [5]. The SF-36 is the most widely used health-related quality-of-life measure, and it has norms available for several patient groups. Eight areas of social functioning are assessed: physical function, role physical, bodily pain, general health, vitality, social function, role emotional, and mental health.

Impact of Weight on Quality of Life—Lite (IWQOL-Lite) [6]. This is an obesity-specific health related quality-of-life measure with excellent psychometric properties. This inventory provides scores on five domains (physical function, self-esteem, sexual life, public distress, work) and a total score.

The Beck Depression Inventory (BDI) [7]. This is an extensively used 21-item measure of depression with very good reliability and validity.

may wish to review the questions included in these assessments and use this information to help guide the clinical interview.

Psychosocial factors

Comorbid psychopathology

Before approaching weight loss, the practitioner should have a full understanding of the patient's comorbid psychopathology. This information can be gathered informally by means of the clinical interview or can be assessed with a specific psychometric instrument such as the BDI for depression. Some comorbidities may necessitate a delay in initiating weight loss treatment, while others may be improved or even exacerbated as a result of treatment. Mood disorders, substance use/abuse, sexual abuse, and binge eating will be reviewed here briefly.

Dysthymia often is endorsed by individuals seeking weight loss and tends to improve over the course of treatment [8], possibly because of the impact of exercise on mood [9]. Research also shows that such individuals lose weight at a rate similar to peers without depressive symptomatology. On the other hand, the 10% of patients with clinically significant levels of depression (BDI-II score of greater than 29) should be encouraged to focus first on improving their mood before attempting to lose weight, as depression can interfere with treatment compliance, and weight loss interventions can worsen depression [10].

As one would expect, there is evidence that active substance abuse/dependence is detrimental to weight loss success [11]. Although substance problems are not common among obese individuals, when present, they should be addressed independently before starting a weight loss program. Practitioners also may wish to assess for a history of sexual abuse, as there is some evidence that it may be more common in very obese females than in average-weight peers [12]. If the patient indicates that she has been a victim of sexual abuse, probe for treatment seeking and current impact. Refer the patient for counseling if the patient continues to be distressed by these events. In contrast to substance abuse or dependence, a history of abuse does not need to delay weight loss treatment. Practitioners should keep in mind, however, that these patients may feel vulnerable when they lose weight and may be more likely to drop out of treatment.

In addition, approximately a third of patients who seek weight loss treatment endorse binge eating, defined as a loss of control while eating a large amount of food in a short period of time [13]. About half of these meet criteria for BED, which is defined further by marked distress about binge eating in the absence of compensatory behaviors and three or more of the following behaviors: (1) eating rapidly, (2) eating until uncomfortably full, (3) eating even when not hungry, (4) eating alone due to embarrassment, and (5) feeling disgusted, depressed or guilty about their eating [14].

The presence of BED is associated with a higher incidence of depression and anxiety [4,13,15], but this does not necessarily result in less weight loss. In fact, most studies show that obese individuals with BED lose the same amount of weight as non-BED individuals seeking weight loss, and that binge eating tends to decrease simply as a result of behavioral weight loss methods [8,15,16]. Yet practitioners should be aware that individuals with BED are more likely to drop out of treatment and may experience increased difficulties during the maintenance phase of treatment [8,15]. In the latter case, it may be helpful to offer more frequent booster sessions to monitor potential increases in binge eating to intervene as early as possible.

Availability of food

Rates of obesity in the United States have soared in recent years, and now more than one out of every two Americans is considered overweight. Some of this is attributed to the increasing availability of palatable, calorie-dense food [17]. Also, families increasingly are eating outside of the home at a rate that parallels the rise in obesity [18,19]. A patient's socioeconomic status can provide information about potential problems, since healthier, lower fat foods tend to be more expensive. In developed countries, low socioeconomic status is an obesity risk factor for women in particular, possibly because of the larger number of fast food restaurants and fewer recreational facilities [20].

It also can be helpful to determine who does the grocery shopping, meal preparation and food serving to get a better understanding of the context in which eating episodes occur. If the patient is not responsible for these activities, it may be helpful to obtain collateral information from the family members responsible for these duties. In particular, when assessing a child or adolescent patient, it is wise to obtain information about both the patient and the parents' points of view.

In situations where the patient lives with family members, it can be enlightening to also determine what mealtimes are like. Does the family eat together, or does the patient eat alone? Is there a lot of conflict surrounding mealtimes, or are they a positive social occasion? Last, specific information should be obtained about cooking methods that are used more frequently. Are foods baked, fried, or grilled? Does the patient frequently eat out of the home?

Food intake, amount and pattern

Given the importance of behavioral factors, it is important to have the patient describe a typical day of eating. Does the patient eat breakfast, lunch, and dinner or does he or she eat only one meal each day? Does the patient snack, and are these snacking episodes discrete or prolonged? Research shows that obese individuals tend to skip breakfast and eat a larger meal later in the day, a pattern that is associated with increased hunger and consumption or more energy-rich foods [21,22]. The practitioner also should form a rough estimate of the daily average number of calories and should know what types and amounts of foods the patient is eating. Last, it may be helpful to review a typical weekday versus weekend day, as the latter tends to be associated with a greater degree of disinhibition.

Ideally, this information should be available on the self-monitoring forms of daily food intake that the patient completed as part of the preassessment packet. If completed in a timely manner, the information recorded on these forms likely will be more reliable and valid than the patient's retrospective recall during an office appointment. The practitioner should confirm that these are representative days and should remain aware that obese patients tend to underestimate daily consumption by up to 50% [23–27]. In particular, unhealthy or undesirable foods are most likely to be under-estimated [25,28]. More accurate assessments of energy needs such as double-labeled water are available but cost-prohibitive. Typically, though, enough general information can be gathered from the food logs and clinical interview without resorting to other methods.

Diet composition

Food logs provide invaluable information about dietary composition. These records display the types of foods that the patient is consuming on a routine basis. In particular, attention should be paid to fat content and variety. Although all foods are fine to eat in moderation, a diet high in fat content is more likely to lead to weight gain [29,30]. Alcohol consumption at 7 calories per gram also should be monitored and in most cases reduced, because of decreased control over eating when one is intoxicated or hung over.

Typically, it is best to collaborate with a registered dietitian who can assess and educate the patient better about well-balanced food choices based on the food pyramid. It seems that individuals with highly variable, high-fat diets tend to be more successful when prescribed a structured meal plan with portion-controlled foods and occasionally meal replacements [31].

Binge eating

As mentioned earlier, binge eating does not require a treatment separate from weight loss interventions. Its presence, however, should be assessed carefully to guide treatment follow-up and to communicate to the patient a full understanding of his or her difficulties. Often, patients can be reluctant to record an entire binge episode on their food logs, so it may be helpful to ask patients to "describe exactly what and how much food you ate during your last binge episode." This will allow the practitioner to determine if the amount of food consumed was objectively large, or if the patient was experiencing a subjective binge (ie, a sense of loss of control with a small or normal amount of food). If patients initially deny a loss of control, follow-up questions should include "Did you feel driven or compelled to eat?" and "Could you have stopped yourself from eating?" The QEWP-R is a good assessment tool to screen for BED, whether this is delivered in self-report format, or comparable questions are asked during the clinical interview.

Other pathological eating patterns

In addition to binge eating, the practitioner should assess for symptoms of night eating syndrome. Although not an official *Diagnostic and Statistical Manual of Mental Disorders'* diagnosis, this disorder is thought to affect 8.9% to 27% of obese patients who are seeking interventions for weight loss [31,32]. Night eating syndrome is defined as morning anorexia and night-time snacking with more than half of the day's calories consumed after the evening meal. Helpful questions include: "How would you describe your appetite in the morning?", "What percentage of your total food intake do you consume after your evening meal?", or "Do you sometimes get up in the middle of the night and eat something?"

Physical activity

Sedentary individuals are more likely to gain weight and require weight loss interventions [33]. In addition, one of the best methods to ensure weight loss maintenance is to increase physical activity [34]. Therefore, a comprehensive assessment of activity level should inform the course of treatment. As most obese patients are very inactive, it can be beneficial to first focus questions about exercise on lifestyle versus programmed activity. For example, rather than asking how much time the patient spends at the gym, it might be preferable to start out with questions like, "About how many blocks do you walk on a typical day?" or "Do you take the elevator or stairs at work?" It is also important to determine how much time is spent each day on sedentary activities such as working at a desk job, watching TV, or reading. Activity level also can be assessed by means of self-report instruments, such as the Physical Activity Survey used in the Cross-Cultural Activity Participation Study (CAPS) [35,36].

It can be helpful at this point to reassure patients that weight loss benefits can be reaped from small increases in activity level. Also, patients are more likely to engage in behavior that they enjoy, so it is important to inquire about preferred methods of physical activity. Exercise compliance can be increased when an exercise "buddy" is available, so information about their preferences in this regard should be obtained. Frequently, patients will indicate that a variety of factors keep them from exercising. It can be helpful to remind these individuals that change will be gradual rather than immediate.

Biological factors

There is growing evidence that genetic factors account for much of the variance in adult body weight and body fat distribution, with various studies finding estimated genetic contributions anywhere from 20% to 70% [37–42]. A recent review on the topic concluded that currently more than 300 genes, markers, and chromosomal regions have been associated with obesity phenotypes [37]. Monogenic causes of obesity in people, however, appear to be rare [43]. For example, a defect in the leptin gene has been shown to result in obesity in some rare cases [44], as have mutations of melancortin-4 receptor gene [45]. Therefore, most cases are polygenic, and the number of areas of interest identified thus far on DNA suggests that the genetic factors involved in most cases of obesity in people eventually will be shown to be extremely complex. Currently, with the exception of rare, unusual child-hood-onset cases, there is no precise way to adequately evaluate genetic risk for obesity. Two factors that are associated with genetic risk, however, are age of onset of obesity and family history of obesity. Obtaining detailed information on both of these variables is important. Relative to family history, it is known that obesity runs in families, and the presence of one obese biological parent or two obese biological parents raises the risk exponentially [46]. Therefore, detailed information about weights and heights and ages of onset should be obtained regarding biological mother and father, siblings, and grandparents. Relative to age of onset, in general, the earlier the age of onset of overweight or obesity, the higher the likelihood of severe obesity in adulthood [47,48]. Also, people with early onset of obesity are less likely to achieve a normal body weight through dieting than those with an adult-onset pattern.

A second biological factor that relates to obesity risk is birth weight [43]. Both low and high birth weight infants are at higher risk for obesity, suggesting that the environment in utero influences later body weight.

Another biological variable that may be important in determining the likelihood of successful weight loss among the obese is whether the obesity is accompanied by an increase in fat cell numbers (hyperplasic obesity) or fat cell size (hypertrophic obesity) [49]. In theory, cell hypertrophy is reversible, while fat cell number is not [50]. Little research has been published in this area in the last 20 years, however, and fat cell size and number are not ascertained easily in the usual clinical setting.

Overview of treatment

A panel of obesity treatment experts, brought together by the National Heart, Lung and Blood Institute in 1998, reviewed the literature on the various treatments of obesity and issued recommendations for selecting among the various available interventions. This report was abbreviated and

Table 1
Overview of assessment of the obese

Complete →	Measure →	BMI ≥ 25	Evaluate	→	Decide
Hx and	BMI	or waist	comorbidities		treatment
PE	+	circumference	↓ ↓ ↓		
	waist	>35 in female	↑BP? Type II Dyslipidemia?		
	circumference	>40 in male	DM?		

published as "The Practical Guide to the Identification, Evaluation, and Treatment of Obesity in Adults" [51]. This guide informs the recommendations offered in this article, linking specific treatment recommendations to a specific body mass index (BMI) and the presence or absence of comorbid medical conditions.

The panel used the following classification for BMI:

Underweight (less than 18.5 kg/m^2)
Normal weight (18.5 to 24.9 kg/m^2)
Overweight (25 to 29.9 kg/m^2)
Class 1 obesity (30 to 34.9 kg/m^2)
Class 2 obesity (35 to 39.9 kg/m^2)
Class 3 extreme obesity (greater than or equal to 40 kg/m^2)

The guide also stresses that waist circumference, in addition to BMI, correlates to increased risk for type II diabetes, dyslipidemias, hypertension, and cardiovascular disease in overweight and obese subjects, with a high risk waist circumference being greater than 40 in in men and greater than 35 in in women. A brief evaluation formula is shown in Table 1.

The guide also details other factors that contribute to relative risk. These include established coronary heart disease or other atherosclerotic diseases, type II diabetes, sleep apnea, smoking, hypertension, high levels of low density lipoprotein cholesterol, low levels of high density lipoprotein cholesterol, impaired fasting glucose, family history of premature cardiac disease, and age of at least 45 years in men, and at least 55 years in women. An overview for evaluating risk and choosing treatments is shown in Table 2 [52].

Table 2
Choices of treatment by body mass index and comorbidities

BMI	25–26.9	27–29.9	30–34.9	35–39.9	≥40
Diet + physical activity + behavior therapy	With comorbidities	With comorbidities	+	+	+
Drug therapy		With comorbidities	+	+	+
Bariatric surgery				With comorbidities	+

+, Use regardless of comorbidities.

In selecting treatment options, the patient's involvement in decision making is crucial. One needs to incorporate information about patient's attitude toward various treatments and prior successes and failures.

Summary

Many genetic, environmental, behavioral, and psychological factors intersect to increase or decrease the risk of someone becoming obese. In assessing patients with obesity, however, a supportive, nonjudgmental, and sensitive approach usually leads to the best results and most complete information. Relative to treatment, the options vary depending on the severity of obesity and the presence or absence of obesity-related comorbidities.

References

[1] Wadden TA, Phelan S. Behavioral assessment of the obese patient. In: Wadden TA, Stunkard AJ, editors. Handbook of obesity treatment. New York: Guilford Press; 2002. p. 186–226.

[2] Mitchell JE, Hatsukami D, Eckert ED, et al. 1985 Eating disorders questionnaire. Psychopharmacol Bull 1985;21:1025–43.

[3] Stunkard AJ, Messick S. The three-factor eating questionnaire to measure dietary restraint, disinhibition, and hunger. J Psychosom Res 1985;29:71–83.

[4] Spitzer RL, Devlin M, Walsh TB, et al. Binge eating disorder: a multi-site field trial of the diagnostic criteria. Int J Eat Disord 1992;11:191–203.

[5] Ware JE, Kosinski M, Keller SD. SF-36 physical and mental summary scales: a user's manual. Boston: The Health Institute; 1994.

[6] Kolotikin RL, Crosby RD, Kosloski KD, et al. Development of a brief measure to assess quality of life in obesity. Obes Res 2001;9:102–11.

[7] Beck AT, Ward CH, Mendelson M, et al. An inventory for measuring depression. Arch Gen Psychiatry 1961;4:561–71.

[8] Gladis MM, Wadden TA, Rogt RA, et al. Behavioral treatment of obese binge eaters: do they need different care? J Psychosom Res 1988;44:375–84.

[9] Brosse AL, Sheets ES, Lett HS, et al. Exercise and treatment of clinical depression in adults: recent findings and future directions. Sports Med 2002;32(12):741–60.

[10] Wadden TA, Bartlett SJ. Very low calorie diets: an overview and appraisal. In: Wadden TA, Vanitallie TB, editors. Treatment of the seriously obese patient. New York: Guilford Press; 1992. p. 44–79.

[11] Valley V, Grace M. Psychosocial risk factors in gastric surgery for obesity: identifying guidelines for screening. Int J Obes 1987;11:105–13.

[12] Brewerton TD, O'Neil PM, Dansky BS, et al. Links between morbid obesity, victimization, PTSD, major depression and bulimia in a national sample of women. Obes Res 1999;7:56S.

[13] Marcus MD, Wing RR, Hopkins J. Obese binge eaters: affect, cognitions, and response to behavioral weight control. J Consult Clin Psychol 1988;56:433–9.

[14] American Psychiatric Association. Diagnostic and statistical manual of mental disorders. 4th edition. Washington (DC): American Psychiatric Association; 1994.

[15] Sherwood NE, Jeffery RW, Wing RR. Binge status as a predictor of weight loss treatment. Int J Obes 1999;23:485–93.

[16] Wadden TA, Foster GD, Letizia KA. Response of obese binge eaters to treatment by behavior therapy combined with very low calorie diet. J Consult Clin Psychol 1992;60: 808–11.

[17] Drewnowski A. Nutrition transition and global dietary trends. Nutrition 2000;16:486–7.

[18] French SA, Story M, Jeffery RW. Environmental influences on eating and physical activity. Annu Rev Public Health 2001;22:309–35.

[19] McCrory MA, Fuss PJ, Hays NP, et al. Overeating in America: association between restaurant food consumption and body fatness in healthy adult men and women ages 19 to 80. Obes Res 1999;7:564–71.

[20] Swinburn BA, Caterson I, Seidell JC, et al. Diet, nutrition and the prevention of excess weight gain and obesity. Public Health Nutr 2004;7:123–46.

[21] Morgan KJ, Zabik ME, Stampley GL. The role of breakfast in the diet adequacy of the US population. J Am Coll Nutr 1986;5:551–63.

[22] Schlundt DG, Sbrocco T, Bell C. Identification of high-risk situations in a behavioral weight loss program: application of the relapse prevention model. Int J Obes Relat Metab Disord 1989;13:223–34.

[23] Goris AH, Westerterp-Plantenga MS, Westerterp KR. Undereating and under-recording of habitual food intake in obese men: selective underreporting of fat intake. Am J Clin Nutr 2000;71:130–4.

[24] Heitmann BL, Lissner L. Dietary underreporting by obese individuals—is it specific or nonspecific? BMJ 1994;311:986–9.

[25] Lafay L, Basdevant A, Charles MA, et al. Determinants and nature of dietary underreporting in a free-living population: the Fleurbaix Laventie Ville Sante (FLVS) study. Int J Obes Relat Metab Disord 1997;21:567–73.

[26] Lichtman SW, Pisarka K, Berman ER, et al. Discrepancy between self-reported and actual caloric intake and exercise in obese subjects. N Engl J Med 1992;327:1893–8.

[27] Schoeller DA. Limitations in the assessment of dietary energy intake by self-report. Metabolism 1995;44:18–22.

[28] Mendez MA, Wynter S, Wilks R, et al. Under- and over-reporting of energy is related to obesity, lifestyle factors and food group intakes in Jamaican adults. Public Health Nutr 2003; 7:9–19.

[29] Golay A, Bobbioni E. The role of dietary fat in obesity. Int J Obes Relat Metab Disord 1997; 21:S2–S11.

[30] Stubbs RJ, Harbron CG, Murgatroyd PR. Covert manipulation of dietary fat and energy density: effect of substrate flux and food intake in men eating ad libitum. Am J Clin Nutr 1995;62:316–29.

[31] Raynor HA, Epstein LH. Dietary variety, energy regulation, and obesity. Psychol Bull 2001; 127(3):325–41.

[32] Rand CSW, MacGregor AMC, Stunkard AJ. The night eating syndrome in the general population and among postoperative obesity surgery patients. Int J Eat Disord 1997;22: 65–9.

[33] Brownell KD. Exercise in the treatment of obesity. In: Brownell KD, Fairburn CG, editors. Eating disorders and obesity: a comprehensive handbook. New York: Guilford Press; 1995. p. 437–8.

[34] Pronk NP, Wing RR. Physical activity and long-term maintenance of weight loss. Obes Res 1994;2:587–99.

[35] Henderson KA, Ainsworth BE. A synthesis of perceptions about physical activity among older African American and American Indian women. Am J Public Health 2003;93:313–7.

[36] Henderson KA, Ainsworth BE. Sociocultural perspectives on physical activity in the lives of older African American and American Indian women: a cross cultural activity participation study. Women Health 2000;31:1–20.

[37] Chagnon YC, Rankinen R, Snyder EE, et al. The human obesity gene map: the 2002 update. Obes Res 2003;11(3):313–67.

[38] Considine RV. Leptin and obesity in humans. Eat Weight Disord 1997;2(2):61–6.

[39] Damcott CM, Sack P, Schuldiner AR. The genetics of obesity. Endocrinol Metab Clin North Am 2003;32(4):761–86.

[40] Liu YH, Araujo S, Recker RR, et al. Molecular and genetic mechanisms of obesity: implications for future management. Curr Mol Med 2003;3:325–40.

[41] Loos RJ, Bouchard C. Obesity—is it a genetic disorder? J Intern Med 2003;254:401–24.

[42] Rosmond R. Association studies of genetic polymorphisms in central obesity: critical review. Int J Obes Relat Metab Disord 2003;27(10):1141–51.

[43] Oken E, Gillman MW. Fetal origins of obesity. Obes Res 2003;11(4):496–506.

[44] Montague CT, Farooqi IL, Whitehead JP, et al. Congenital leptin deficiency is associated with severe early onset obesity in humans. Nature 1997;387:903–8.

[45] Lubrano-Berthelier C, Cavazos M, Dubern B, et al. Molecular genetics of human obesity-associated MC4R mutation. Ann N Y Acad Sci 2003;994:49–57.

[46] Lake JK, Power C, Cole TJ. Child to adult body mass index in the 1958 British birth cohort: associations with parental obesity. Arch Dis Child 1997;77:376–81.

[47] Dietz WH. Health consequences of obesity in youth: childhood predictors of adult disease. Pediatrics 1998;101:518–25.

[48] Schoeller DA. Measurement of energy expenditure in free-living humans by using doubly labeled water. J Nutr 1988;118:1278–89.

[49] Bjorntorp P, Carlgren G, Isaksson B, et al. The effect of an energy reducing dietary regime in relation to adipose tissue cellularity in obese women. Am J Clin Nutr 1975;28:445–52.

[50] Krotiewski M, Sjöström L, Bjorntorp P, et al. Adipose tissue cellularity in relation to prognosis for weight reduction. Int J Obes 1977;1:395–416.

[51] National Heart, Lung, and Blood Institute (NHLBI). Clinical guidelines on the identification, evaluation, and treatment of overweight and obesity in adults: the evidence report. Obes Res 1998;6(Suppl 2):51S–209S.

[52] Stunkard AJ. Eating patterns and obesity. Psychiatr Q 1959;33:284–94.

PSYCHIATRIC CLINICS
OF NORTH AMERICA

ELSEVIER
SAUNDERS

Psychiatr Clin N Am 28 (2005) 117–139

Dietary Approaches to the Treatment of Obesity

Angela P. Makris, PhD, RD, Gary D. Foster, PhD*

*Department of Psychiatry, University of Pennsylvania School of Medicine,
3535 Market Street, Philadelphia, PA 19104, USA*

The perennial appearance of diet books on best seller lists underscores Americans' perpetual search for the "best" weight loss diet. This search for novel approaches is driven, in part, by the limited long-term efficacy of the best clinic-based approaches to obesity treatment [1]. It is also fueled by the public's perception that "experts can't make up their minds" when it comes to the best diet.

Currently, the best dietary strategy for tipping the energy balance equation in favor of weight loss is a matter of some debate among professionals and the public alike. During the last 20 years, there has been a focus on decreasing fat intake [2,3]. This recommendation is guided by the high-energy density of all dietary fat and the link between increased risk of chronic disease and saturated fat [4–6]. Although low-calorie, low-fat approaches are effective in the short term, they have not been proven to be sustainable for many living in an environment in which palatable, inexpensive, and high-fat foods are easily accessible [7]. More recently, researchers have explored other means of reducing energy intake (eg, manipulating the amount or type of carbohydrate and protein, altering the energy density of the diet). Although "energy in versus energy out" remains the cornerstone of obesity treatment, it is unclear whether particular macronutrients differentially affect satiety, adherence, and other factors that would reduce energy intake and skirt energy balance.

This article reviews dietary approaches to obesity treatment, with an emphasis on the relative roles of fat, carbohydrate, and protein. It begins with an overview of the general characteristics and functions of macronutrients. The relative effects of these macronutrients on hunger and satiety

---

* Corresponding author.
E-mail address: foster@mail.med.upenn.edu (G.D. Foster).

0193-953X/05/$ - see front matter © 2005 Elsevier Inc. All rights reserved.
doi:10.1016/j.psc.2004.11.001

are then discussed. Finally, the efficacy of various macronutrient-based strategies for weight loss is examined.

General characteristics and functions of macronutrients

Dietary fat

Dietary fat is a term used for a diverse group of water-insoluble compounds (also referred to as lipids) that perform a variety of functions in the body as well as in food. Lipids deliver essential fatty acids that are vital for normal immune function and vision, carry fat-soluble vitamins, comprise cell membranes, provide energy for immediate and long-term use, and contribute to satiety by delaying gastric emptying. In addition, fats add flavor and texture to foods.

The most abundant type of fat in food (eg, triglyceride) consists of a variety of fatty acids that differ in chain length and degree of saturation. Fatty acids are divided into two basic categories: saturated and unsaturated. Saturated fat is generally solid at room temperature and is most commonly found in animal sources (eg, fat in whole milk, cheese, butter). High saturated fat intake can raise low-density cholesterol levels and increase the risk for cardiovascular disease [8,9]. Monounsaturated and polyunsaturated fats are examples of unsaturated fats. Sources of monounsaturated fat include olive, canola (rapeseed), and peanut oils; nuts; and avocados. Polyunsaturated fats can be found in corn, soybean, sunflower, safflower, and flaxseed oil as well as fish. Replacing saturated fat with unsaturated fat, particularly monounsaturated fat, seems to lower cholesterol (ie, low-density lipoprotein) and reduce the risk for cardiovascular disease [10]. Two polyunsaturated fatty acids, linoleic acid and linolenic acid, are considered essential, because the body cannot produce them. Thus, if not consumed in adequate amounts, symptoms of deficiency begin to appear. Consumption of approximately 4% of total energy intake from plant oils (eg, approximately 1 tablespoon of oil) prevents essential fatty acid deficiency [11].

Dietary fat can affect body weight regulation in a variety of ways. First, dietary fat (9 kcal/g) has more than twice the energy of carbohydrate and protein (4 kcal/g each). Thus, reducing fat intake is an efficient way to reduce energy intake and create an energy deficit [12]. This is the underlying concept behind low-fat diets and reduced-fat foods.

Second, dietary fat is palatable. Although good taste enhances the enjoyment of eating, it may undermine weight control. Flavor and taste are strong mediators of food intake [13]. In one study, taste was rated as the most important determinant of food selection, followed by cost, nutrition, convenience, and weight control [14]. It has been demonstrated that intake of palatable high-fat foods can lead to passive overconsumption [15–19] without appropriate compensation [20,21]. Moreover, high-fat preloads have been shown to increase the amount of fat consumed at a subsequent meal [22].

Protein

Protein is a unique macronutrient in that, unlike fat or carbohydrate, it provides the body with a useable form of nitrogen. Nitrogen is found in amino acids, the building blocks of protein. The amino acids consumed from food are used to synthesize a variety of proteins that have diverse functions in the body (ie, enzymes, hormones, structural components, antibodies).

As with some fatty acids, the body cannot produce certain amino acids; therefore, they are considered essential and must be obtained from the diet. Protein requirements vary as a function of one's age and health status. The goal for healthy adults is to maintain protein equilibrium. Assuming high-quality protein is consumed, protein equilibrium can be achieved, on average, by consuming protein at a rate of 0.8 g/kg of body weight per day [23]. Requirements are generally greater for infants, children, adolescents, pregnant and lactating women, and athletes. The average American consumes approximately 1.2 g/kg/d [24].

Although protein seems to be an important promoter of satiety, excessive consumption can be associated with increased intake of saturated fat and cholesterol and with reduced consumption of carbohydrate-rich foods, including whole grains, fruits, and vegetables, which are good sources of fiber, vitamins, and minerals [25]. Reductions in potassium, calcium, and magnesium may have a negative effect on blood pressure [26,27]. Individuals with a family history of osteoporosis may also be at heightened risk, because high-protein consumption increases urinary calcium excretion when phosphorus intake is held constant [28,29]. It has been suggested that calcium losses are minimized when there is a parallel increase in phosphorus intake (a pattern typically observed in the United States) and consumption of potassium is adequate [30,31]. Although it is unclear whether high-protein intake adversely affects kidney function in healthy adults, high-protein intake is contraindicated for those with mild renal insufficiency, renal disease, and diabetes, who are at risk of developing the condition [32].

Carbohydrate

Like fat, various forms of carbohydrate exist in food. Sugars (eg, glucose, fructose, sucrose) are the simplest form of carbohydrate. More complex carbohydrates are both digestible (ie, multiple glucose units linked together like starch) and indigestible (ie, fiber). Although simple sugars are readily consumed in the form of table sugar, soft drinks, and baked goods, they are also found in healthier foods, such as fruits and milk. Fruits and vegetables also contain complex carbohydrates and dietary fiber. Whole grains and beans are also sources of dietary fiber. Most carbohydrates add flavor (eg, sweetness) to food. Carbohydrates play an important role in inducing satiety; however, the primary function of dietary carbohydrate is to provide energy. Certain cells use glucose for energy exclusively (eg, red blood cells, brain cells). As a survival mechanism during times of carbohydrate insufficiency, these cells (eg, brain, heart) adapt to using ketones for energy, a condition referred to as ketosis. Consumption of 50 to 100 g of carbohydrate per day prevents ketosis [33]. Because protein, glycerol, and some organic acids can be converted to glucose, there is no absolute dietary requirement for carbohydrate [31]. A carbohydrate-free diet is not recommended, however, because it is associated with adverse effects, including tissue breakdown, dehydration, and electrolyte imbalance [31]. Like dietary fat, carbohydrate can positively and negatively affect weight regulation. Increased intake of fiber-rich foods can promote satiety; however, excess intake of digestible carbohydrate, like any other macronutrient, results in energy storage in adipose tissue.

Glycemic index

Carbohydrates vary in the degree to which they raise blood glucose and insulin levels. The term *glycemic index* (GI) refers to a property of carbohydrate-containing food that affects the change in blood glucose after food consumption [34]. The GI is a value calculated by dividing the incremental area under the glucose response curve after consumption of a standard 50-g portion of a test food (during a 2-hour period) by the area under the curve after consumption of an equal portion of a control substance (eg, white bread, glucose) [34,35]. Carbohydrate-containing foods are ranked in relation to glucose or white bread, which have a GI of 100. Thus, foods with a GI between 0 and 55 are considered low-GI foods (eg, apple, beans), those with a GI of 70 or greater are considered high-GI foods (eg, corn flakes, potatoes), and those that fall between these two ranges are categorized as intermediate GI foods (eg, raisins, boiled long-grain rice). A variety of factors, such as carbohydrate type, amount and type of fiber, degree of processing, cooking, storage, acidity, food structure, and macronutrient content, can all affect the GI.

Some investigators believe high-GI foods or meals disrupt homeostatic mechanisms and spawn undesirable endocrine and metabolic responses, such as hyperinsulinemia, hypoglycemia, increased hunger, and hyperphagia [36]. More specifically, the high insulin/glucagon ratio (caused by the rapid spike in glucose from a high GI meal) causes metabolic processes to shift from oxidation toward nutrient storage and blood sugar levels to drop below normal physiologic ranges. Together, these effects are thought to increase hunger and result in weight gain.

Energy density

A concept that crosses all macronutrient categories is energy density. The energy density of a food is calculated simply by dividing energy content by amount. For example, the energy density of 80 g (ie, ~0.5 cup) of grapes would be 0.75 (ie, 60 kcal per 80 g). The energy density of the same portion of cheese would be 320 kcal per 80 g or 4.0. Cheese is more energy dense than grapes because it contains more energy for a similar weight of food.

Reducing the energy density of a diet may be an effective strategy, considering that individuals tend to eat a constant volume of food [37–39]. Increasing the water and fiber content and reducing the fat of meals are two strategies for decreasing the energy content of a diet. Unfortunately, reducing the fat content also affects the flavor of food; thus, manufacturers often replace fat with significant amounts of carbohydrate in the form of sugar, often high-fructose corn syrup. Adding large amounts of carbohydrate maintains or increases the energy density of a product. Some low-fat foods (eg, melba toast, pretzels) can be as energy dense as high-fat foods (eg, cheddar cheese) because of their low moisture content [40]. Thus, in terms of energy density, factors that affect the weight of food, including moisture and fiber content, must be considered along with the caloric content. Otherwise, there is no benefit in eating certain low-fat foods, because the end result is the same—consumption of a significant amount of calories for a small weight of food.

Effects of macronutrients, glycemic index, and energy density on satiety

Macronutrients

Although hunger is only one of the many factors that influences food consumption, it is an important factor in terms of weight control. An individual who is satisfied is more likely to limit food intake and maintain body weight than one who is constantly hungry. A variety of short-term feeding studies have investigated the effects of macronutrients on satiety and subsequent food intake but have not controlled for confounding factors, such as energy density, fiber content, palatability, prior food intake, and interval between preload and ad libitum meal [41]. Therefore, it is difficult to make comparisons among studies. It seems, however, that protein has the greatest potential to enhance satiety, followed by carbohydrate and fat. Findings from four studies are presented to illustrate this point.

Rolls et al [42] found that protein (cooked chicken breast) and starch (pasta shells in tomato sauce) preloads were more satiating relative to high-fat (cream cheese on celery), simple sugar (lemon-flavored confectionery), and mixed sugar and fat (chocolate confectionery) preloads in normal-weight women. Similarly, Holt et al [43,44] found significant differences in energy consumption after individuals consumed six categories of foods varying in macronutrient content (eg, fruits, bakery products, snack foods, carbohydrate-rich foods, protein-rich foods, breakfast cereals) but similar in energy content. Foods high in protein, fiber, and water content were more satiating than foods high in fat [43], and high-fat test foods were associated with higher daily fat and energy intakes than carbohydrate-rich test foods [44]. The caloric content of the preloads was controlled, and the weight of each preload was matched by adjusting water intake. Other factors, such as orosensory characteristics and visual cues, were not controlled in these studies, however, which may have affected the results. To control for sensory characteristics (ie, texture, taste) and cognitive factors (ie, expectancy), Latner and Schwartz [45] and Rolls et al [15] used liquid and yogurt preloads, respectively, varying in macronutrient composition but similar in flavor. Intake and subjective ratings of hunger after the high-protein (72% protein) liquid meal were significantly less than intake after a high-carbohydrate (99% carbohydrate) but not the mixed macronutrient (36% protein, 55% carbohydrate) meal [45]. In addition, high-carbohydrate yogurt preloads suppressed subsequent intake more than high-fat yogurt preloads [15]. Considering that dietary fat is energy dense and has weak effects on satiety as well as the greatest potential to trigger overeating, decreasing the proportion of fat in the diet is theoretically a logical strategy for managing appetite and caloric intake.

Glycemic index

In addition to macronutrients, it has been suggested that low-GI foods (ie, those that produce smaller changes in glucose and insulin response) are more desirable, in part, because they prolong satiety. Roberts [34] reported that compared with low-GI meals, individuals consume approximately 29% more energy after high-GI meals. Ludwig et al [46] compared the effects of three isocaloric breakfasts varying in GI on subsequent food intake and a variety of metabolic parameters, including glycemic response. The area under the glycemic response curve of the high-GI meal was two times higher than that of the medium-GI meal and four times higher than that of the low-GI meal. Energy intake during a subsequent meal (lunch) was significantly higher after the high-GI meal compared with the medium- and low-GI meals. Furthermore, latency to the next meal request after lunch was significantly less after the high-GI lunch compared with the low-GI lunch. These findings suggest that low-GI diets may potentially be efficacious in reducing energy intake and frequency of eating. In contrast to these findings, Ball et al [47] did not observe any significant differences in energy consumed after a high-GI meal replacement, low-GI meal replacement, or low-GI whole food meal. The authors did observe a decreased latency between the test meal and the next request for food after the high-GI meal replacement.

Dumesnil et al [48] compared an ad libitum low-GI, high-protein diet with a pair-fed or ad libitum American Heart Association (AHA) phase I diet (eg, 55% carbohydrate, 15% protein, 30% fat) in 12 overweight men. Participants followed each dietary condition for 6 days, with a washout period of 2 weeks between conditions. Compared with energy intake in the ad libitum AHA condition, energy intake was less in the ad libitum low-GI condition. Interestingly, participants did not report any changes in hunger or desire to eat during either ad libitum condition; however, increased hunger and desire to eat were reported when participants consumed the pair-fed AHA diet. These findings suggest that isocaloric low-GI, high-protein, and low-fat diets are effective in producing weight loss but that a low-GI, high-protein combination may be more satisfying. If poor compliance to a low-fat diet and weight regain are associated with hunger and discontent with food choice, a low-GI, high-protein diet may be a more appealing and sustainable strategy for weight management. Further research is needed before any conclusions can be made regarding the efficacy of low-GI diets for weight loss.

Energy density

In addition to macronutrient content and type, satiety seems to be influenced by energy density. There are a number of mechanisms by which energy density can affect satiety. One is through visual cues. Individuals make judgments regarding how full they feel when they see a portion of food on a plate. A small portion may appear inadequate to some individuals, even if it is energy dense and packed with calories. This response is based on past eating experiences and learned behaviors. Another mechanism by which energy density can affect satiety is through volume and its effects on gastrointestinal distention and rate of gastric emptying. Mechanical (eg, gastric stretch receptors) and chemical (eg, peptides, hormones) signals from the gastrointestinal tract, in combination with dietary factors (eg, caloric, macronutrient, fiber, and water content of food), can influence an individual's subjective evaluation of fullness as well as physiologic mechanisms that regulate food intake [49–51].

Several laboratory-based studies have evaluated the short-term effects of energy density on energy intake. These studies suggest that lowering the energy density, particularly by incorporating water into a food or recipe (as opposed to simply drinking water with a meal), is a more effective strategy for reducing food intake than altering the proportion of macronutrients in a meal [43,52–54]. In a study in which macronutrient and energy content of a preload were held constant but energy density differed (by varying the water content), energy intake at a subsequent meal was significantly lower after consumption of a low-energy dense preload compared with a high-energy dense preload [52]. Ratings of fullness corresponded with intake, and participants did not compensate for the reduced energy intake later in the day. Moreover, others have shown that energy intake increased with increasing energy density [38,54]. Duncan et al [38] found that energy intake after consumption of energy-dense foods (eg, meats, desserts) was twice as high as intake after consumption of low-energy dense foods (eg, fruit, vegetables, beans). These findings suggest that individuals can feel satisfied eating fewer calories when they eat a standard weight of food.

Dietary approaches for the treatment of obesity

The following section describes various dietary approaches to weight loss (ie, low-, very low–, and moderate-fat diets; high-protein diets; low-carbohydrate diets; and low-glycemic index diets). Descriptions of each approach are followed by a review of short- and long-term efficacy data.

Low-fat diets

The *Dietary Guidelines for Americans* (with the Food Guide Pyramid) provides one example of a low-fat eating plan [55]. The guidelines are based on the premise that a low-fat (20%–30%), high-carbohydrate (55%–60%) diet results in optimal health [56]. By consuming a variety of foods and the recommended number of servings from each food group, individuals meet their protein requirements as well as their recommended dietary allowances (RDA) for vitamins and minerals and consume adequate amounts of fiber. In addition, healthy limits on total fat, saturated fat, cholesterol, and sodium are encouraged. Other examples of a low-fat diet are the Dietary Approaches to Stop Hypertension (DASH) diet and those recommended by the American Diabetes Association [57], American Heart Association [58], and American Cancer Society [59] as well as commercial programs like Weight Watchers.

Efficacy of low-fat diets on weight loss

Low-fat diets are the best studied of all approaches to weight loss. Three large, multicenter, randomized studies (ie, the PREMIER trial, Diabetes Prevention Program, and Finnish Diabetes Prevention study) have demonstrated that greater weight loss is achieved in groups consuming low-fat diets compared with controls receiving standard lifestyle recommendations [60–62]. Findings from these studies are summarized in Table 1.

The PREMIER trial investigated the effects of the DASH diet, a diet high in fruits and vegetables as well as fiber and mineral content (eg, calcium, magnesium, potassium) and low in total and saturated fat, cholesterol, and refined sugar. This diet was combined with recommendations known individually to lower blood pressure (ie, sodium and alcohol restriction, exercise, weight loss) and evaluated for reductions in weight and hypertension [46]. A total of 810 participants were randomly assigned to a control group (single advice-giving session for consuming a DASH diet) or one of two intervention groups. One intervention group instructed participants to reduce calories through the DASH diet (established intervention plus DASH diet) and exercise. The other encouraged calorie restriction and exercise (established intervention) alone. Both intervention groups included behavior modification instruction.

There were significant differences in dietary intake and weight loss between the control and intervention groups at 6 months. The established intervention plus DASH diet group consumed more fruits and vegetables

Table 1
Summary of findings from low- and moderate-fat studies

	PREMIER (6-month data)	DPP (6-month data)	Finnish Diabetes Prevention (12-month data)	McManus et al [72] (18-month data)
Sample size (n)	810	3234	522	101
Control	273	1082	257	51
Intervention 1	268	1079	265	50
Intervention 2	269	1073	N/A	N/A
Sex				
Male	310	1043	172	10
Female	500	2191	350	91
Age (years)				
Control	49.5	50.3	55	44
Intervention 1	50.2	50.9	55	44
Intervention 2	50.2	50.6	N/A	N/A
Baseline BMI (kg/m^2)				
Control	32.9	34.2	31.0	33
Intervention 1	33.0	33.9	31.3	34
Intervention 2	33.3	33.9	N/A	N/A
Weight loss (kg)				
Control	−1.1	−0.1	−0.8	2.9
Intervention 1	−4.9	−5.6	−4.2	−4.1
Intervention 2	−5.8	−2.1	N/A	N/A

Abbreviations: BMI, body mass index; DASH, Dietary Approaches to Stop Hypertension; DPP, Diabetes Prevention Program; N/A, not applicable.

PREMIER: Intervention 1, established Intervention; Intervention 2, established Intervention plus DASH; Control, advice only.

DPP: Intervention 1, intensive lifestyle group; Intervention 2, metformin; Control, placebo.

Finnish Diabetes Prevention: Intervention 1, detailed diet and exercise instruction in seven sessions during year 1; Control, diet and exercise information at baseline and annual visit.

McManus et al: Intervention 1, moderate-fat; Control, low-fat.

and dairy products than the other two groups. Significantly greater weight losses were observed in the established intervention and the established intervention plus DASH diet groups compared with the control group at 6 months (see Table 1). There were no significant differences in weight loss between the established intervention and established intervention plus DASH diet groups.

The Diabetes Prevention Program was a 27-center, randomized, clinical trial that evaluated the effects of lifestyle intervention and pharmacotherapy on the incidence of type 2 diabetes in individuals with impaired glucose tolerance [61]. In this study, 3234 overweight participants were randomly assigned to one of three groups: (1) placebo plus standard lifestyle recommendations, (2) metformin plus standard lifestyle recommendations, and (3) intensive lifestyle intervention. Participants in the medication and placebo groups were provided written information on the Food Guide Pyramid and the National Cholesterol Education Program Step 1 diet and were seen annually in individual sessions. Participants in the lifestyle intervention group were prescribed fat and calorie goals and were asked to monitor their intake daily. Calorie levels were based on initial body weight and were designed to produce a weight loss of 0.5 to 1.0 kg/wk.

Participants in the intensive lifestyle group lost significantly more weight than those in the metformin and placebo groups (see Table 1). The intensive lifestyle group also had a significantly lower incidence of type 2 diabetes than the placebo or metformin group at 1 year (see Table 1).

Similar to the Diabetes Prevention Program, the Finnish Diabetes Prevention study investigated the ability of lifestyle intervention to prevent or delay the onset of type 2 diabetes in 522 overweight participants with impaired glucose tolerance [62]. Participants were randomly assigned to a control group, which received verbal and written diet and exercise information at baseline and at annual visits, or to an intervention group, which was provided detailed dietary and exercise instructions in seven sessions with a nutritionist during the first year and every 3 months after the first year. These latter participants were instructed to consume less than 30% of energy from fat (ie, consuming low-fat dairy and meat products), less than 10% from saturated fat (ie, increase consumption of vegetable oils rich in monounsaturated fat), and 15 g per 1000 kcal of fiber from whole-grain products, vegetables, berries, and other fruits. They also were told to engage in moderate activity for 30 minutes or more per day.

Results showed that there was a significantly greater reduction in the incidence of type 2 diabetes and greater weight loss in the intervention group. Greater reductions in mean body weight were observed in the intervention group compared with the control group in the first year and remained significantly greater in the intervention group after 2 years (see Table 1).

Taken together, these findings suggest that consumption of a low-fat, low-calorie diet in the context of intensive group or individual counseling is an effective strategy for weight management. A major limitation of these studies is that the control and intervention groups did not receive the same number of treatment visits. Participant-clinician contact and instruction were greater in the intervention groups. It also can be also argued that these studies do not resemble treatment in the "real" world because of their high intensity and frequency. Although not effectiveness studies, these well-designed efficacy studies show that low-calorie, low-fat, and high-fiber diets have positive effects on weight control and, more importantly, on comorbid conditions.

Very low–fat diets

Some argue that a reduction in fat greater than 20% to 35% of calories is necessary for optimal health [63]. Diets that provide less than 10% fat are defined as very low–fat diets [64]. The Pritikin and Ornish diets are examples of very low–fat diets. The Ornish diet is a plant-based diet and thus encourages consumption of high–complex carbohydrate, high-fiber foods (eg, fruits, vegetables, whole grains, beans, soy) as well as moderate amounts of reduced-fat dairy foods and eggs and limited amounts of sugar and white flour [64]. The Pritikin diet is similar; however, limited quantities of lean meats and fish are also allowed. The major difference between low- and very low–fat diets is that the latter are more restrictive in terms of the types of foods permitted. Unlike low-fat plans, which incorporate all foods, the very low–fat diets strongly discourage consumption of foods containing high amounts of refined carbohydrate or fat, such as sugar, high-fructose corn syrup, white flour, and rice.

Efficacy of very low–fat diets on weight loss

The Lifestyle Heart Trial was a long-term randomized trial in 48 patients with coronary atherosclerosis that evaluated the effects of a very low–fat diet and intensive lifestyle modification on the progression of this disease [65]. Twenty participants were randomly assigned to an intervention group, and 28 were assigned to a control group. The intervention group consumed a very low–fat vegetarian diet and was prescribed a behavior modification program that included moderate aerobic activity, stress management, and smoking cessation. Those in the control group followed recommendations consistent with conventional guidelines for a healthy lifestyle (provided by their primary care physician).

Participants in the intervention group reduced their fat intake from 29.7% to 6.22% at 1 year. The decrease in the control group (eg, from 30.5% to 28.8%) was less dramatic. Participants in the two groups lost 10.8 kg and 1.5 kg, respectively, at 1 year. Furthermore, there were significant differences in coronary artery outcomes. The average coronary artery percent diameter stenosis in the intervention group decreased (ie, 1.75 absolute percentage points) at 1 year, whereas it increased (ie, 2.3 absolute percentage points) in the control group. These data suggest that a very low–fat diet, in combination with lifestyle change, can result in regression of coronary atherosclerosis. Adherence to these dietary and lifestyle recommendations outside of clinical trials is unknown, however.

Moderate-fat diets

Although many argue that intake of 30% fat or less is the most favorable approach for treating obesity and preventing chronic disease, others note that many European countries with relatively high percentages of fat intake (eg, France, Italy) have a low prevalence of obesity [66] and lower rates of cardiovascular disease [67,68] and mortality [69–71]. Moreover, there is evidence to suggest that individuals who adhere to a diet higher in fat may be better able to sustain weight losses over the long term compared with those who adhere to a diet lower in fat [72].

Efficacy of moderate-fat diets on weight loss

McManus et al [72] examined the effects of a moderate-fat diet (35% of total energy) and a lower fat control diet (eg, 20% of total energy) in 101 overweight men and women. Women were instructed to consume 1200 kcal/d, whereas men were asked to consume 1500 kcal/d in both groups. All subjects participated in weekly behavior modification sessions. There were no differences between the moderate-fat and low-fat groups in weight loss at 6 and 12 months. At 18 months, however, they were significantly different, because participants in the intervention group maintained their weight loss, whereas the low-fat group regained weight (see Table 1). Furthermore, there were greater reductions in percent body fat and waist circumference in the intervention group.

In summary, many studies have assessed the effects of fat intake on weight loss. Compared with very low–fat and moderate-fat diets, low-fat diets are the best studied. These diets have been shown to be effective in treating obesity and preventing disease. Although the low-fat diet is an effective weight loss strategy, there are questions concerning long-term adherence. The moderate-fat Mediterranean diet is less studied for weight loss but has impressive effects on the prevention of disease [70]. Shifting the focus from low-fat to healthy fat (eg, eating more nuts, fish, unsaturated oils) and focusing on portion control may be a more enjoyable and sustainable approach to weight management for some people. Additional studies comparing the effects of low-fat and moderate-fat diets on weight loss, satiety, and adherence would help to clarify the amount of fat that is most effective for long-term weight control in the context of an energy-deficit diet.

High-protein diets

There is no standard definition of a "high-protein diet"; however, intakes greater than 25% of total energy or 1.6 g/kg/d can be considered high [73]. The Zone diet (30% protein, 40% carbohydrate, and 30% fat) is an example of a high-protein diet. The most prominent difference between a high-protein diet like the Zone diet and a low-carbohydrate diet like the Atkins New Diet Revolution is that a high-protein diet is typically low in fat.

Efficacy of high-protein diets on weight loss

A limited number of studies have investigated the effects of high-protein diets on weight loss. In a recent investigation, 50 overweight and obese (body mass index [BMI] of 25–35 kg/m^2) individuals were randomly assigned to an ad libitum low-protein diet (12% protein, 30% fat, and 58% carbohydrate) or high-protein regimen (25% protein, 30% fat, and 45% carbohydrate) [74]. During the first 6 months of the study, foods were provided to ensure that the prescribed diet was consumed. Between months 6 and 12, foods were no longer provided but participants were asked to maintain their dietary prescription and attend biweekly group behavior therapy sessions.

The high-protein group lost significantly more weight than the low-protein group after 6 months (−9.4 kg versus −5.9 kg). Not surprisingly, the high-protein group had a greater decrease than the low-protein group in waist circumference, waist-to-hip ratio, and intra-abdominal adipose tissue (assessed by dual-energy x-ray absorptiometry). At the 24-month assessment, the former group continued to have a greater weight loss than the latter group (−6.4 kg versus −3.2 kg), but this difference was not significant, because a large number of participants were lost to follow-up.

These findings suggest that although participants in the high-protein group regained weight after 6 months, there was a trend toward better weight maintenance in these individuals. The authors speculated that the greater weight loss in the high-protein group may have been attributable to the satiating effect of protein, smaller reductions in resting energy expenditure, or greater diet-induced thermogenesis. In addition to weight loss, there was a greater reduction in waist circumference, waist-to-hip ratio, and intra-abdominal adipose tissue even after weight was regained, which is important, because these measures are highly correlated with certain chronic conditions, such as cardiovascular disease. Similarly, Skov et al [75] and Parker et al [76] reported greater total fat and intra-abdominal fat losses in individuals after high-protein diets for 3 to 6 months, whereas others reported no differences in total or intra-abdominal fat as a function of diet condition [77,78].

Other studies have also reported that high-protein diets are superior to high-carbohydrate diets in reducing body weight, preserving lean body mass, and promoting fat loss [75,79–81]. In one study in which macronutrient composition was controlled but quantity was unrestricted, reductions in body weight (ie, 8.7 kg versus 5.0 kg) and intra-abdominal adipose tissue (33.0 cm^2 versus 16.8 cm^2) were significantly greater in the high-protein group (ie, 46% carbohydrate, 25% protein, and 29% fat) compared with the high-carbohydrate group (eg, 59% carbohydrate, 12% protein, and 29% fat) at 6 months [75]. Similar to reports in the Dumesnil et al study [48], the decrease in energy intake in this study was not associated with increased ratings of hunger. Farnsworth et al [79] found that women who consumed a high-protein diet lost significantly less lean body mass after 16 weeks than women who ate a standard protein diet. The researchers stated that the high-protein diet provided women approximately 1.4 g of protein per kilogram of ideal body weight, a level sufficient to suppress proteolysis in women but not in men, because it only provided approximately 1.1 g of protein per kilogram of ideal body weight for men. Intakes of 1.5 g of protein per kilogram of ideal body weight have also been shown to prevent loss of lean body mass [81,82].

Low-carbohydrate diets

Currently, one of the most popular approaches to weight loss is the low-carbohydrate diet. Many versions of the low-carbohydrate diet exist (ie, Atkins New Diet Revolution, South Beach diet), each with a unique interpretation of optimal low-carbohydrate eating. Unlike low-fat diets, the US Food and Drug Administration (FDA) has not established a clear definition for "low carbohydrate." Much attention has focused on the high-fat and high-protein content of the diet. Nevertheless, the focus of low-carbohydrate diets, as the name implies, is on carbohydrate rather than on fat or protein. Low-carbohydrate approaches encourage consumption of controlled amounts of nutrient-dense carbohydrate-containing foods (ie, low-GI vegetables, fruits, whole-grain products) and eliminate intake of carbohydrate-containing foods based on refined carbohydrate (ie, white bread, rice, pasta, cookies, chips). Although consumption of foods that do not contain carbohydrate (ie, meats, poultry, fish, butter, oil) is not restricted, the emphasis is on moderation and quality rather than on quantity.

Efficacy of low-carbohydrate diets on weight loss

Four randomized studies have now compared the short-term (≤ 12 months) effects of a low-carbohydrate diet and a calorie-controlled, low-fat diet on weight, body composition, and cardiovascular risk factors in obese adults [83–87]. With the exception of one study that prescribed nutritional supplements, including vitamins, minerals, essential oils, and chromium picolinate to the low-carbohydrate group but not to the low-fat group [87], diet prescriptions in these studies were comparable (eg, a low-carbohydrate diet containing less than 60 g of carbohydrate). BMIs and ages ranged from 33 to 43 kg/m^2 and 43 to 54 years, respectively, in all four studies. Although there were many similarities in diet prescriptions and participant character-istics, a few differences emerged. Most of the studies were predominantly of women [83–87], except one that was primarily of men [86]. Comorbidities and amount of clinician contact also differed slightly between these studies. Two of the investigations evaluated effects in healthy adults [83,84], one examined effects in adults primarily with diabetes or metabolic syndrome [86], and one studied hyperlipidemic individuals [86]. Treatment occurred primarily in a self-help setting in one study [82] and in individual or group treatment in the others [84,86,87]. Only two studies evaluated these effects at 1 year [83,86]. Findings of these studies are summarized in Table 2.

Across all four studies, participants who followed a low-carbohydrate diet lost significantly more weight than those who adhered to a low-fat diet during the first 6 months of treatment [83–87]. Differences in weight loss did not persist at 1 year (see Table 2), however [83,86]. One study [83] observed weight regain in both groups after 6 months, with a greater regain in the low-carbohydrate group. Although participants in the low-carbohydrate

Table 2
Summary of findings from low-carbohydrate studies

	Brehm et al [84] (6-month data)	Yancy et al [87] (6-month data)	Stern et al [86] (12-month data)	Foster et al [83] (12-month data)
Sample size (n)	53	119	132	63
LC	26	59	64	33
C	27	60	68	30
Sex				
Male	N/A	28 (15 LC/13 C)	109 (51 LC/58 C)	20 (12 LC/8 C)
Female	53 (26 LC/27 C)	91 (44 LC/47 C)	23 (13 LC/10 C)	43 (21 LC/22 C)
Age (years)				
LC	44.2	44.2	53.0	44.0
C	43.1	45.6	54.0	44.2
Baseline BMI (kg/m^2)				
LC	33.2	34.6	42.9	33.9
C	34.0	34.0	42.9	34.4
Weight loss (% change)				
LC	−9.3	−12.9	−3.9	−7.3
C	−4.2	−6.7	−2.3	−4.5

Abbreviations: BMI, body mass index; C, conventional diet; LC, low-carbohydrate diet; N/A, not applicable.

group did not regain weight in the study by Stern et al [86], those in the low-fat group continued to lose weight after 6 months, resulting in similar weight losses at 1 year.

These data suggest that although participants in the low-carbohydrate group were not instructed to limit their energy intake, as were individuals in the conventional group, the low-carbohydrate group consumed fewer calories [84,87]. It is interesting to note that at 6 months, subjects who were instructed to count carbohydrates consumed fewer calories than those who were instructed to count calories across all four studies. The reason for this is unknown but may include greater satiety on a higher protein, low-GI diet. Greater weight loss may also be the result of the increased structure (ie, clear boundaries about what foods are allowed). Structured approaches, including meal replacements and food provision, have been shown to increase the magnitude of weight loss [88–95].

Although few in number, it is interesting to note that findings are remarkably consistent despite differences across studies (eg, gender, comorbid conditions, clinician contact). These initial results are encouraging but preliminary and do not signal a call for revised dietary guidelines. Limitations of these studies include small sample sizes, high attrition, short duration of treatment, and assessments limited to glycemic control and lipids. These preliminary data need to be replicated in larger and longer trials that include more comprehensive assessment of safety, including measures of bone, kidney, endothelial, and cognitive function.

Low-glycemic index diets

As carbohydrate consumption has increased, more attention has been focused on the impact of high- and low-GI foods on food intake and obesity. The low-GI diet is an example of a unique blend of low-fat, low-carbohydrate, and low-energy density concepts. Recommendations for this dietary approach are based not only on the GI values of foods but on the overall nutritional content of the diet [96]. Like the low-fat diet, a low-GI diet should consist of a variety of foods that are low in saturated fat and sodium and high in fiber, vitamins, and minerals. The main focus, however, is increased consumption of low-GI foods, such as whole grains, legumes, vegetables, and fruit. Refined and highly processed grains should be replaced with whole-grain versions. Unlike the low-carbohydrate diet, this approach allows foods that may be relatively high on the GI scale as long as they are nutrient dense. Individuals following this dietary plan are also encouraged to consume foods low in energy density (eg, number of calories in a given weight of food) and to recognize that "low fat" does not necessarily mean that a food is healthy. By making wise GI choices, individuals should feel satisfied without having to restrict food intake extensively, which should make adherence to this weight loss approach easier [96].

Effects of low–glycemic index diets on hunger and weight loss

There is considerable discussion regarding whether clinicians should recommend low-GI diets to overweight and obese patients [97–99]. Some suggest that low-GI diets produce greater decreases in weight and fat [100–102] better preservation of lean body mass [103] and a smaller reduction in resting energy expenditure (REE) during weight loss [104]. Others argue that these findings are not consistently observed and that there is insufficient evidence to conclude that low-GI diets are more effective than high-GI, low-fat diets in reducing food intake and producing weight loss [98]. The effects of low-GI diets on weight loss have not been extensively studied. Two studies have examined outcomes in obese but otherwise healthy children [101] and adolescents [102]. Three small crossover studies have compared the effects of low- and high-GI diets in obese hyperinsulinemic women [100], patients with non–insulin-dependent diabetes [105], and overweight but healthy nondiabetic men. One large multicenter randomized trial evaluated the effects of diets consisting of simple versus complex carbohydrates on body weight in obese adults [106]. Although all studies evaluated the effects of increased intake of low-GI foods, these studies differed in study duration and dietary instruction and macronutrient composition, making it difficult to compare studies.

In a nonrandomized study, Speith et al [101] compared the effects of an ad libitum low-GI diet (45%–50% carbohydrate, 20%–25% protein, and 30%–35% fat) with an energy-restricted low-fat diet (55%–60%

carbohydrate, 15%–20% protein, and 25%–30% fat) in 107 children (mean age of 10 years) attending an outpatient obesity program. Participants in the low-GI group were instructed to follow the Low GI Pyramid and focus on food selection rather than on energy restriction, whereas those in the low-fat group were prescribed a calorie-controlled diet based on the Food Guide Pyramid. Children who consumed a low-GI diet had a significantly larger decrease in BMI (-1.53 kg/m^2) compared with children who followed a low-fat diet (-0.06 kg/m^2).

Ebbeling et al [102] found similar effects on weight in a study comparing an ad libitum reduced glycemic load diet with an energy-restricted low-fat diet in 16 obese adolescents (age range: 13–21 years). Macronutrient distributions were the same as those in the Speith et al study [101]. Participants also received behavior therapy during treatment. The study consisted of a 6-month intervention phase and 6-months of follow up. Significantly greater reductions in BMI (-1.3 kg/m^2 versus 0.7 kg/m^2) and fat mass (-3.0 kg versus 1.8 kg) were observed in the low-GI group at 12 months.

Taken together, these studies suggest that children who follow an ad libitum low-GI diet are more successful in losing weight than those who adhere to a standard low-fat diet. It is unclear whether these effects are a result of differences between diets in GI or macronutrient composition, however.

Slabber et al [100] compared the effects of low- and high-GI energy-restricted diets on weight loss and plasma insulin concentrations in 42 obese hyperinsulinemic women during a 12-week period. Both diets were similar in macronutrient composition (50% carbohydrate, 20% protein, and 30% fat) and differed primarily in the types of carbohydrate-containing foods permitted (ie, high-GI foods were excluded from the low-GI food plan). The Exchange List for Meal Planning was used in both groups to aid in meal selection. Participants in the low-GI group lost 9.3 kg, whereas those in the high-GI group lost 7.4 kg after 12 weeks of treatment. Despite similar weight loss, fasting insulin concentrations dropped significantly more in the low-GI group than in the high-GI group.

Similarly, Bouche et al [103] examined whether differences in glucose and lipid metabolism as well as in total fat mass could be observed in nondiabetic men who adhered to a low-GI or high-GI diet for 5 weeks. With the exception of the type of carbohydrate prescribed, total energy and macronutrient intakes of the experimental diets were similar to those of the regular diet for each participant. Participants in the low-GI group were instructed to consume foods with a GI less than 45, whereas those in the high-GI group were asked to consume foods with a GI greater than 60. Each participant was provided a substitution list allowing exchanges within food groups and a list of commonly consumed foods. No significant changes in body weight were observed during the 5 weeks in either group; however, participants who consumed a low-GI diet had lower postprandial plasma glucose and insulin profiles as well as lower postprandial cholesterol and triglycerides compared with those in the high-GI group. In another small

6-week study that compared low- and high-GI diets, overall blood glucose and lipid control were improved in patients with non-insulin dependent diabetes (NIDDM) after a low-GI diet. Similar amounts of weight were lost on both diets (ie, 1.8 kg on the low-GI diet, 2.5 kg on the high-GI diet) [105]. Similarly, Saris et al [106] found that simply substituting simple carbohydrate for complex carbohydrate in the context of a low-fat diet does not result in significant differences in weight after 6 months of treatment. In a recent randomized study comparing the effects of low-fat and low-GI diets on REE and metabolic parameters in adults achieving a 10% weight loss, Pereira et al [104] reported that a low-glycemic index diet decreased REE less than a low-fat diet. In addition, the low-GI diet produced greater improvements in insulin resistance, serum triglycerides, and C-reactive protein. Participants in this study also reported less hunger on the low-glycemic index diet. However, the diets in this study differed in both macronutrient composition and glycemic index, which may have confounded the effects on hunger.

Findings from the studies in children and adolescents suggest that ad libitum low-GI diets that provide slightly higher percentages of protein and fat may be more efficacious in reducing weight than standard energy-restricted diets. Based on these limited findings in adults, however, there seems to be no advantage in terms of weight loss when the GI is altered and energy and macronutrient composition are held constant. Findings in adults do suggest, however, that low-GI diets may play an important role in the prevention and treatment of metabolic and cardiovascular disease.

Clinical implications future directions for research

Popular dietary approaches for weight loss have generated widespread interest and considerable debate. Despite the publicity surrounding the myriad of dietary approaches to weight loss, little is known about their comparative short- and long-term effects.

It seems that in our results-oriented society, more attention has been devoted to the potential for "success" of various weight loss approaches, traditionally measured by the general public in terms of pounds lost, rather than to their potential health effects and long-term sustainability. As such, overweight and obese individuals often find themselves in a vicious cycle of weight loss and regain looking for the next "best" diet.

More effective weight loss options are needed to support healthy and sustainable eating behaviors. Energy balance remains the cornerstone of weight control (ie, calories still count). Randomized control weight loss trials have been designed to assess which diet is best, but perhaps researchers have been asking the wrong question. The "winner takes all" mentality does not serve the field or patients well. Rather than asking which is the best diet, investigators should be asking for which type of patients do certain diets work best. Future research might focus more on how macronutrients affect cravings, satiety, hunger, and other behavioral factors that often undermine dieters in the long term. These studies require large samples that allow examination of various behavioral and metabolic subtypes.

References

[1] Wadden TA, Foster GD. Behavioral treatment of obesity. Med Clin N Am 2000;84(2): 441–61.

[2] NHLBI Obesity Education Initiative Expert Panel. Clinical guidelines on the identification, evaluation, and treatment of overweight and obesity in adults. The evidence report. Bethesda: National Institutes of Health; 1998. p. 1–228.

[3] Lauber RP, Sheard NF, for the American Heart Association. The American Heart Association dietary guidelines for 2000: a summary report. Nutr Rev 2001;59(9):298–306.

[4] Tanasescu M, Cho E, Manson JE, et al. Dietary fat and cholesterol and the risk of cardiovascular disease among women with type 2 diabetes. Am J Clin Nutr 2004;79: 999–1005.

[5] Wolfram G. Dietary fatty acids and coronary heart disease. Eur J Med Res 2003;8:321–4.

[6] Minehira K, Tappy L. Dietary and lifestyle interventions in the management of the metabolic syndrome: present status and future perspective. Eur J Clin Nutr 2002;56:1264–9.

[7] Wadden TA, Brownell KD, Foster GD. Obesity: responding to the global epidemic. J Consult Clin Psychol 2002;70(3):510–25.

[8] Henkin Y, Shai I. Dietary treatment of hypercholesterolemia: can we predict long-term success? J Am Coll Nutr 2003;22(6):555–61.

[9] Jakobsen MU, Overvad K, Dyerberg J, et al. Dietary fat and risk of coronary heart disease: possible effect modification by gender and age. Am J Epidemiol 2004;160(2):141–9.

[10] Hu FB, Manson JE, Willett WC. Types of dietary fat and risk of coronary heart disease: a critical review. J Am Coll Nutr 2001;20(1):5–19.

[11] Wardlaw GM. What nourishes you? In: Wardlaw GM, editor. Perspectives in nutrition. 4th edition. Boston: McGraw-Hill Company; 1999. p. 1–31.

[12] Bray GA, Popkin BM. Dietary fat intake does affect obesity!. Am J Clin Nutr 1998;68(6): 1157–73.

[13] Nasser J. Taste, food intake and obesity. Obes Rev 2001;2(4):213–8.

[14] Glanz K, Basil M, Maibach E, et al. Why Americans eat what they do: taste, nutrition, cost, convenience, and weight control concerns as influences on food consumption. J Am Diet Assoc 1998;98(10):1118–26.

[15] Rolls BJ, Kim-Harris S, Fischman MW, et al. Satiety after preloads with different amounts of fat and carbohydrate: implications for obesity. Am J Clin Nutr 1994;60(4):476–87.

[16] Blundell JE, MacDiarmid JI. (a). Passive overconsumption. Fat intake and short-term energy balance. Ann NY Acad Sci 1997;827:392–407.

[17] Blundell JE, MacDiarmid JI. (b). Fat as a risk factor for overconsumption: satiation, satiety, and patterns of eating. J Am Diet Assoc 1997;97(7 Suppl):S63–9.

[18] Green SM, Burley VJ, Blundell JE. Effect of fat- and sucrose-containing foods on the size of eating episodes and energy intake in lean males: potential for causing overconsumption. Eur J Clin Nutr 1994;48(8):547–55.

[19] Green SM, Wales JK, Lawton CL, et al. Comparison of high-fat and high-carbohydrate foods in a meal or snack on short-term fat and energy intakes in obese women. Br J Nutr 2000;84(4):521–30.

[20] Green SM, Blundell JE. Effect of fat- and sucrose-containing foods on the size of eating episodes and energy intake in lean dietary restrained and unrestrained females: potential for causing overconsumption. Eur J Clin Nutr 1996;50(9):625–35.

[21] Tremblay A, Lavallee N, Almeras N, et al. Nutritional determinants of the increase in energy intake associated with a high-fat diet. Am J Clin Nutr 1991;53(5):1134–7.

[22] Johnson J, Vickers Z. Effects of flavor and macronutrient composition of food servings on liking, hunger and subsequent intake. Appetite 1993;21(1):25–39.

[23] Institutes of Medicine. Dietary reference intakes for energy, carbohydrate, fiber, fat, fatty acids, cholesterol, protein, and amino acids. Washington, DC: National Academy Press; 2002. p. 465–608.

[24] Smit E, Nieto FJ, Crespo CJ, et al. Estimates of animal and plant protein intake in US adults: results from the Third National Health and Nutrition Examination Survey, 1988–1991. J Am Diet Assoc 1999;99(7):813–20.

[25] St. Jeor ST, Howard BV, Prewitt TE, et al. Dietary protein and weight reduction. Circulation 2001;104:1869–74.

[26] Gums JG. Magnesium in cardiovascular and other disorders. Am J Health Syst Pharm 2004;61:1569–76.

[27] McCarron DA, Reusser ME. Are low intakes of calcium and potassium important causes of cardiovascular disease? Am J Hypertens 2001;14(Suppl):206S–12S.

[28] Barzel US, Massey LK. Excess dietary protein can adversely affect bone. J Nutr 1998;128: 1051–3.

[29] Massey LK. Dietary animal and plant protein and human bone health: a whole foods approach. J Nutr 2003;133(Suppl):862S–5S.

[30] Whiting SJ, Boyle JL, Thompson A, et al. Dietary protein, phosphorus and potassium are beneficial to bone mineral density in adult men consuming adequate dietary calcium. J Am Coll Nutr 2002;21(5):402–9.

[31] National Research Council. Protein and amino acids. In: Recommended dietary allowances. 10th edition. Washington, DC: National Academy Press; 1989. p. 52–77.

[32] Knight EL, Stampfer MJ, Hankinson SE, et al. The impact of protein intake on renal function decline in women with normal renal function or mild renal insufficiency. Ann Intern Med 2003;138(6):460–7.

[33] Mahan LK, Arlin MT. Carbohydrates. In: Krause's food, nutrition and diet therapy. 8th edition. Philadelphia: WB Saunders; 1992. p. 29–43.

[34] Roberts SB. High-glycemic index foods, hunger, and obesity: is there a connection? Nutr Rev 2000;58(6):163–9.

[35] Ludwig DS. Dietary glycemic index and obesity. J Nutr 2000;130(Suppl):280S–3S.

[36] Ludwig DS. The glycemic index: physiological mechanisms relating to obesity, diabetes, and cardiovascular disease. JAMA 2002;287(18):2414–23.

[37] Rolls BJ, Bell EA. Dietary approaches to the treatment of obesity. Med Clin N Am 2000; 84(2):401–18.

[38] Duncan KH, Bacon JA, Weinsier RL. The effects of high and low energy density diets on satiety, energy intake, and eating time of obese and nonobese subjects. Am J Clin Nutr 1983;37:763–7.

[39] Stubbs RJ, Ritz P, Coward WA, et al. Covert manipulation of the ratio of dietary fat to carbohydrate and energy density: effect on food intake and energy balance in free-living men eating ad libitum. Am J Clin Nutr 1995;62:330–7.

[40] Rolls BJ, Barnett RA. The volumetrics weight control plan. New York: Harper Collins Publishers; 2000.

[41] Reid M, Hetherington M. Relative effects of carbohydrate and protein on satiety—a review of methodology. Neurosci Biobehav Rev 1997;21(3):295–308.

[42] Rolls BJ, Hetherington M, Burley VJ. The specificity of satiety: the influence of foods of different macronutrient content on the development of satiety. Physiol Behav 1988;43: 145–53.

[43] Holt SH, Miller JC, Petocz P, et al. A satiety index of common foods. Eur J Clin Nutr 1995; 49(9):675–90.

[44] Holt SH, Brand Miller JC, Petocz P. Interrelationships among postprandial satiety, glucose and insulin responses and changes in subsequent food intake. Eur J Clin Nutr 1996;50(12): 788–97.

[45] Latner JD, Schwartz M. The effects of a high-carbohydrate, high-protein or balanced lunch upon later food intake and hunger ratings. Appetite 1999;33:119–28.

[46] Ludwig DS, Majzoub JA, Al-Zahrani A, et al. High glycemic index foods, overeating, and obesity. Pediatrics 1999;103:26–32.

[47] Ball SD, Keller KR, Moyer-Mileur LJ, et al. Prolongation of satiety after low versus moderately high glycemic index meals in obese adolescents. Pediatrics 2003;111: 488–94.

[48] Dumesnil JG, Turgeon J, Tremblay A, et al. Effect of a low-glycaemic index-low-fat-high-protein diet on the atherogenic metabolic risk profile of abdominally obese men. Br J Nutr 2001;86:557–68.

[49] Hellstrom PM, Geliebter A, Naslund E, et al. Peripheral and central signals in the control of eating in normal, obese and binge-eating human subjects. Br J Nutr 2004;92(1 Suppl 1): 47–57.

[50] Gerstein DE, Woodward-Lopez G, Evans AE, et al. Clarifying concepts about macronutrients' effects on satiation and satiety. J Am Diet Assoc 2004;104:1151–3.

[51] Geliebter A, Westreich S, Gage D. Gastric distention by balloon and test-meal intake in obese and lean subjects. Am J Clin Nutr 1988;48:592–4.

[52] Rolls BJ, Castellanos VH, Halford JC, et al. Volume of food consumed affects satiety in men. Am J Clin Nutr 1998;67(6):1170–7.

[53] van Stratum P, Lussenburg RN, van Wezel LA, et al. The effect of dietary carbohydrate: fat ratio on energy intake by adult women. Am J Clin Nutr 1978;31(2):206–12.

[54] Stubbs RJ, Prentice AM. The effect of covertly manipulating the dietary fat: CHO ratio of isoenergetically dense diets on ad libitum intake in "free-living" humans. Proc Nutr Soc 1993;52:341A.

[55] US Department of Agriculture and the US Department of Health and Human Services. Dietary guidelines for Americans. 5th edition. Washington, DC: Home and Garden Bulletin No. 232. 2000.

[56] Johnson RK, Kennedy E. The 2000 dietary guidelines for Americans. What are the changes and why were they made? J Am Diet Assoc 2000;100:769–74.

[57] Irwin T. New dietary guidelines from the American Diabetes Association. Diabetes Care. 2002;25:1262; author reply, 1262–3.

[58] Kinsella A. American Heart Association issues new dietary guidelines. Home Healthc Nurse 2002;20:86–8.

[59] Byers T, Nestle M, McTiernan A, et al. American Cancer Society 2001 Nutrition and Physical Activity Guidelines Advisory Committee. American Cancer Society guidelines on nutrition and physical activity for cancer prevention: reducing the risk of cancer with healthy food choices and physical activity. CA Cancer J Clin 2002;52:92–119.

[60] Svetkey LP, Harsha DW, Vollmer WM, et al. Premier: a clinical trial of comprehensive lifestyle modification for blood pressure control: rationale, design and baseline character-istics. Ann Epidemiol 2003;13(6):462–71.

[61] Knowler WC, Barrett-Connor E, Fowler SE, et al. Diabetes Prevention Program Research Group. Reduction in the incidence of type 2 diabetes with lifestyle intervention or metformin. N Engl J Med 2002;346(6):393–403.

[62] Lindstrom J, Eriksson JG, Valle TT, et al. Prevention of diabetes mellitus in subjects with impaired glucose tolerance in the Finnish Diabetes Prevention Study: results from a randomized clinical trial. J Am Soc Nephrol 2003;14(7 Suppl):S108–13.

[63] Ornish D. Low-fat diets. N Engl J Med 1998;338: 127; author reply, 128–9.

[64] Freedman MR, King J, Kennedy E. Popular diets: a scientific review. Obes Res 2001; 9(1 Suppl):1S–40S.

[65] Ornish D, Scherwitz LW, Billings JH, et al. Intensive lifestyle changes for reversal of coronary heart disease. JAMA 1998;280:2001–7.

[66] Marques-Vidal P, Ruidavets JB, Cambou JP, et al. Trends in overweight and obesity in middle-aged subjects from southwestern France, 1985–1997. Int J Obes Relat Metab Disord 2002;26(5):732–4.

[67] Willett WC, Sacks F, Trichopoulou A, et al. Mediterranean diet pyramid: a cultural model for healthy eating. Am J Clin Nutr 1995;61(6 Suppl):1402S–6S.

[68] Kok FJ, Kromhout D. Atherosclerosis epidemiological studies on the health effects of a Mediterranean diet. Eur J Nutr 2004;43(Suppl 1):I2–5.

[69] Trichopoulou A, Costacou T, Bamia C, et al. Adherence to a Mediterranean diet and survival in a Greek population. N Engl J Med 2003;348(26):2599–608.

[70] Knoops KT, de Groot LC, Kromhout D, et al. Mediterranean diet, lifestyle factors, and 10-year mortality in elderly European men and women: the HALE project. JAMA 2004; 292:1433–9.

[71] Esposito K, Marfella R, Ciotola M, et al. Effect of a Mediterranean-style diet on endothelial dysfunction and markers of vascular inflammation in the metabolic syndrome: a randomized trial. JAMA 2004;292:1440–6.

[72] McManus K, Antinoro L, Sacks F. A randomized controlled trial of a moderate-fat, low-energy diet compared with a low-fat, low-energy diet for weight loss in overweight adults. Int J Obes Relat Metab Disord 2001;25:1503–11.

[73] Eisenstein J, Roberts SB, Dallal G, et al. High-protein weight-loss diets: are they safe and do they work? A review of the experimental and epidemiologic data. Nutr Rev 2002;1:189–200.

[74] Due A, Toubro S, Skov AR, et al. Effect of normal-fat diets, either medium or high in protein, on body weight in overweight subjects: a randomised 1-year trial. Int J Obes Relat Metab Disord 2004;28:1283–90.

[75] Skov AR, Toubro S, Ronn B, et al. Randomized trial on protein vs carbohydrate in ad libitum fat reduced diet for the treatment of obesity. Int J Obes Relat Metab Disord 1999; 23:528–36.

[76] Parker B, Noakes M, Luscombe N, et al. Effect of a high-protein, high-monounsaturated fat weight loss diet on glycemic control and lipid levels in type 2 diabetes. Diabetes Care 2002;25:425–30.

[77] Luscombe ND, Clifton PM, Noakes M, et al. Effects of energy-restricted diets containing increased protein on weight loss, resting energy expenditure, and thermic effect of feeding in type 2 diabetes. Diabetes Care 2002;25:652–7.

[78] Golay A, Eigenheer C, Morel Y, et al. Weight-loss with low or high carbohydrate diet? Int J Obes Relat Metab Disord 1996;20(12):1067–72.

[79] Farnsworth E, Luscombe ND, Noakes M, et al. Effect of a high-protein, energy-restricted diet on body composition, glycemic control, and lipid concentrations in overweight and obese hyperinsulinemic men and women. Am J Clin Nutr 2003;78:31–9.

[80] Layman DK, Boileau RA, Erickson DJ, et al. A reduced ratio of dietary carbohydrate to protein improves body composition and blood lipid profiles during weight loss in adult women. J Nutr 2003;133(2):411–7.

[81] Piatti PM, Monti F, Fermo I, et al. Hypocaloric high-protein diet improves glucose oxidation and spares lean body mass: comparison to hypocaloric high-carbohydrate diet. Metabolism 1994;43(12):1481–7.

[82] Hoffer LJ, Bistrian BR, Young VR, et al. Metabolic effects of very low calorie weight reduction diets. J Clin Invest 1984;73(3):750–8.

[83] Foster GD, Wyatt HR, Hill JO, et al. A randomized trial of a low-carbohydrate diet for obesity. N Engl J Med 2003;348:2082–90.

[84] Brehm BJ, Seeley RJ, Daniels SR, et al. A randomized trial comparing a very low-carbohydrate diet and a calorie-restricted low-fat diet on body weight and cardiovascular risk factors in healthy women. J Clin Endocrin Metab 2003;88:1617–23.

[85] Samaha FF, Iqbal N, Seshadri P, et al. A low-carbohydrate as compared with a low-fat diet in severe obesity. N Engl J Med 2003;348:2074–81.

[86] Stern L, Iqbal N, Seshadri P, et al. The effects of low-carbohydrate versus conventional weight loss diets in severely obese adults: one-year follow-up of a randomized trial. Ann Intern Med 2004;140:778–85.

[87] Yancy WS, Olsen MK, Guyton JR, et al. A low-carbohydrate, ketogenic diet versus a low-fat diet to treat obesity and hyperlipidemia. Ann Intern Med 2004;140:769–77.

[88] Jeffery RW, Wing RR, Thorson C, et al. Strengthening behavioral interventions for weight loss: a randomized trial of food provision and monetary incentives. J Consult Clin Psychol 1993;6:1038–45.

[89] Wing RR, Jeffery RW, Burton LR, et al. Food provision vs structured meal plans in the behavioral treatment of obesity. Int J Obes Relat Metab Disord 1996;20:56–62.

[90] Ditschuneit HH, Flechtner-Mors M. Value of structured meals for weight management: risk factors and long-term weight maintenance. Obes Res 2001;9(Suppl 4):284S–9S.

[91] Ditschuneit HH, Flechtner-Mors M, Johnson TD, et al. Metabolic and weight loss effects of a long-term dietary intervention in obese patients. Am J Clin Nutr 1999;69:198–204.

[92] Rothacker DQ, Staniszewski BA, Ellis PK. Liquid meal replacement vs traditional food: a potential model for women who cannot maintain eating habit change. J Am Diet Assoc 2001;101(3):345–7.

[93] Ashley JM, St. Jeor ST, Perumean-Chaney S, et al. Meal replacements in weight intervention. Obes Res 2001;9(Suppl):312S–20S.

[94] Hannum SM, Carson L, Evans EM, et al. Use of portion-controlled entrees enhances weight loss in women. Obes Res 2004;12:538–46.

[95] Metz JA, Stern JS, Kris-Etherton P, et al. A randomized trial of improved weight loss with a prepared meal plan in overweight and obese patients. Arch Intern Med 2000;160:2150–8.

[96] Brand-Miller J, Wolever TMS, Foster-Powell K, et al. The new glucose revolution. New York: Marlowe and Company; 1996. p. 71–94, 173–95.

[97] Pawlak DB, Ebbeling CB, Ludwig DS. Should obese patients be counseled to follow a low-glycaemic index diet? Yes. Obes Rev 2002;3:235–43.

[98] Raben A. Should obese patients be counseled to follow a low-glycaemic index diet? No. Obes Rev 2002;3:245–56.

[99] Pi-Sunyer FX. Glycemic index and disease. Am J Clin Nutr 2002;76(Suppl):290S–8S.

[100] Slabber M, Barnard HC, Kuyl JM, et al. Effects of a low-insulin-response, energy-restricted diet on weight loss and plasma insulin concentrations in hyperinsulinemic obese females. Am J Clin Nutr 1994;60:48–53.

[101] Speith LE, Harnish JD, Lenders CM, et al. A low-glycemic index diet in the treatment of pediatric obesity. Arch Pediatr Adolesc Med 2000;154:947–51.

[102] Ebbeling CB, Leidig MM, Sinclair KB, et al. A reduced-glycemic load diet in the treatment of adolescent obesity. Arch Pediatr Adolesc Med 2003;157:773–9.

[103] Bouche C, Rizkalla SW, Luo J, et al. Five-week, low-glycemic index diet decreases total fat mass and improves plasma lipid profile in moderately overweight nondiabetic men. Diabetes Care 2002;25:822–8.

[104] Pereira MA, Swain J, Goldfine AB, Rifai N, Ludwig DS. Effects of a low-glycemic load diet on resting energy expenditure and heart disease risk factors during weight loss. JAMA 2004;292:2482–90.

[105] Wolever TM, Jenkins DJ, Vuksan V, et al. Beneficial effect of low-glycemic index diet in overweight NIDDM subjects. Diabetes Care 1992;15:562–4.

[106] Saris WH, Astrup A, Prentice AM, et al. Randomized controlled trial of changes in dietary carbohydrate/fat ratio and simple vs complex carbohydrates on body weight and blood lipids: the CARMEN study. The Carbohydrate Ratio Management in European National diets. Int J Obes Relat Metab Disord 2000;24(10):1310–8.

ELSEVIER
SAUNDERS

PSYCHIATRIC
CLINICS
OF NORTH AMERICA

Psychiatr Clin N Am 28 (2005) 141–150

Physical Activity Recommendations in the Treatment of Obesity

John M. Jakicic, PhD*, Amy D. Otto, PhD, RD, LDN

University of Pittsburgh, Department of Health and Physical Activity,
Physical Activity and Weight Management Research Center,
140 Trees Hall, Pittsburgh, PA 15261, USA

Overweight and obesity are linked to increased health risks because of numerous chronic diseases, including heart disease, diabetes, and various forms of cancer [1]. This is of concern because of the increasing rates of obesity in the United States over the past 30 to 40 years [2]. To address this concern, effective interventions are needed to induce weight loss, prevent weight regain, and prevent weight gain in persons of normal weight.

Results of weight loss interventions have shown that the most rapid weight loss is achieved by reducing energy intake. To maximize weight loss, enhance the maintenance of weight loss, and potentially reduce the onset of overweight and obesity, however, energy expenditure in the form of physical activity should be incorporated into interventions [3]. Moreover, physical activity can have a significant independent impact on risk factors (ie, lipids, blood pressure, insulin) that are commonly present in overweight individuals [1]. Therefore, adequately incorporating physical activity into a comprehensive weight management program may prove beneficial for improving weight loss outcomes and reducing associated risk factors for chronic diseases. The following information should be considered when incorporating physical activity in weight control interventions for overweight and obese individuals.

Preactivity screening

It has been demonstrated repeatedly that physical activity can have acute and chronic effects on risk factors for numerous chronic diseases. For example, insulin is decreased following acute periods of physical activity,

---

* Corresponding author.
E-mail address: jjakicic@pitt.edu (J.M. Jakicic).

0193-953X/05/$ - see front matter © 2005 Elsevier Inc. All rights reserved.
doi:10.1016/j.psc.2004.09.003   *psych.theclinics.com*

and this reduction is sustainable with repeated bouts of activity. Exercise also has been shown to decrease the onset of chronic diseases such as heart disease, diabetes, and cancer [1]. Acute bouts of physical activity, however, may be associated with a certain level of health risk that typically is associated with increases in cardiovascular load (eg, increased blood pressure, heart rate, stroke volume, cardiac output) or altered energy requirements (eg, hypoglycemia). Therefore, the health benefits of physical activity must be weighed against the potential risks before recommending physical activity to overweight and obese individuals.

The degree of medical screening required to assess the potential risk of physical activity for obese adults may vary from a detailed medical history, to a physical examination, to clinical tests to determine the presence of underlying disease that may increase health risk. The American College of Sports Medicine [4] has provided guidelines to determine the degree of preactivity screening that may be required based on classifying individuals into one of the following categories:

- Low-risk participant: asymptomatic of cardiovascular, pulmonary, or metabolic disease; no more than one risk factor
- Moderate-risk participant: male at least 45 years of age or women at least 55 years of age; at least two risk factors
- High-risk participant: signs/symptoms or known cardiovascular, pulmonary, or metabolic disease

Based on these guidelines, it is recommended that individuals who are classified as high-risk should undergo a medical examination or a clinical exercise test before undertaking a physical activity program that is of moderate intensity (40% to 60% of maximal oxygen uptake) [4]. Before undertaking a vigorous-intensity activity program (greater than 60% of maximal oxygen uptake), it is recommended that both moderate-risk and high-risk individuals undergo a medical examination or a clinical exercise test [4]. When properly screened, the risk of a significant clinical event during moderate-to-vigorous physical activity is less than one event per 20,000 adults [4]. Clinicians and health care professionals should consider these recommendations when incorporating physical activity in interventions for overweight and obese adults.

Factors that impede physical activity participation

Despite the known benefits of exercise, adoption and maintenance of physical activity are less than optimal. National surveys have shown that the prevalence of individuals who engage in adequate levels of physical activity to promote health has remained relatively stable at approximately 25% to 30% of adults. Moreover, despite the importance of physical activity in maximizing weight loss [3], rates of long-term adherence in overweight and obese adults are suboptimal. Therefore, before prescribing physical activity to overweight and obese adults, clinicians should consider factors that may impair the adoption of their recommendations.

One approach is to consider the patient's stage of motivational readiness for behavior change. Targeting and tailoring interventions to match the individual's stage of motivational readiness may improve the adoption and maintenance of physical activity behaviors. Stages of motivational readiness include the following: precontemplation, contemplation, preparation, action, and maintenance. At the levels of precontemplation or contemplation, the intervention should focus on educating the individual about the benefits of physical activity and addressing the potential barriers to becoming more active. Transition from the preparation to the action stage is a critical step. This step involves providing specific information regarding the components of adequate levels of physical activity for weight management and continued education to address the barriers that impact the transition to the action stage. Interventions targeting individuals in the action or maintenance stages should focus on addressing factors that may contribute to an individual being unable to sustain adequate physical activity behaviors long-term and regressing to the precontemplation, contemplation, or preparation stage. Specific information on tailoring interventions to the stage of motivational readiness for change is presented in Table 1.

Numerous potential barriers to physical activity should be considered with overweight and obese adults. Survey results from participants before enrolling in weight loss interventions in the authors' research studies are presented in Fig. 1. Identifying factors that may increase motivation for physical activity, or developing strategies for overcoming the perceived lack of time identified by many individuals, may improve rates of adoption and maintenance of the targeted level of physical activity. Moreover, because unpublished analysis of these data indicates a significant and positive

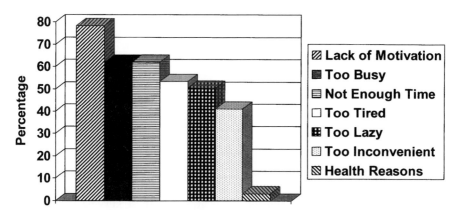

Fig. 1. Prevalence of reported barriers to physical activity adoption in overweight adult women. (Unpublished data from John M. Jakicic, PhD, University of Pittsburgh.)

Table 1
Stages of motivational readiness for change related to physical activity for overweight adults

Stage	Defining stage	Intervention approach within stage
Precontemplation	Participant currently does not exercise and is not considering beginning an exercise program.	Provide information related to the health and weight control benefits of exercise that may be effective for progressing beyond this stage.
Contemplation	Participant currently does not exercise but is considering beginning an exercise program.	The individual may recognize the health and weight loss benefits of exercise. Discussion of the potential barriers that the patient perceives that are prohibiting the adoption of an exercise program may be beneficial.
Preparation	Participant currently does not exercise but is taking steps to begin an exercise in the near future.	Discussion about the specific plan for beginning a program and the steps that will be implemented to facilitate this process may be beneficial.
Transition from preparation to action	Participant currently exercises, however participates in fewer than 150 minutes of exercise per week.	Commend the patient for engaging in his or her current level of exercise and address the barriers that are prohibiting this patient from engaging in higher levels or more regular episodes of exercise.
Action	Participant currently engages in at least 150 minutes of exercise per week but has been doing this level of exercise for less than 6 months.	The first step is to commend the patient for engaging in this level of exercise, and query the patient regarding specifics of their exercise program to determine if there are any anticipated barriers that may impact the ability to maintain this level of exercise.
Maintenance	Participant currently engages in at least 150 minutes of exercise per week and has been doing this level of exercise for greater than 6 months.	Discuss anticipated barriers that may impact the ability of the patient to continue to maintain this level of exercise, and potentially discuss with the patient the ability to progressively increase to a higher level of exercise, as this may impact long-term weight control.

Adapted from ref. [23]. Jakicic JM. Exercise in the treatment of obesity. Endocrinol Metab Clin North Am 2003;32:967–80.

association between the number of barriers to physical activity participation and participation in physical activity, reducing the total number of barriers may be critical. Few overweight or obese adults in these surveys report that health limitations affect their ability to adopt and maintain a physically active lifestyle.

Physical activity prescription considerations for the overweight or obese adult

The minimal dose of physical activity for overweight or obese adults

The minimal recommended dose of physical activity for overweight adults may vary based on the desired clinical outcome. For example, the minimal dose of activity needed to reduce health risks may differ from that required to maximize weight loss and long-term weight maintenance. Clinicians should help patients understand the benefits of different types and doses of activity.

Physical activity interventions for overweight and obese adults initially should focus on progressing to activity levels that are consistent with the minimal public health recommendations to improve health-related outcomes. To achieve these improvements, it is recommended that individuals engage in at least 30 minutes of moderate-intensity physical activity, on most, preferably all days of the week, which typically is interpreted as achieving at least 150 minutes of moderate intensity physical activity per week [5]. This level of physical activity is consistent with the recommendations of the Centers for Disease Control and Prevention (CDC) and the American College of Sports Medicine (ACSM) [5], and with the Surgeon General's recommendations for physical activity and health [1].

Although of benefit for improving health, there is limited evidence to support the 150-minute-per-week goal for maximizing weight loss and preventing weight regain. Much higher levels of physical activity appear to be needed. The Institute of Medicine (IOM) [6] has recommended 45 to 60 minutes of physical activity per day, whereas the International Association for the Study of Obesity (IASO) [7] has recommended 60 to 90 minutes per day to successfully control body weight long-term. These levels are consistent with the 60 minutes per day (300 minutes per week) that have been recommended by the ACSM [8]. These recommendations are supported by several recent studies [9–12]. What remains unclear is the optimal level of physical activity for preventing initial weight gain in normal-weight individuals (body mass index = 20 to 24.9 kg/m^2).

Intensity of physical activity

Recommendations for physical activity for overweight or obese adults should consider the intensity of the prescribed activity. This is important for two primary reasons. First, because cardiovascular disease risk factors are present in many overweight adults, the intensity of the activity should be selected to minimize potential risks for the participant. Second, the impact of physical activity intensity on weight loss outcomes needs to be considered. The interaction between these two factors should be considered when recommending physical activity intensity to overweight and obese individuals.

Current public health recommendations call for levels of activity that are at least moderate in intensity [1,5]. Moderately intense activity may provide significant health benefits while presenting low-to-moderate health risks to patients. In contrast, low-intensity physical activity may elicit the lowest health risk but may also result in the lowest health benefit. Vigorous-intensity activity may maximize health benefits, but it is coupled with more significant acute health risks for the participant. The continuum of health risks and health benefits resulting from varying intensities of physical activity is illustrated in Fig. 2.

In addition to improving risk factors associated with obesity, the benefits of varying intensities of physical activity on weight loss outcomes should be considered. Studies suggest that the intensity of physical activity may have limited impact on weight control efforts when total energy expenditure is fixed across different activity intensities. Following a 24-week intervention, Duncan et al [13] reported similar reductions in percent body fat for overweight participants engaging in different intensities of physical activity while energy expenditure remained constant across the different conditions. Jakicic et al [9] recently conducted a comprehensive behavioral weight control program and compared the effect of moderate- versus vigorous-intensity physical activity on weight loss outcomes at two different levels of energy expenditure. Results showed no difference in 12-month weight loss between the moderate- and vigorous-intensity physical activity groups for a given energy expenditure. Regardless of intensity, however, higher levels of energy expenditure modestly improved weight loss compared with lower

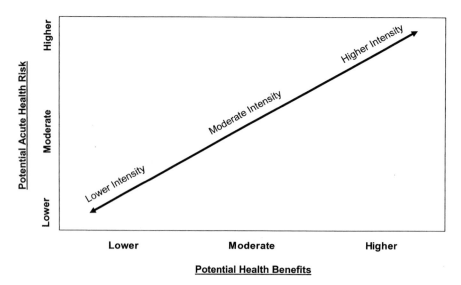

Fig. 2. Relationship between potential health risk and potential health benefit for varying intensities of physical activity.

levels of physical activity. Therefore, more vigorous levels of physical activity will only improve weight loss outcomes if there is a concurrent increase in overall energy expenditure. These findings appear to suggest that overweight and obese individuals can benefit from moderate-intensity physical activity provided that overall energy expenditure is sufficiently high.

Clinicians should educate overweight and obese individuals regarding the regulation of physical activity intensity. Intensity traditionally has been monitored using physiological parameters such as heart rate, with moderate intensity typically defined as 40% to 59% of heart rate reserve or 55% to 70% of maximal heart rate [4]. Some individuals may have difficulty monitoring their heart rate during periods of activity, however, and while available, many will not have access to portable heart rate monitoring systems. Therefore, clinicians should consider training participants to monitor activity intensity using perceptual techniques such as ratings of perceived exertion (RPE). The most commonly used RPE scale is the Borg 15 category scale [4,14], with an RPE of 12 to 13 on this scale reflecting moderate-intensity physical activity. Recently, however, the OMNI pictorial scale has been proposed [15], with moderate-intensity activity reflected by an RPE of 4 to 5 on this scale. Studies have shown that overweight and obese individuals can regulate activity intensity using RPE and that it elicits expected levels of physiological parameters (eg, heart rate).

Alternative physical activity considerations

Resistance exercise

Resistance exercise is recommended commonly in health-fitness settings for overweight and obese adults. This may be a reflection of the perceived physiological changes that may occur with resistance training that could impact weight loss outcomes. Theoretically, resistance exercise may increase muscle mass (lean body mass or fat-free mass), which ultimately may increase energy expenditure at rest and during periods of physical activity. Despite the theoretical benefits of resistance exercise for weight control, however, there are few data to support the belief that this form of exercise improves weight loss and body composition in overweight and obese adults. A recent literature review concluded that resistance training alone, without caloric restriction, resulted in minimal changes in body weight and body composition [16]. Results of this review also concluded that combined with reductions in energy intake, the addition of resistance exercise did not appear to enhance weight loss outcomes [16]. Few studies reported that resistance exercise was successful in preserving fat-free mass or metabolic rate, which have been targeted as physiological parameters that will improve weight loss outcomes. Therefore, the benefit of resistance exercise for overweight and obese individuals may be the improvement of muscular strength and function rather than physiological enhancements that may impact body weight.

Intermittent physical activity

Perceived lack of time is a commonly reported barrier to physical activity, and clinicians need to consider strategies to address this barrier [17]. One potential strategy is to incorporate intermittent bouts of activity into the day to complement or replace traditional, continuous bouts of physical activity. For example, rather than walking for 30 continuous minutes, a patient could participate in two 15-minute sessions, three 10-minute sessions, or the combination of one 20-minute session plus one 10-minute session performed throughout the day. This strategy has been shown to increase the adoption of physical activity in overweight women during the initial 20 to 24 weeks of a weight loss intervention [10,17]. However, long-term results of this intervention have been less promising [10,18]. Therefore, intermittent periods of activity should be considered as a strategy to complement additional behavioral approaches for promoting adoption and maintenance of adequate levels of physical activity in overweight and obese adults.

Lifestyle approaches to physical activity

Interventions that increase energy expenditure throughout the course of the day (ie, lifestyle activity) also may be beneficial [19,20]. Studies suggest that lifestyle activity may be as effective as more traditional structured exercise in improving fitness and weight control [19,20]. A limitation of this research, however, has been the lack of information regarding how participants interpret the message of lifestyle physical activity, which would involve understanding the type and intensity of the activity that they chose to perform. Therefore, clinicians should interpret the results of these studies with caution when developing activity interventions. Although modest changes in lifestyle activity may increase energy expenditure and contribute to weight control, the optimal type, intensity, or pattern of lifestyle physical activity for weight control has not been determined.

Using pedometers to modify physical activity

Pedometers, which are also known has step counters, may be useful tools to promote physical activity in overweight and obese individuals. Current public health campaigns recommend the accumulation of at least 10,000 steps per day, a level that is associated with improved health outcomes [21]. This is encouraging, because the accumulation of steps can be achieved in a number of ways, including both lifestyle and structured bouts of physical activity. It appears that usual daily physical activity results in approximately 6000 to 7000 steps per day, (although obese individuals may take significantly fewer steps) [21]. This suggests that an additional 3000 to 4000 steps per day would be required to achieve the goal of 10,000 steps per day. It is estimated that approximately 2000 steps is the equivalent of 1 mile of walking, and this would require an additional two miles of walking per day for most sedentary adults to achieve the goal of 10,000 steps per day. This is remarkably consistent with the public health recommendation to achieve at least 30 minutes of moderate intensity physical activity per day, which is the equivalent of approximately 2 miles of brisk walking [1,5]. A higher step goal may be required, or a concurrent reduction in energy intake may be necessary, however, to significantly reduce body weight in overweight or obese individuals [22].

Summary

The inclusion of physical activity in behavioral weight control programs may enhance long-term weight loss significantly. Moreover, physical activity may have independent effects on risk factors that impact morbidity and mortality rates of overweight and obese individuals. Therefore, it is important that overweight individuals engage in at least 150 minutes per week of moderate-intensity physical activity to promote health. It may be necessary for daily activity to reach 45 to 90 minutes per day to enhance weight loss outcomes, however. To achieve these higher levels of physical activity, it may be necessary to include numerous behavioral strategies, including intermittent activity, lifestyle activity, and pedometer-based interventions to complement traditional forms of structured physical activity. This may improve the adoption and maintenance of physical activity and, thus, contribute to the effective management of body weight.

References

[1] US Department of Health and Human Services. Physical activity and health: a report of the Surgeon General. Atlanta (GA): US Department of Health and Human Services, Centers for Disease Control and Prevention, National Center for Chronic Disease Prevention and Health Promotion; 1996.

[2] Flegal KM, Carroll MD, Ogden CL, et al. Prevalence and trends in obesity among US adults, 1999–2000. JAMA 2002;288(14):1723–7.

[3] National Institutes of Health. Clinical guidelines on the identification, evaluation, and treatment of overweight and obesity in adults—the evidence report. Obes Res 1998;6 (Suppl 2).

[4] American College of Sports Medicine. Guidelines for exercise testing and prescription. Philadelphia: Lippincott, Williams and Wilkins; 2000.

[5] Pate RR, Pratt M, Blair SN, et al. Physical activity and public health: a recommendation from the Centers for Disease Control and Prevention and the American College of Sports Medicine. JAMA 1995;273(5):402–7.

[6] Institute of Medicine. Dietary reference intakes for energy, carbohydrates, fiber, fat, protein and amino acids (macronutrients): a report of the Panel on Macronutrients, Subcommittees on Upper Reference Levels of Nutrients and Interpretation and Uses of Dietary Reference Intakes, and the Standing Committee on the Scientific Evaluation of Dietary Reference Intakes. Washington (DC): The National Academies Press; 2002.

[7] Saris WHM, Blair SN, van Baak MA, et al. How much physical activity is enough to prevent unhealthy weight gain? Outcome of the IASO 1st Stock Conference and consensus statement. Obes Rev 2003;4:101–14.

[8] Jakicic JM, Clark K, Coleman E, et al. American College of Sports Medicine position stand: appropriate intervention strategies for weight loss and prevention of weight regain for adults. Med Sci Sports Exerc 2001;33(12):2145–56.

[9] Jakicic JM, Marcus BH, Gallagher KI, et al. Effect of exercise duration and intensity on weight loss in overweight, sedentary women. A randomized trial. JAMA 2003;290:1323–30.

[10] Jakicic JM, Winters C, Lang W, et al. Effects of intermittent exercise and use of home exercise equipment on adherence, weight loss, and fitness in overweight women: a randomized trial. JAMA 1999;282(16):1554–60.

[11] Klem ML, Wing RR, McGuire MT, et al. A descriptive study of individuals successful at long-term maintenance of substantial weight loss. Am J Clin Nutr 1997;66:239–46.

[12] Schoeller DA, Shay K, Kushner RF. How much physical activity is needed to minimize weight gain in previously obese women? Am J Clin Nutr 1997;66:551–6.

[13] Duncan JJ, Gordon NF, Scott CB. Women walking for health and fitness: how much is enough? JAMA 1991;266(23):3295–9.

[14] Borg GAV. Psychophysical bases of perceived exertion. Med Sci Sports Exerc 1982;14: 377–87.

[15] Robertson RJ. Perceived exertion for practitioners: rating effort with the OMNI picture system. Champaign (IL): Human Kinetics; 2004.

[16] Donnelly JE, Jakicic JM, Pronk NP, et al. Is resistance exercise effective for weight management? Evidenced Based Preventive Medicine 2004;1(1):21–9.

[17] Jakicic JM, Wing RR, Butler BA, et al. Prescribing exercise in multiple short bouts versus one continuous bout: effects on adherence, cardiorespiratory fitness, and weight loss in overweight women. Int J Obes 1995;19:893–901.

[18] Jacobsen DJ, Donnelly JE, Snyder-Heelan K, et al. Adherence and attrition with intermittent and continuous exercise in overweight women. Int J Sports Med 2003;24: 459–64.

[19] Andersen R, Wadden T, Bartlett S, et al. Effects of lifestyle activity vs structured aerobic exercise in obese women: a randomized trial. JAMA 1999;281:335–40.

[20] Dunn A, Marcus B, Kampert J, et al. Comparison of lifestyle and structured interventions to increase physical activity and cardiorespiratory fitness. JAMA 1999;281:327–34.

[21] Tudor-Locke C, Bassett DR. How many steps/day are enough? Preliminary pedometer indices for public health. Sports Med 2004;34(1):1–8.

[22] Yamanouchi K, Takashi T, Chikada K, et al. Daily walking combined with diet therapy is a useful means for obese NIDDM patients not only to reduce body weight but also to improve insulin sensitivity. Diabetes Care 1995;18(6):775–8.

[23] Jakicic JM. Exercise in the treatment of obesity. Endocrinol Metab Clin North Am 2003;32: 967–80.

ELSEVIER
SAUNDERS

Psychiatr Clin N Am 28 (2005) 151–170

PSYCHIATRIC
CLINICS
OF NORTH AMERICA

Behavioral Treatment of Obesity

Thomas A. Wadden, PhD*, Canice E. Crerand, PhD,
Johanna Brock, BA

*Department of Psychiatry, University of Pennsylvania School of Medicine,
3535 Market Street, Philadelphia, PA 19104, USA*

Numerous studies have demonstrated the health benefits of modest weight loss combined with increased physical activity. The Diabetes Prevention Program (DPP), for example, examined more than 3200 overweight or obese individuals with impaired glucose tolerance [1]. It found that a lifestyle intervention, designed to induce a 7% reduction in initial weight and to increase physical activity to 150 minutes a week, reduced the risk of developing type 2 diabetes by 58% compared with placebo. The intervention also was more effective than metformin, a medication for type 2 diabetes. Results of a similar study from Finland yielded the same results. Individuals who lost 4.3 kg with diet and exercise reduced their risk of developing type 2 diabetes by 58% compared with a control group [2]. These studies leave little doubt that small weight losses can have big health benefits [3].

This article reviews the behavioral treatment of obesity, its short- and long-term results, and methods to improve long-term weight loss. The terms "behavioral treatment," "lifestyle modification," and "behavioral weight control" often are used interchangeably [4]. They all encompass three principal components: diet, physical activity, and behavior therapy. This latter term, as applied to weight control, refers to a set of principles and techniques used to help patients adopt new habits.

Preparation of this article was supported, in part, by National Institutes of Health grants DK57135 and DK065018, and by an unrestricted educational grant from Abbott Laboratories.

* Corresponding author.

E-mail address: wadden@mail.med.upenn.edu (T.A. Wadden).

Principles and characteristics of behavioral treatment

Behavioral treatment, as applied to obesity, seeks to modify eating, activity, and thinking habits that contribute to a patient's weight problem. This approach recognizes that body weight is affected by factors other than behavior. These include genetic, metabolic, and hormonal influences [5–8] that likely predispose some persons to obesity and may set the range of possible weights that an individual can achieve. Behavioral treatment helps obese individuals develop a set of skills (eg, consuming a low-calorie diet and adopting a high-activity lifestyle) to regulate weight at the lower end of this range, even though patients may remain overweight after treatment [9].

Principles

The principle of classical conditioning plays a central role in behavioral treatment. It holds that stimuli that repeatedly are presented before or simultaneously with a given behavior will become associated with that behavior [10,11]. For example, eating often is associated with watching television. The more often two events are paired, the stronger the association between them, so that eventually the presence of one automatically triggers the other. For example, after repeatedly eating salty snacks while watching TV, simply turning on the set may trigger a craving for potato chips. Behavioral treatment attempts to identify and extinguish cues (ie, antecedent events) that trigger overeating (or inactivity). Although eating can be triggered by a single cue, more typically, several events, linked together, lead to overeating, as illustrated in the behavior chain in Fig. 1 [12].

Behavioral analysis examines the consequences (ie, reinforcement value) of eating and physical activity [11,13]. Behaviors, such as eating favorite foods, that are rewarded with pleasant consequences are likely to be repeated. Those that yield negative effects, such as exercising to exhaustion, are unlikely to be practiced regularly. An obese sedentary woman, for example, who tries to run 4 miles a day, is likely to experience soreness and other discomfort that will lead her to abandon her activity program. If she had begun by walking 10 minutes a day, she might have felt more successful and, thus, been motivated to continue exercising.

Thoughts and images are internal cues that can affect behavior. Negative thoughts frequently are associated with negative outcomes, as in the case of a man who overeats, tells himself he's blown his diet, and then proceeds to eat triple the original amount because of feelings of disgust and despair [14]. Cognitive therapy teaches patients to correct negative thoughts that occur when they do not meet their goals [15,16].

The examination of antecedent events, behaviors, and consequences (ie, the ABC model) provides a functional analysis of behavior, a key tool of behavioral weight control [9,11]. Such analysis identifies events (ie, times, places, events, and people) that are associated with inappropriate eating and

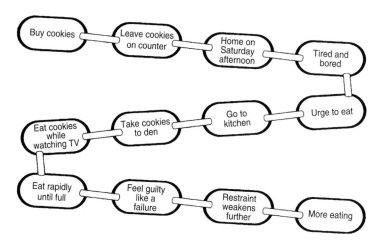

Fig. 1. A behavior chain, illustrating how one behavior, linked to another, can contribute to an overeating episode. What appears to be an unexpected dietary lapse can be traced to a whole series of small decisions and behaviors. The behavior chain also reveals where the individual can intervene in the future to prevent unwanted eating. Thus, the individual might avoid bringing cookies into the house or at least store them out of sight to reduce impulse eating. (*From* Brownell KD. The LEARN program for weight management 2000. Dallas (TX): American Health Publishing Company; 2000; with permission.)

activity behaviors, and the cognitive and emotional consequences of these behaviors. The analysis identifies opportunities for intervention.

Characteristics

Behavioral treatment has three distinctive characteristics [17]. First, it is goal-oriented. It specifies clear goals in terms that can be measured easily. This is true whether the goal is walking 10,000 steps a day (as assessed by a pedometer), lengthening meal duration by 10 minutes, or decreasing the number of self-critical thoughts about one's appearance. Specific goals allow a clear assessment of progress.

Second, treatment is process-oriented [17]. It is more than helping people decide what they want to accomplish; it helps them identify how to do so. Patients are encouraged to identify the specific behavior they wish to adopt and to then specify when, where, and how (and with whom) they will practice it. In cases in which the behavior is not adopted, attention is devoted to finding new strategies or to removing barriers. This skill-building philosophy views weight management as a set of skills that can be learned, in the same manner that people can learn a new sport or musical instrument.

Third, behavioral treatment advocates small rather than large changes [17]. This is based on the learning principle of successive approximation (or shaping), in which incremental steps are taken to achieve demanding or complex goals. Making small changes gives patients successful experiences upon which to build rather than attempting drastic changes, which typically are short-lived.

Components and structure of behavioral treatment

Over the past 30 years, the behavioral treatment of obesity has evolved into a package that includes several components such as self-monitoring, nutrition education, stimulus control, slowing the rate of eating, physical activity, problem solving, and relapse prevention [9]. This approach has been summarized in several manuals, including the *LEARN Program for Weight Management 2000* [12]. Given the availability of such manuals and reviews of the literature [9,11,13], this section will review only three components of behavioral treatment: self-monitoring, stimulus control, and cognitive restructuring. Diet and physical activity, the principal targets of behavioral treatment, are discussed in later sections of the article.

Self-monitoring

Self-monitoring (ie, recording one's behavior) is perhaps the most important component of behavioral treatment [11,12]. Patients keep detailed records of their food intake, physical activity, and weight throughout treatment. In the initial weeks, they record daily the types, amounts, and caloric value of foods eaten. In a traditional behavioral program, they try to reduce hidden sources of fat and sugar from their diet, with a goal of decreasing energy intake by approximately 2100 to 4200 kJ (500–1000 kcal) per day. Record keeping is increased over time to include information about times, places, and feelings associated with eating. Self-monitoring records often reveal patterns of which patients were previously unaware, such as consuming 2100 kJ (500 kcal) per day from sodas or fruit juices. The records also yield targets for intervention, as suggested by the behavior chain in Fig. 1 [12]. Record keeping decreases, but does not eliminate, obese individuals' tendency to underestimate their food intake (by approximately 40% to 50% a day) [18,19].

Frequent self-monitoring correlates with long-term weight loss [20–22]. It may be a particularly effective strategy during periods of heightened risk for weight gain [23,24]. In addition, recording food intake contributes favorably to treatment with weight loss medications [25,26]. Among obese adolescents treated with sibutramine, for example, those who completed the most food records had the greatest decrease in body mass index (BMI) during the first 6 months of treatment [27].

Stimulus control

Stimulus control techniques help patients manage cues associated with inappropriate eating [10–12]. Chief among these are avoiding high-risk venues such as fast-food restaurants, all-you-can-eat buffets, convenience stores, and certain aisles of the grocery store. Reducing exposure to problem foods is likely to reduce their consumption. Shopping from a list also aids this effort. At home, strategies such as storing foods out of sight, serving modest portion sizes, keeping serving dishes off the table, and cleaning plates immediately after eating (to decrease nibbling on leftovers) may help to reduce inappropriate eating [12]. All of these interventions capitalize on the premise of "out of sight, out of mind, out of mouth." Despite their common-sense appeal, there have been no specific studies of stimulus control techniques. These techniques only have been tested as part of the larger behavioral package.

Positive cues can be used to increase physical activity. These might include placing a treadmill in a frequently used room (ie, the bedroom rather than the basement), placing walking shoes at the front door, or keeping an activity calendar on the refrigerator [12]. Two studies showed that the use of large colorful signs in public areas increased the use of stairs in lieu of escalators [28,29].

Cognitive restructuring

Cognitive restructuring teaches patients to modify irrational thoughts that frequently undermine weight control efforts [11,12]. Thoughts typically fall into one of three categories: the impossibility of successful weight control (in view of previous failures), unrealistic eating and weight loss goals, and self-criticism in response to overeating or gaining weight [9,12]. Patients identify their negative thoughts through self-monitoring and role play their rational responses to them [12]. A common cognitive distortion involves catastrophizing, as captured by the statement, "I've blown my diet so I might as well eat whatever I want."

Several investigators have proposed the use of cognitive therapy to help patients accept (and value) the modest weight losses they are able to achieve [30,31]. Most obese individuals lose only about one-third of the weight they would like, which may lead to disappointment and abandonment of continued weight loss efforts [16,26,32]. Acceptance of modest weight losses could be facilitated by improving patients' satisfaction with their body image. Several studies found that cognitive therapy improved body image in obese individuals in the absence of weight loss [33–35]. It also is effective in the treatments of depression, bulimia nervosa, and other psychiatric conditions [36–39]. There have been no specific studies, however, of its efficacy with obesity. Cooper et al are conducting such an investigation [30].

Structure of treatment

Behavioral treatment usually is provided weekly for an initial period of 16 to 26 weeks [9,13]. This time-limited approach provides a clear starting and finishing line that helps patients pace their efforts. In hospital- and university-based clinics, therapy usually is provided to groups of 10 to 20 individuals (during 60- to 90-minute sessions) by registered dietitians, behavioral psychologists, or related health professionals. Group sessions provide a combination of social support and friendly competition [9]. The weekly weigh-in appears to be a major motivator for participants, who compare weight losses (either formally or informally) with each other. A well-controlled study found that group treatment induced a larger initial weight loss (ie, approximately 2 kg) than did individual treatment [40]. This was true even in patients who indicated they preferred individual treatment but were assigned randomly to receive group care (Fig. 2). They lost more weight than people who preferred individual treatment and received it. Group treatment also is more cost-effective.

Treatment sessions usually are conducted following a structured curriculum, as provided by the LEARN Program [12] or the protocol for the DPP [1]. The practitioner typically reviews patients' completion of their food and activity records, helps them identify strategies to cope with problems identified, and then introduces a new topic for the week. Lecturing is held to a minimum in favor of participants asking questions or discussing their progress in completing assignments. Visits conclude with discussion of homework for the coming week.

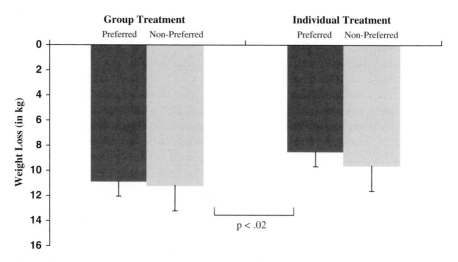

Fig. 2. Comparison of individual versus group treatment for obesity. Participants indicated whether they preferred individual or group treatment and then were assigned to conditions randomly. Participants who received group treatment lost significantly more weight, regardless of which approach they preferred. (*Data from* Renjilian DA, Perri MG, Nezu AM, et al. Individual vs. group therapy for obesity: effects of matching participants to their treatment preference. J Consult Clin Psychol 2001;69:717–21.)

Short-term results of behavioral treatment

Table 1 presents the results of behavioral treatment from 1974 to 2002, as determined from randomized controlled trials published in four journals: *Addictive Behaviors, Behavior Research and Therapy, Behavior Therapy,* and *Journal of Consulting and Clinical Psychology.* Only studies representative of standard behavioral treatment are included in the table. No interventions prescribed a diet providing fewer than 3780 kJ (900 kcal) per day.

Patients treated with a comprehensive group behavioral approach lose approximately 10.7 kg (about 10% of initial weight) in 30 weeks of treatment. In addition, about 80% of patients who begin treatment complete it. Thus, behavior therapy yields very favorable results as judged by the criteria for success (ie, a 5% to 10% reduction in initial weight) proposed by the National Institutes of Health (NIH)/National Heart Lung and Blood Institute, [41] the World Health Organization [42], and the Dietary Guidelines for Americans [43].

Examination of early (ie, 1974) and more recent (1996 to 2002) studies shows that weight losses have increased almost three-fold over the past 30 years as treatment duration has increased by the same amount. In 1974, for example, treatment of 8.4 weeks was associated with a mean loss of 3.8 kg, while treatment from 1996 to 2002 averaged 31.6 weeks and produced a mean loss of 10.7 kg. Although several new components, including cognitive restructuring, have been added to the behavioral approach since 1974, the most parsimonious explanation for the larger weight losses is the longer duration of treatment. The rate of weight loss has remained constant at about 0.4 to 0.5 kg per week.

Table 1
Summary of behavior therapy for obesity

	1974	1985–1987	1991–1995	1996–2002*
Number of studies	15	13	5	9
Sample size	53.1	71.6	30.2	28.0
Initial weight (kg)	73.4	87.2	94.9	92.2
Length of treatment (wk)	8.4	15.6	22.2	31.4
Weight loss (kg)	3.8	8.4	8.5	10.7
Loss per week (kg)	0.5	0.5	0.4	0.4
Attrition (%)	11.4	13.8	18.5	21.2
Length of follow-up (wk)	15.1	48.3	47.7	41.8
Loss at follow-up (kg)	4.0	5.3	5.9	7.2

All values, except for number of studies, are weighted means; thus, studies with larger sample sizes had a greater impact on mean values than did studies with smaller sample sizes. *Data updated from ref.* [87]. Brownell KD, Wadden TA. The heterogeneity of obesity: fitting treatments to individuals. Behav Ther 1991;22:153–77.

* Studies included in 1996–2002 sample are found in refs. [88–96].

Dietary options to increase short-term weight loss

Women in behavioral weight loss programs usually are prescribed a 5040 to 6300 kJ (1200–1500 kcal) per day diet of conventional foods and men a diet of 6300 to 7560 kJ (1500–1800 kcal) per day. Dietary recommendations are based on the Food Guide Pyramid and include limiting fat to no more than 30% of calories (with no more than 10% from saturated fat). Patients, however, are encouraged to eat foods they like, including sweets and salty foods, to avoid feeling deprived. Calorie counting is critical to this approach; it allows patients to eat desired foods, provided they fall within the daily calorie allotment.

Although behavioral treatment recommends modest and flexible dietary changes that can be maintained long-term, the behavioral approach can be used with several dietary interventions. This section briefly describes the use of more structured or restrictive diets that have been used to induce larger initial weight losses.

Very low calorie diets

Very low calorie diets (VLCDs), providing fewer than 3360 kJ (800 kcal) per day, were very popular in the 1980s and are still available today [44]. VLCDs may be consumed as either liquid shakes or as servings of lean meat, fish, and fowl. Both approaches provide large amounts of dietary protein (70 to 100 g per day) to prevent the loss of lean body mass. VLCDs are safe when provided to appropriately selected patients under careful medical supervision [45,46]; however, they are associated with an increased risk of gallstones. VLCDs induce reductions of approximately 20% of initial weight in 12 to 16 weeks of treatment, losses nearly double the size of those produced by a conventional 5050 to 6300 kJ (1200–1500 kcal) per day reducing diet. All but one [47] of seven [47–53] randomized trials that compared the two diets, however, found no differences in weight losses between the two approaches 1 year after treatment. This is because VLCD-treated patients regained 35% to 50% of their lost weight during this time. This finding, and the high cost of VLCDs (ie, approximately $3000 for a 6-month program), has reduced demand for this approach.

Meal replacements

Very low calorie diets have been replaced by 4200 to 5040 kJ (1000–1200 kcal) per day diets that combine two servings or more a day of a liquid diet with a meal of conventional foods. Dietschuneit et al [54] found that patients who replaced two meals and two snacks a day with a liquid supplement (ie, SlimFast) lost 8% of initial weight during 3 months of treatment, compared with a loss of only 1.5% for patients who were prescribed the same number of calories (5040 to 6300 kJ (1200–1500 kcal)) but who consumed a self-selected diet of conventional foods. Patients who continued to replace one meal and one snack a day with liquid supplements maintained a loss of 11% at 27 months and 8% at 51 months [55]. A meta-analysis by Heymsfield et al [56] recently confirmed the superiority of meal replacements to isocaloric diets comprised of conventional foods. Meal replacements provide patients a fixed amount of food with a known calorie content. They also simplify food choices, require little preparation, and allow dieters to avoid contact with problem foods. All of these factors would appear to facilitate patients' adherence to their targeted calorie goals [46].

Portion-controlled diets

Portion-controlled servings of conventional foods also improve the induction of weight loss. Patients in one study, for example, who were prescribed a diet of 4200 kJ (1000 kcal) per day and were provided the actual foods for five breakfasts and five dinners a week, lost significantly more weight at 6 and 18 months than people who were prescribed the same number of calories but consumed a diet of self-selected table foods [57]. A second study [58] compared weight loss among groups that received standard behavioral treatment plus: (1) no additional structure; (2) structured meal plans and grocery lists; (3) meal plans with food provided at reduced cost; and (4) meal plans with free food provision. Although the calorie goals were equivalent across groups, participants in groups 2, 3, and 4 lost significantly more weight after 6 months of treatment and maintained greater losses at the 18-months follow-up than did those in group 1. There were no differences in weight loss among groups 2, 3, or 4. This finding indicates that specifying the foods (and amounts) patients should eat improves weight loss significantly, but it is not necessary to provide the foods.

High-protein, low-carbohydrate diets

High-protein, low-carbohydrate diets, as recommended by Atkins [59], also appear to facilitate dietary adherence and weight loss. Such diets simplify food choices by eliminating an entire class of macronutrients (ie, carbohydrates). In addition, the high protein intake may increase feelings of fullness (ie, satiety) [60]. A recent study of severely obese patients, many of whom had diabetes or metabolic syndrome, found that those assigned randomly to consume a low-carbohydrate diet for 6 months lost more weight (5.8 kg versus 1.9 kg) and had greater improvements in triglyceride levels and insulin sensitivity compared with those assigned to a low-fat diet [61]. Weight losses of the two groups did not differ significantly at 1 year [62]. A second study similarly found significantly greater weight losses for a low-carbohydrate diet at 6 months (6.9 kg versus 3.2 kg, respectively), but differences between groups were not significant at 1 year (4.3 kg versus 2.5 kg, respectively), as a result of weight regain with both diets [60]. Two additional 6-month trials confirmed the short-term superiority of low-carbohydrate diets with adults [63,64], as did a randomized trial with adolescents [65]. As discussed in the article by Makris and Foster in this issue, additional studies are needed of long-term (at least 2 years) changes in weight and health outcomes to determine the ultimate benefit of high-protein, low-carbohydrate diets [60].

Long-term results of behavioral treatment

Weight regain remains the Achilles' heel of virtually all dietary and behavioral interventions. As shown in Table 1, patients treated by behavior therapy for 20 to 30 weeks typically regain about 30% to 35% of their lost weight in the year following treatment. Weight regain slows after the first year, but by 5 years, 50% or more of patients are likely to have returned to their baseline weight [51].

Obesity increasingly is being recognized as a chronic disorder that requires long-term care [41]. When considered from this perspective, the long-term results of obesity treatment are not entirely surprising. Few practitioners, for example, would expect 30 weeks of antihypertensive medication to provide adequate control of blood pressure 1 year, or even 1 month, after medication was terminated [66]. Continuous, long-term care is needed [67]. When long-term treatment—in the form of behavior therapy—is applied to obesity, the maintenance of weight loss improves significantly. There are several methods of providing continued care including on-site, telephone, and Internet/e-mail contact.

Long-term on-site treatment

Numerous studies have shown the benefits of patients continuing to attend weight maintenance classes after completing an initial 16- to 26-week weight-loss program [57,68,69]. Perri et al [68], for example, found that individuals who attended every-other-week group maintenance sessions for 1 year following weight reduction maintained 13.0 kg of their 13.2 kg end-of-treatment weight loss, whereas those who did not receive such therapy maintained only 5.7 kg of a 10.8 kg loss. Maintenance sessions appear to provide patients the support and motivation needed to continue to practice weight control skills, such as keeping food records and exercising regularly [68]. In reviewing 13 studies on this topic, Perri et al found that patients who received long-term treatment, which averaged 41 sessions over 54 weeks, maintained 10.3 kg of their initial 10.7 kg weight loss [69]. Fig. 3 illustrates the difference in weight loss produced by standard and long-term treatment, as determined from three randomized trials [68,70,71], in which all participants received behavioral weight control for the first 20 weeks. Thereafter, half the patients continued to have every-other-week treatment for 1 year, while the other half received no further care.

Figure 3 shows a clear limitation of long-term behavioral treatment; it appears only to delay rather than to prevent weight regain. Patients

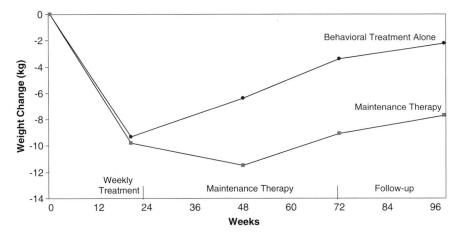

Fig. 3. Long-term results of standard behavioral treatment with or without biweekly maintenance therapy. Note, data for week 98 are available for Perri et al's 1986 and 1988 studies only. (*Data from* Perri MG, McAllister DA, Gange JJ, et al. Effects of four maintenance programs on the long-term management of obesity. J Consult Clin Psychol 1988;56:529–34. Perri MG, Nezu AM, McKelvey WF, et al. Relapse prevention training and problem-solving therapy for obesity. J Consult Clin Psychol 2001;69:722–6. Perri MG, McAdoo WG, McAllister DA, et al. Enhancing the efficacy of behavior therapy for obesity: effects of aerobic exercise and a multi-component maintenance program. J Consult Clin Psychol 1986;54:670–5.)

maintain their full end-of-treatment weight loss as long as they participate in biweekly maintenance sessions. In fact, they lose additional weight during the first 6 months of extended treatment but regain the additional loss during the second 6 months of therapy. Weight gain continues with the termination of maintenance therapy. The optimal frequency of maintenance therapy is not known. Patients eventually tire of attending sessions twice monthly (and 50% drop out), but monthly visits do not appear to be sufficient to maintain end-of-treatment weight loss [57].

Telephone and mail contact

Long-term contact also may be provided by telephone or mail, which is likely to be more convenient than on-site visits. Perri et al [72] demonstrated that therapist contact by either of these modalities significantly improved weight maintenance, compared with no further intervention. When scheduling telephone calls, the same therapist optimally should contact the patient on each occasion. A study in which patients were contacted by staff members unknown to them failed to produce weight maintenance results superior to those of a no-contact group [22].

Internet and e-mail

Recent studies indicate that the Internet and e-mail can be used to provide short- and long-term behavioral treatment. In an initial study, Tate et al [73] assigned participants to one of two 6-month weight loss programs delivered over the Internet: an education intervention, which provided a directory of on-line resources for weight control, and a behavior therapy intervention, which provided Internet resources and 24 weekly lessons conducted by e-mail, weekly submission of self-monitoring diaries, and an on-line bulletin board. The behavior therapy participants lost significantly more weight at 6 months (4.1 kg versus 1.6 kg, respectively). In a 1-year study, Tate et al [74] randomly assigned individuals to an Internet weight loss program or to the same intervention with the addition of weekly behavioral counseling, delivered by e-mail. Participants in the latter group lost significantly more weight at 1 year (4.4 kg versus 2.0 kg, respectively). These studies, taken together, underscore the importance of completing behavioral assignments (eg, food and activity records) and suggest that even the most effective Internet interventions are likely to produce only half the weight loss of traditional on-site behavioral programs.

Several studies [75–77] have examined the use of the Internet as a means of facilitating weight maintenance. Harvey-Berino et al [75] randomly assigned patients to one of three 22-week maintenance programs: an on-site therapist-led program; an Internet therapist-led program; or a control condition. There were no significant differences among the three maintenance groups in total weight loss. Participants in the on-site program, however, were more satisfied with their treatment and attended more sessions than those in the Internet program.

A more recent study [77] that investigated the efficacy of a 12-month Internet weight maintenance program found no significant differences in long-term weight losses between participants who received an Internet program and those who were provided with either frequent or minimal in-person and telephone support (7.6 kg versus 5.5 kg versus 5.1 kg, respectively). Individuals assigned to the Internet condition completed significantly more self-monitoring diaries compared with those who participated in the frequent support condition. There was greater attrition during the maintenance program, however, among those assigned to the Internet condition.

Internet-delivered interventions, for both the induction and maintenance of weight loss, currently are not as effective as traditional face-to-face behavioral interventions. Nonetheless, Internet-based programs do induce clinically significant weight losses and potentially could be provided to the millions of overweight and obese Americans who do not have access to behavioral weight control, as delivered at academic medical centers. Further research likely will improve upon these initial promising findings.

National Weight Control Registry

Long-term behavioral treatment encourages patients to practice four key behaviors: exercise regularly, consume a low-calorie diet, monitor weight regularly, and record food intake and physical activity. The importance of these behaviors is underscored by findings from the National Weight Control Registry (NWCR). The NWCR, directed by Wing et al [78,79], identifies individuals nationwide who have lost a minimum of 13.6 kg (and maintained the loss for at least 1 year. It consists of over 2900 members who have lost an average of 32.4 kg and maintained the loss for 5.5 years. These losses clearly are not representative of obese individuals in the general population who diet. Moreover, investigators have not identified the specific factors that contribute to NWCR members' success after numerous previous failures to control their weight. The NWCR, however, provides valuable descriptive information about the behaviors practiced by successful weight loss maintainers. As shown in Table 2, NWCR members consume a low-calorie, low-fat diet. Women report eating only 5443.2 kJ (1302 kcal) per day, and men report eating 7240.8 kJ (1732 kcal) per day. They also engage in high levels of physical activity, expending approximately 11,865 kJ (2838 kcal) a week, the equivalent of walking about 28 miles. NWCR members also weigh themselves regularly; 44% do so at least once a day, and an additional 33% do so at least once a week.

The importance of physical activity

Increased physical activity plays a critical role in managing obesity, as suggested by findings from the NWCR. Practitioners and their patients, however, should understand that exercise has different short- and long-term effects. On a short-term basis, increased physical activity has minimal effects on weight loss. The addition of 30 minutes of walking, five times a week, to a behavioral weight-loss program increases weight loss by an average of 2 kg over 16 to 26 weeks, a modest amount considering the effort involved [41,80]. This is not unexpected, given that approximately 70 miles of walking

Table 2
Eating habits of National Weight Control Registry members

	Women ($n = 629$)	Men ($n = 155$)
Maximum weight (kg)	94.6	121.0
Maximum BMI (kg/m^2)	34.6	37.2
Current weight (kg)	66.0	85.6
Current BMI (kg/m^2)	24.1	26.4
Energy intake (kJ/d)	5443.2	1724
Energy from fat (%)	24	23
Energy from protein (%)	19	18
Energy from carbohydrate (%)	55	56
Number of meals or snacks/d	5.0	4.5
Number of meals at fast food restaurants/wk	0.7	0.8
Number of meals at non fast food restaurants/wk	2.4	2.9

Data from Klem ML, Wing RR. McGuire MT, et al. A descriptive study of individuals successful at long-term maintenance of substantial weight loss. Am J Clin Nutr 1997;66:239–46.

is required to burn 1 kg of fat. Thus, realistic expectations are critical to prevent patients from becoming disappointed when they do not see a weight loss after having walked 5 miles on a hot summer's day.

Long-term effects

On a long-term basis, increased physical activity is the single best predictor of weight loss maintenance, as discussed in the article by Jakicic and Otto in this issue. Numerous studies have shown that people who continue to exercise regularly after losing their weight are more likely to keep the weight off than are individuals who lapse in their physical activity [4,20]. Additional studies have revealed the importance of high levels of activity, as demonstrated in a recent randomized trial by Jeffery et al [81]. Patients in a high-activity group were instructed to expend 10500 kJ (2500 kcal) per week, while those in a low-activity group were prescribed a goal of 4200 kJ (1000 kcal) per week. As shown in Fig. 4, weight losses of the two treatment conditions did not differ significantly at the end of 6 months, during which participants attended weekly group meetings. Participants, however, in the high-activity group maintained their losses significantly better at both the 12- and 18-month follow-up assessments than did patients in the low-activity group. Jakicic et al [82] similarly found, in secondary analyses of results of a randomized trial, that obese individuals who exercised 200 or more minutes a week achieved significantly greater weight losses at 18 months than persons who exercised less than 150 minutes a week.

Mechanisms of action

The mechanisms by which exercise facilitates weight maintenance are not understood well. The simplest explanation is that increased physical activity

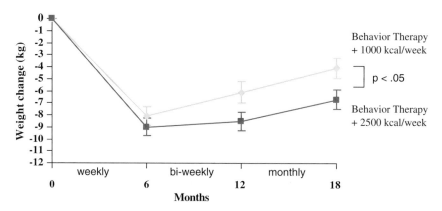

Fig. 4. Short- and long-term weight losses for participants assigned to low-intensity exercise (ie, 4200 kJ per week) or high-intensity exercise (ie, 10,500 kJ per week). (*Data from* Jeffery RW, Wing RR, Sherwood NE, et al. Physical activity and weight loss: does prescribing higher physical activity goals improve outcome? Am J Clin Nutr 2003;78:684–9.)

helps to keep patients in energy balance. Walking 2 or 3 miles a day may help to compensate for occasional dietary indiscretions that are associated with weight regain (in persons who do not exercise regularly). Alternatively, exercise spares the loss of fat-free mass during diet-induced weight loss, an occurrence that could help minimize undesired reductions in resting energy expenditure [83]. Increased physical activity also could be associated with improved mood which, in turn, could facilitate long-term adherence to a low-calorie diet [83]. Regardless of the mechanism of action, the message remains the same. Patients should increase their physical activity by whatever means possible, including increasing lifestyle activity, incorporating short bouts of exercise throughout the day, and decreasing sedentary behaviors (which are discussed in the article by Jakicic and Otto in this issue).

Health benefits

Regular physical activity confers important health benefits, including reducing lipid levels, blood pressure, and the risks of osteoporosis [84]. In patients with type 2 diabetes, exercise also improves insulin sensitivity, abdominal adiposity, and glycemic control [85]. Increased physical activity may decrease the risk of cardiovascular morbidity and mortality, even in the absence of achieving normal body weight. Lee et al [86] found in a longitudinal study of over 21,000 men that those who were fit but obese had lower rates of death from cardiovascular disease than those who were lean but unfit (Fig. 5). Collectively, these findings indicate that obese

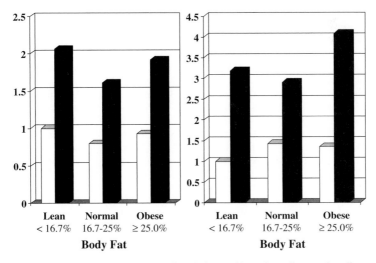

Fig. 5. Relative risks for all-cause mortality (left graph) and cardiovascular disease (right graph) by stratum of percent body fat and cardiorespiratory fitness level in 21,925 men. (*Data from* Lee CD, Blair SN, Jackson AS. Cardiorespiratory fitness, body composition, and all-cause and cardiovascular disease mortality in men. Am J Clin Nutr 1999;69:373–80.)

individuals should increase their physical activity to improve their health, regardless of its impact on their weight [84].

Looking ahead

This article has shown that behavioral treatment is effective in inducing a loss of 10% of initial weight and that losses of this size are associated with significant improvements in health, as shown by the DPP [1]. The NIH is conducting a follow-up investigation to determine whether a weight loss of at least 7% of initial weight, combined with increased physical activity, will decrease morbidity and mortality in overweight individuals who already have developed type 2 diabetes. This Look AHEAD (ie, Action for Health in Diabetes) study will enroll 5000 participants at 16 sites nationwide and evaluate patients for up to 12 years. The results will provide the most definitive assessment to date of the health consequences of intentional weight loss.

References

[1] Diabetes Prevention Program Research Group. Reduction in the incidence of type 2 diabetes with lifestyle intervention or metformin. N Engl J Med 2002;346:393–403.

[2] Tuomilehto J, Lindstrom J, Eriksson JG, et al. Prevention of type 2 diabetes mellitus by changes in lifestyle among subjects with impaired glucose tolerance. N Engl J Med 2001;344: 1343–50.

[3] Blackburn GL. Effect of degree of weight loss on health benefits. Obes Res 1995;3: 211S–6S.

[4] Wadden TA, McGuckin BG, Rothman RA, et al. Lifestyle modification in the management of obesity. J Gastrointest Surg 2003;7:452–63.

[5] Stunkard AJ, Harris JR, Pederson NL, et al. The body-mass index of twins who have been reared apart. N Engl J Med 1990;322:1483–7.

[6] Ravussin E, Lillioja S, Knowler WC, et al. Reduced rate of energy expenditure as a risk factor for body weight gain. N Engl J Med 1988;318:467–72.

[7] Campfield LA, Smith FJ, Guisez Y, et al. Recombinant mouse OB protein: evidence for a peripheral signal linking adiposity and central neural networks. Science 1995;269: 475–6.

[8] Considine RV, Sinha MK, Heiman ML, et al. Serum immunoreactive-leptin concentrations in normal-weight and obese humans. N Engl J Med 1996;334:292–5.

[9] Wadden TA, Butryn ML. Behavioral treatment of obesity. Endocrinol Metab Clin North Am 2003;32:981–1003.

[10] Stuart RB. Behavioral control of overeating. Behav Ther 1967;5:357–65.

[11] Wing RR. Behavioral approaches to the treatment of obesity. In: Bray GA, Bouchard C, James WPT, editors. Handbook of obesity. New York: Marcel Dekker; 1998. p. 855–73.

[12] Brownell KD. The LEARN program for weight management 2000. Dallas (TX): American Health Publishing Company; 2000.

[13] Wing RR. Behavioral weight control. In: Wadden TA, Stunkard AJ, editors. Handbook of obesity treatment. New York: Guilford; 2002. p. 301–16.

[14] Beck AT. Cognitive therapy and the emotional disorder. New York: International Universities Press; 1976.

[15] Foster GD. Goals and strategies to improve behavior-change effectiveness. In: Bessesen DH, Kushner RF, editors. Evaluation and management of obesity. Philadelphia: Hanley & Belfus; 2002. p. 29–32.

[16] Foster GD, Wadden TA, Vogt RA, et al. What is a reasonable weight loss? Patients' expectations and evaluations of obesity treatment outcomes. J Consult Clin Psychol 1997;65: 79–85.

[17] Wadden TA, Foster GD. Behavioral treatment of obesity. Med Clin North Amer 2000;84: 441–61.

[18] Lichtman SW, Pisarka K, Berman ER, et al. Discrepancy between self-reported and actual caloric intake and exercise in obese subjects. N Engl J Med 1992;327:1893–8.

[19] Prentice AM, Black AE, Coward WA, et al. Energy expenditure in overweight and obese adults in affluent societies: an analysis of 319 doubly-labeled water experiments. Eur J Clin Nutr 1996;50:93–7.

[20] Wadden TA. Characteristics of successful weight loss maintainers. In: Allison DB, Pi-Sunyer FX, editors. Obesity treatment: establishing goals, improving outcomes, and reviewing the research agenda. New York: Plenum Press; 1995. p. 103–11.

[21] Head S, Brookhart A. Lifestyle modification and relapse-prevention training during treatment for weight loss. Behav Ther 1997;28:307–21.

[22] Wing RR, Jeffery RW, Hellerstedt WL, et al. Effect of frequent phone contact and optional food provision on maintenance of weight loss. Ann Behav Med 1996;18:172–6.

[23] Baker RC, Kirschenbaum DS. Weight control during the holidays: highly consistent self-monitoring as a potentially useful coping mechanism. Health Psychol 1998;17:367–70.

[24] Boutelle KN, Kirschenbaum DS, Baker RC, et al. How can obese weight controllers minimize weight gain during the high risk holiday season? By self-monitoring very consistently. Health Psychol 1999;18:364–8.

[25] Wadden TA, Berkowitz RI, Vogt RA, et al. Lifestyle modification in the pharmacologic treatment of obesity: a pilot investigation of a primary care approach. Obes Res 1997;5: 218–25.

[26] Wadden TA, Berkowitz RI, Sarwer DB, et al. Benefits of lifestyle modification in the pharmacologic treatment of obesity. A randomized trial. Arch Intern Med 2001;161:218–27.

[27] Berkowitz RI, Wadden TA, Tershakovec AM, et al. Behavior therapy and sibutramine for the treatment of adolescent obesity. JAMA 2003;289:1805–12.

[28] Brownell KD, Stunkard AJ, Albaum JM. Evaluation and modification of exercise patterns in the natural environment. Am J Psychiatry 1980;137:1540–5.

[29] Andersen RE, Franckowiak SC, Snyder SW, et al. Can inexpensive signs encourage the use of stairs?: Results from a community intervention. Ann Intern Med 1998;129:363–9.

[30] Cooper Z, Fairburn CG, Hawker DM. Cognitive–behavioral treatment of obesity. New York: Guilford; 2003.

[31] Cooper Z, Fairburn CG. Cognitive–behavioral treatment of obesity. In: Wadden TA, Stunkard AJ, editors. Handbook of obesity treatment. New York: Guilford; 2002. p. 465–79.

[32] Wadden TA, Womble LG, Sarwer DB, et al. Great expectations: "I'm losing 25% of my weight no matter what you say.". J Consult Clin Psychol 2003;71:1084–9.

[33] Ciliska D. Evaluation of two nondieting interventions for obese women. West J Nurs Res 1998;20:119–35.

[34] Rosen JC, Orosan P, Reiter J. Cognitive–behavior therapy for negative body image in obese women. Behav Ther 1995;26:25–42.

[35] Polivy J, Herman CP. Undieting: a program to help people stop dieting. Int J Eat Disord 1992;11:261–8.

[36] Fairburn CG, Norman PA, Welch SL, et al. A prospective study of outcome in bulimia nervosa and the long-term effects of three psychological treatments. Arch Gen Psychiatry 1995;52:304–12.

[37] Fairburn CG, Jones R, Peveler RC, et al. Three psychological treatments for bulimia nervosa. Arch Gen Psychiatry 1991;48:463–9.

[38] Fairburn CG, Jones R, Peveler RC, et al. Psychotherapy and bulimia nervosa: the longer-term effects of interpersonal psychotherapy, behavior therapy, and cognitive–behavior therapy. Arch Gen Psychiatry 1993;50:419–28.

[39] Beck AT, Rush AJ. Cognitive therapy. In: Kaplan HI, Sadock BJ, editors. Comprehensive textbook of psychiatry. Baltimore (MD): Williams & Wilkins; 1995. p. 1847–57.

[40] Renjilian DA, Perri MG, Nezu AM, et al. Individual vs. group therapy for obesity: effects of matching participants to their treatment preference. J Consult Clin Psychol 2001;69:717–21.

[41] National Institutes of Health/National Heart, Lung, and Blood Institute. Clinical guidelines on the identification, evaluation, and treatment of overweight and obesity in adults: the evidence report. Obes Res 1998;6:51S–210S.

[42] World Health Organization. Obesity: preventing and managing the global epidemic. Geneva (Switzerland): World Health Organization; 1998.

[43] Agricultural Research Service. Report of the Dietary Guidelines Advisory Committee on the dietary guidelines for Americans. 1995.

[44] Wadden TA, Stunkard AJ, Brownell KD. Very low calorie diets: their efficacy, safety, and future. Ann Intern Med 1983;99:675–84.

[45] National Task Force on the Prevention and Treatment of Obesity. Very low calorie diets. JAMA 1993;270:967–74.

[46] Wadden TA, Berkowitz RI. Very low calorie diets. In: Fairburn CG, Brownell KD, editors. Eating disorders and obesity. 2nd edition. New York: Guilford Press; 2002. p. 534–8.

[47] Miura J, Arai K, Ohno M, et al. The long-term effectiveness of combined therapy by behavior modification and very low calorie diet: 2-year follow-up. Int J Obes 1989;13:73–7.

[48] Ryttig KR, Flaten H, Rossner S. Long-term effects of a very low calorie diet (Nutrilett) in obesity treatment. A prospective, randomized comparison between VLCD and a hypocaloric diet + behavior modification and their combination. Int J Obes 1997;21:574–9.

[49] Togerson JS, Lissner L, Lindross AK, et al. VLCD plus dietary and behavioral support versus support alone in the treatment of severe obesity: a randomized two-year clinical trial. Int J Obes 1997;21:987–94.

[50] Wadden TA, Foster GD, Letizia KA. One-year behavioral treatment of obesity: Comparison of moderate and severe caloric restrictions and the effects of weight maintenance therapy. J Consult Clin Psychol 1994;62:165–71.

[51] Wadden TA, Sternberg JA, Letizia KA, et al. Treatment of obesity by very low calorie diet, behavior therapy, and their combination: A five-year perspective. Int J Obes 1989;51:167–72.

[52] Wing RR, Blair E, Marcus MD, et al. Year-long weight loss treatment for obese patients with type II diabetes: does inclusion of intermittent very low calorie diet improve outcome? Am J Med 1994;97:354–62.

[53] Wing RR, Marcus MD, Salata R, et al. Effects of a very-low-calorie diet on long-term glycemic control in obese type II diabetic subjects. Arch Intern Med 1991;151:1334–40.

[54] Ditschuneit HH, Flechtner-Mors M, Johnson TD, et al. Metabolic and weight loss effects of long-term dietary intervention in obese subjects. Am J Clin Nutr 1999;69:198–204.

[55] Flechtner-Mors M, Ditschuneit HH, Johnson TD, et al. Metabolic and weight loss effects of long-term intervention in obese patients: four-year results. Obes Res 2000;8:399–402.

[56] Heymsfeld SB, van Mierlo CA, van der Knaap HC, et al. Weight management using a meal replacement strategy: meta- and pooling analysis from six studies. Int J Obes 2003;27:537–49.

[57] Jeffery RW, Wing RR, Thornson C, et al. Strengthening behavioral interventions for weight loss: a randomized trial of food provision and monetary incentives. J Consult Clin Psychol 1993;61:1038–45.

[58] Wing RR, Jeffery RW, Burton LR, et al. Food provision vs. structured meal plans in the behavioral treatment of obesity. J Consult Clin Psychol 1996;20:56–62.

[59] Atkins RC. Dr. Atkins' new diet revolution. New York: Avon Books; 1998.

[60] Foster GD, Wyatt HR, Hill JO, et al. A randomized trial of a low-carbohydrate diet for obesity. N Engl J Med 2003;348:2082–90.

[61] Samaha FF, Iqbal N, Seshadri P, et al. A low-carbohydrate as compared with a low-fat diet in severe obesity. N Engl J Med 2003;348:2074–81.

[62] Stern L, Iqbal N, Seshadri P, et al. The effects of low-carbohydrate versus conventional weight loss diets in severely obese adults: one-year follow-up of a randomized trial. Ann Intern Med 2004;140:778–85.

[63] Yancy W, Olsen MK, Guyton JR, et al. A low-carbohydrate, ketogenic diet versus a low-fat diet to treat obesity and hyperlipidemia: a randomized, controlled trial. Ann Intern Med 2004;140:769–77.

[64] Brehm BJ, Seeley RJ, Daniels SR, et al. A randomized trial comparing a very low carbohydrate diet and a calorie-restricted low fat diet on body weight and cardiovascular risk factors in healthy women. J Clin Endocrinol Metab 2003;88:1617–23.

[65] Sondike SB, Copperman N, Jacobson MS. Effects of a low-carbohydrate diet on weight loss and cardiovascular risk factor in overweight adolescents. J Pediatr 2003;142:253–8.

[66] Bray GA. Use and abuse of appetite-suppressant drugs in the treatment of obesity. Ann Intern Med 1993;119:707–13.

[67] Perri MG, Nezu AM, Viegener BJ. Improving the long-term management of obesity: theory research and clinical guidelines. New York: John Wiley and Sons; 1992.

[68] Perri MG, McAllister DA, Gange JJ, et al. Effects of four maintenance programs on the long-term management of obesity. J Consult Clin Psychol 1988;56:529–34.

[69] Perri MG, Corsica JA. Improving the maintenance of weight lost in behavioral treatment of obesity. In: Wadden TA, Stunkard AJ, editors. Handbook of obesity treatment. New York: Guilford Press; 2002. p. 357–79.

[70] Perri MG, Nezu AM, McKelvey WF, et al. Relapse prevention training and problem-solving therapy in the long-term management of obesity. J Consult Clin Psychol 2001;69:722–6.

[71] Perri MG, McAdoo WG, McAllister DA, et al. Enhancing the efficacy of behavior therapy for obesity: Effects of aerobic exercise and a multi-component maintenance program. J Consult Clin Psychol 1986;54:670–5.

[72] Perri MG, Shapiro RM, Ludwig WW, et al. Maintenance strategies for the treatment of obesity: An evaluation of relapse prevention training and post-treatment contact by telephone and mail. J Consult Clin Psychol 1984;52:404–13.

[73] Tate D, Wing RR, Winett R. Development and evaluation of an internet behavior therapy program for weight loss. JAMA 2001;285:1172–7.

[74] Tate DF, Jackvony EH, Wing RR. Effects of internet behavioral counseling on weight loss in adults at risk for type 2 diabetes. JAMA 2003;289:1833–6.

[75] Harvey-Berino J, Pintauro SJ, Gold EC. The feasibility of using Internet support for the maintenance of weight loss. Behav Modif 2002;26:103–16.

[76] Harvey-Berino J, Pintauro S, Buzzell P, et al. Does using the Internet facilitate the maintenance of weight loss? Int J Obes 2002;26:1254–60.

[77] Harvey-Berino J, Pintauro S, Buzzell P, et al. Effect of Internet support on the long-term maintenance of weight loss. Obes Res 2004;12:320–9.

[78] Klem ML, Wing RR, McGuire MT, et al. A descriptive study of individuals successful at long-term maintenance of substantial weight loss. Am J Clin Nutr 1997;66:239–46.

[79] Wing RR, Hill JO. Successful weight loss maintenance. Annu Rev Nutr 2001;21:323–41.

[80] Wing RR. Physical activity in the treatment of adulthood overweight and obesity: current evidence and research issues. Med Sci Sports Exerc 1999;31:547S–52S.

[81] Jeffery RW, Wing RR, Sherwood NE, et al. Physical activity and weight loss: does prescribing higher physical activity goals improve outcome? Am J Clin Nutr 2003;78:684–9.

[82] Jakicic JM, Winters C, Lang W, et al. Effects of intermittent exercise and use of home exercise equipment on adherence, weight loss, and fitness in overweight women: a randomized trial. JAMA 1999;16:1554–60.

[83] Wadden TA, Vogt RA, Andersen RE, et al. Exercise in the treatment of obesity: effects of four interventions on body composition, resting energy expenditure, appetite and mood. J Consult Clin Psychol 1997;65:269–77.

[84] Blair SN, Leermakers EA. Exercise and weight management. In: Wadden TA, Stunkard AJ, editors. Handbook of obesity treatment. New York: Guilford Press; 2002. p. 283–300.

[85] Foreyt JP, Poston WSC. The challenge of diet, exercise, and lifestyle modification in the management of the obese diabetic patient. Int J Obes Relat Metab Disord 1999;23:S5–11.

[86] Lee CD, Blair SN, Jackson AS. Cardiorespiratory fitness, body composition, and all-cause and cardiovascular disease mortality in men. Am J Clin Nutr 1999;69:373–80.

[87] Brownell KD, Wadden TA. The heterogeneity of obesity: fitting treatments to individuals. Behav Ther 1991;22:153–77.

[88] Meyers AW, Graves TJ, Whelan JP, et al. An evaluation of a television-delivered behavioral weight loss program: are the ratings acceptable. J Consult Clin Psychol 1996;64:172–8.

[89] Fuller PR, Perri MG, Leermakers EA, et al. Effects of a personalized system of skill acquisition and an educational program in the treatment of obesity. Addict Behav 1998;23: 97–100.

[90] Perri MG, Martin AD, Leermakers EA, et al. Effects of group- versus home-based exercise in the treatment of obesity. J Consult Clin Psychol 1997;65:278–85.

[91] Wadden TA, Vogt RA, Andersen RE, et al. Exercise in the treatment of obesity: effects of four interventions on body composition, resting energy expenditure, appetite and mood. J Consult Clin Psychol 1997;65:269–77.

[92] Harvey-Berino J. Changing health behavior via telecommunications technology: using interactive television to treat obesity. Behav Ther 1998;29:505–19.

[93] Sbrocco T, Nedegaard R, Stone JM, et al. Behavioral choice treatment promotes continuing weight loss: preliminary results of a cognitive-behavioral decision-based treatment for obesity. J Consult Clin Psychol 1999;67:260–6.

[94] Wing RR, Jeffery RW. Benefits of recruiting participants with friends and increasing social support for weight loss and maintenance. J Consult Clin Psychol 1999;67:132–8.

[95] Perri MG, Nezu AM, Mckelvey WF, et al. Relapse prevention training and problem-solving therapy in the long-term management of obesity. J Consult Clin Psychol 2001;69:722–6.

[96] Ramirez EM, Rosen JC. A comparison of weight control and weight control plus body image therapy for obese men and women. J Consult Clin Psychol 2001;69:440–6.

ELSEVIER
SAUNDERS

Psychiatr Clin N Am 28 (2005) 171–192

PSYCHIATRIC
CLINICS
OF NORTH AMERICA

Commercial and Self-help Programs for Weight Control

Adam Gilden Tsai, MD, Thomas A. Wadden, PhD*, Leslie G. Womble, PhD, Kirstin J. Byrne, MS

Department of Psychiatry, University of Pennsylvania School of Medicine, Weight and Eating Disorders Program, Philadelphia, PA 19104, USA

Each year, millions of Americans participate in commercial and self-help weight loss programs. Health care providers, including psychiatrists, need information about these programs so that they can advise patients appropriately. This article describes the components, costs, and efficacy of the major commercial (nonmedical, medically supervised, and Internet-based) and organized self-help programs. Among nonmedical programs, Weight Watchers is the only one that has sponsored a randomized trial. Participants in their largest study lost 5.3% of initial weight at 12 months and maintained a loss of 3.2% at 2 years. Uncontrolled studies and one randomized trial of medically supervised programs, sponsored by Health Management Resources (HMR) and OPTIFAST, found that participants who completed treatment lost approximately 15% to 25% of initial weight in 4 to 6 months. These programs, however, were associated with high costs, high attrition, and the high probability of regaining 50% or more of lost weight in 1 to 2 years. No studies were found to support the use of commercial Internet programs or organized self-help programs, although the latter interventions present few financial or health risks. Psychiatrists can assist obese individuals by identifying an appropriate weight loss program and then supporting participation by inquiring regularly about progress.

Psychiatrists traditionally have not played a major role in the management of obesity. They are likely to devote more attention to this problem in years to come, because of its increasing prevalence and also

Preparation of this manuscript was supported, in part, by NIH grants T32-HP-010026 and K24-DK-065018. Dr. Wadden serves as a consultant to Novartis Nutrition, which manufactures OPTIFAST. He previously received grant support from the company.

* Corresponding author.

E-mail address: wadden@mail.med.upenn.edu (T.A. Wadden).

because of the realization that many psychiatric medications are associated with undesirable weight gain. Practitioners who are unfamiliar with obesity management can begin by reviewing guidelines for assessment and treatment published by a joint task force of the National Heart, Lung, and Blood Institute and the North American Association for the Study of Obesity [1]. Clinical evaluation includes calculation of the body mass index (BMI), measurement of the waist circumference, and assessment of cardiovascular risk factors. Obesity-related complications are more likely as BMI and waist circumference increase [2]. Weight losses of 5% or more of initial weight, combined with increased physical activity, may be adequate to prevent such complications, as shown by the Diabetes Prevention Program and other studies [2–6].

Several articles in this issue describe methods to manage obesity using diet, exercise, and behavior modification. These three interventions, which together are referred to as lifestyle modification, are the cornerstone of all weight management therapies and may be supplemented by pharmacotherapy or surgery, as described elsewhere [1,2]. Psychiatrists and other physicians, however, may not have the time or skills to provide intensive lifestyle modification strategies for weight loss [7]. Although these skills may be acquired readily, psychiatrists still may not wish to take valuable treatment time to address obesity, when it is not the patient's presenting problem and may seem marginal compared with the distress associated with psychiatric illness. In addition, it is sometimes difficult to integrate the highly structured demands of behavioral weight loss therapy with the more patient-oriented focus of psycho-dynamically oriented psychotherapy.

Psychiatrists may wish to refer obese patients to programs (or colleagues) specializing in weight management. They can support participation in such programs by periodically inquiring about patients' satisfaction with the care they receive, by reviewing success in modifying eating and activity habits, and by assessing whether weight loss has affected mood or self-image. In this manner, psychiatrists can facilitate patients' weight management efforts while not being responsible for providing weekly weight counseling sessions.

Practitioners may wish to consider referring obese patients to a commercial or self-help weight loss program in areas where the local medical community lacks professionals who specialize in weight management. Although there are numerous proprietary and self-help programs for obesity [8], there is little information to guide providers' (or patients') choice of a program.

Drawing upon two prior publications [8,10], this article evaluates the largest commercial and self-help weight loss programs in the United States, using criteria proposed by an expert panel convened by the Federal Trade Commission [9]. The panel recommended that commercial weight loss providers disclose information about four aspects of their interventions: (1) central program components, (2) staff qualifications, (3) costs, and (4) risks of treatment (Table 1). Several panel members also called for disclosure of outcome data, but some members from industry suggested that they did not

Table 1
Voluntary guidelines for disclosure by commercial weight loss programs

Criteria	Description
Program content	Major components of weight loss program (educational format, specifics of diet, physical activity programs, behavior counseling)
Staff qualifications	Program staff training, certification, and experience
Costs	One-time costs (entry or termination fees)
	Recurring costs (weekly fees or meals)
	Optional costs (long-term maintenance program)
	Refundable costs (based on weight loss)
Program risks	Specific program risks (risk of medications, supplements, or physical activity provided in the program)
	Risk of rapid weight loss (cholelithiasis)

Data from Womble L, Wang S, Wadden T. Commercial and self-help weight loss programs. In: Wadden T, Stunkard A, editors. Handbook of obesity treatment. New York: Guilford Press; 2002. p. 395–415.

have adequate resources or expertise to provide such data. This article describes program components and costs and evaluates published efficacy data. The authors searched for randomized trials, and, when these were not available, for prospective case series, and lastly, for retrospective case series reports (ie, studies that obtain long-term follow-up on a subset of participants and report end-of-treatment weight loss for only those patients). Descriptions are provided of several programs that have not been evaluated formally, simply because they treat such large numbers of individuals. The article includes only programs that require in-person or online visits. Thus, diet books and foods are not considered.

Nonmedical commercial programs

Nonmedical programs use nonphysician providers to facilitate clients' weight loss. Staff at such programs usually includes former clients and/or peer counselors trained by the company. Clinicians (dietitians, psychologists, exercise specialists, or nurses) occasionally assist, often as a backup to lay providers. Because these programs do not have physician supervision, people with obesity-related conditions need to be followed by their own primary care provider. Nonmedical programs aim for a weight loss of 1 to 2 lb/week (0.4 to 0.9 kg/wk), which is considered safe [1,2]. The largest nonmedical programs are Weight Watchers, Jenny Craig, and LA Weight Loss.

Weight Watchers

Program components

Weight Watchers provides dietary counseling and group support in 1-hour weekly meetings (Table 2). Dietary education is based on a system that assigns point values to foods. Clients consume a moderately restricted

Table 2
Central program components of selected commercial and self-help weight loss programs

Program	Staff qualifications	Diet	Physical activity	Behavior modification	Support
Weight Watchers	Successful lifetime member	LCD; exchange diet; clients prepare own meals	"Get Moving" booklet	Behavioral weight control methods	Group sessions, weekly meetings
Jenny Craig	Company-trained counselor	LCD; Jenny Craig meals required	Audiotapes for walking	Manual on weight loss strategies provided	Individual sessions, weekly contact
LA Weight Loss	Company-trained counselor	LCD; clients prepare own meals	Optional walking videotape	Included in counseling sessions	Individual sessions, three times weekly
HMR	Licensed physician and other healthcare providers	LCD/VLCD using meal replacement products; three-phase program	Walking and calorie charts provided in lifestyle classes	Included in lifestyle classes; accountability and skill acquisition emphasized	Group format; weekly classes; some telephone support
OPTIFAST	Licensed physician and other healthcare providers	LCD using meal replacement products; three phase program	Physical activity modules taught in lifestyle classes	Included in lifestyle classes; stress management and social support emphasized	Group sessions, weekly classes; some telephone support
Medifast/ TSFL	Not applicable	LCD/VLCD using meal replacement products; three-phase program	May be included in TSFL	May be included in TSFL	Included in TSFL
eDiets.com	Company-trained counselor and company dietitians	LCD using virtual dietitian program; clients prepare own meals	Physical activity seminar as part of eDiets.com "U" (University)	Included in eDiets.com U; stress management emphasized	Individual and group Internet support
TOPS	Group leader elected by local chapter	LCD exchange plan recommended	Members make plan with their healthcare provider	Included in TOPS curriculum	Group format; weekly sessions
OA	Volunteer chapter leaders	No specific recommendation	Members make plan with their healthcare provider	12-step program	Group format; weekly sessions; sponsors

Abbreviations: LCD, low-calorie diet; VLCD, very-low-calorie diet; TSFL, Take Shape for Life; TOPS, Take Off Pounds Sensibly; OA, Overeaters Anonymous.

Data from Tsai AG, Wadden TA. An evaluation of major commercial weight loss programs in the United States. Ann Intern Med, in press.

hypocaloric diet and may expect to lose up to 2 lb (0.9 kg) per week [11]. Group sessions provide social support, instruction in traditional behavioral weight control techniques [12], and educational materials that encourage clients to increase their physical activity. Clients are encouraged to select a final goal weight, within a BMI range of 20 to 25 kg/m^2, and may take as many weeks as needed to reach it [11]. Persons who reach their goal and maintain it for 6 weeks become "Lifetime Members," which entitles them to free meetings as long as they maintain their weight loss to within 2 pounds of goal (see Table 2).

Costs

Weight Watchers costs approximately $167 for 12 weeks. This includes a $35 membership fee and a $12 weekly fee, pay-as-you-go (Table 3).

Outcomes

Weight Watchers has sponsored three controlled evaluations of its program [13–15]. The strongest study was a multi-center trial in which 426 subjects were randomly assigned to weekly Weight Watchers visits or to a self-help intervention. Weight Watchers participants lost 5.3% of initial weight at year 1 and 3.2% at year 2, while self-help participants lost 1.5% and 0%, respectively (p < 0.001 at both times). Attrition was 27% and was similar in the two arms.

In a second study, 48 women with a history of breast cancer at a single site were randomized to: usual care, Weight Watchers (ie, weekly group counseling), individual counseling provided by a dietitian, or the two latter interventions combined. A 1-year follow-up showed that people in usual care gained 0.9 kg, and participants in the other groups lost 2.6, 8.0, and 9.4 kg, respectively. Total attrition in the study was 19%, but the authors did not specify whether it differed by group. Those in groups 3 and 4 lost significantly more weight than those in group 1 (p < 0.05 for both), and there were no other differences between groups [14]. Thus, in this small study, Weight Watchers did not have any incremental benefit compared with usual care or as an adjunct to individual counseling. In a third study, 80 women, also at a single site, were assigned randomly to Weight Watchers or to usual care. At 12 weeks, participants lost 7.5% and 1.6% of initial weight (p < 0.001), and attrition was 25% and 65%, respectively. No long-term data were reported [15].

There are two published case series reports of Weight Watchers [16,17]. They are not reviewed here, given the availability of randomized trials.

Jenny Craig

Program components

Individualized dietary counseling and prepackaged meals are the principal components of Jenny Craig (see Table 2) [18]. Counselors meet

Table 3
Estimated program costs for commercial and self-help weight loss programs[a,b]

Program	Costs			Other	Estimated cost for 12-week program[c]
	Membership fee/ initial cost	Periodic fees	Meal plan		
Weight Watchers	$35 for first week (membership fee)	$12/week, pay-as-you-go	Not required	None	$167
Jenny Craig	$199 for 1 year, $399 for 3 year	None	$70–$105/wk ($10–$15/d)	$10 for second of two weight loss manuals	$1249
LA Weight Loss	$79	Upfront costs of $7/wk × number of weeks calculated to reach goal weight	None	$10 for optional walking videotape	Not calculated[d]
HMR	$150–$300 for medical evaluation	$35/wk for medical visits and lab tests; $35/week for behavior modification	$68–86/wk for very-low-calorie-diet plan	Maintenance visits at extra cost	$1800–$2000
OPTIFAST	$150–$300 for medical evaluation	$35/wk for physician visits; $10/wk for behavior modification	$97/wk for "full fast" meal replacement	Laboratory tests, EKGs, and maintenance visits at extra cost	$1800–$2000
Medifast/TSFL	None	Not required	$70 or $56/wk (full or partial meal replacement)	Physician visits at extra cost	$840[e]

				Individual counseling with experts at extra cost
eDiets.com	None		None	$65
TOPS	$20/yr	$65/3 mo	$0.50 to $1.00/wk	None	$26–$32
OA	None		Donations	None	$0

Abbreviations: TSFL, Take Shape for Life; TOPS, Take Pounds Off Sensibly; OA, Overeaters Anonymous.

a Costs were estimated from discussions with company representatives and calls to programs in the Philadelphia area. Costs also may vary within the same program from site to site and with geographic region.

b Costs were provided by individual companies between Sept. 1 and Oct. 1, 2003, and should be considered approximate and subject to change (with special offers, incentives, and other considerations). For sake of comparison, the authors estimated the total cost of participating in each program for 3 months.

c The estimated cost includes charges for the first visit (eg, membership fee or initial evaluation) and 12 weeks' worth of subsequent visit. Other costs are not included in the estimated cost for the 3 months.

d Costs for LA Weight loss were not estimated because of insufficient information. Applicants are provided a weight loss goal at their initial evaluation and are requested (at this visit) to pay for the number of weeks (of consultation) required to reach their goal (at a cost of $7 a week). Persons who withdraw early are reimbursed for unused visits, minus a fee of $149.

e Costs are estimated for full meal replacement plan.

Data from Tsai AG, Wadden TA. An evaluation of major commercial weight loss programs in the United States. Ann Intern Med, in press.

weekly with clients, either on location or by phone, to help them plan their menus [18]. Additional telephone support is offered 24 hours a day, 7 days a week. All clients are required to purchase Jenny Craig prepackaged meals. The meals provide a standard hypocaloric diet of 5040 to 9660 kJ (1200 to 1500 kcal) per day, designed to induce a loss of approximately 1 to 2 lb (0.5 to 0.9 kg) per week [18]. Clients select a goal weight between a BMI of 20 to 25 kg/m^2. The standard plan (ie, gold membership) lasts 1 year. Clients who purchase the platinum membership (typically 3 years or more) also receive monthly maintenance counseling sessions after the first year [18].

Costs

Jenny Craig costs approximately $1249 for 12 weeks, which includes the $199 sign-up fee for the 1-year standard plan, and $10 to $15 per day for food (Table 3). The platinum plan would cost $1549, including the sign-up fee.

Outcomes

There has been one published report of the Jenny Craig program [19]. It was a retrospective case series of 517 clients who completed the program and reached or nearly reached their goal weight. A total of 256 clients participated in a 1-year follow-up evaluation (conducted by telephone). They lost 19% and 20% of initial weight during treatment and maintained losses of 16.3% and 15.4%, respectively, 1 year after treatment [19]. This study overestimated the efficacy of Jenny Craig, because it did not include any participants who failed to reach their goal weight.

LA Weight Loss

Program components

The major program component of LA Weight Loss is in-person counseling sessions, conducted three times weekly, that emphasize dietary education and behavior modification (see Table 2). The program is divided into three phases: (1) a variable-length weight loss phase in which clients aim to lose 2 lbs (0.9 kg) per week on a moderately restricted hypocaloric diet, (2) a stabilization program of approximately 6 weeks, and (3) a long-term maintenance phase [20]. The length of counseling sessions is variable, based on client need. Clients consume a calorie-restricted diet of conventional foods; no prepackaged meals are required [20]. Dieters select a goal weight, but it does not have to fall in the BMI range of 20 to 25 kg/m^2 (see Table 2).

Costs

Costs for LA Weight Loss are difficult to determine. Participants are asked to pay, in advance, $7 per week, times the number of weeks estimated to reach their goal weight (Table 3). There is also a sign-up fee of $79. Those who drop out early are reimbursed their costs, minus $149.

Outcomes

The authors' search revealed no published articles on the efficacy of LA Weight Loss.

Summary of nonmedical commercial programs

Weight Watchers is the only nonmedical program whose efficacy has been evaluated in randomized trials [13–15]. Participants who adhere to the program can expect to lose approximately 5% of initial weight, the goal recommended by several scientific panels [2,4,5]. Subjects in the Weight Watchers study by Heshka et al [13] regained weight from year 1 to year 2. This is typical for people treated with lifestyle modification [12,21]. People who attended the most group sessions during the 2 years of the study, however, maintained the largest weight losses, demonstrating the importance of adherence.

Controlled studies of Jenny Craig and LA Weight Loss are needed. Naturalistic studies on all three programs would be useful. Such a study would follow a large group of participants who entered a program and determine attrition at 1, 3, 6, and 12 months, and weight loss at the time of discontinuation. These data would provide a realistic estimate of weight loss in commercial programs. For example, one older study (not described in detail here, because average weight loss could not be calculated) found that 50% of participants stopped attending Weight Watchers meetings in the first 6 weeks, and 70% stopped attending within the first 12 weeks [22].

In terms of cost, Weight Watchers is moderately priced at $12/week, although still beyond the reach of many persons who need to lose weight (ie, minority groups and individuals of low socioeconomic status). The cost of prepackaged meals renders Jenny Craig an expensive program. As described previously, the costs of LA Weight Loss are difficult to determine, as they depend on the weight loss goal.

Finally, Weight Watchers may be preferable for persons who prefer group support, while Jenny Craig or LA Weight Loss may be better suited for those who desire individual counseling. The quality and ultimate benefit of the individual counseling provided by these latter two programs, however, cannot be evaluated in the absence of data.

Medically supervised proprietary programs

Medically supervised programs include physician care and, thus, are appropriate for people with obesity-related conditions. Such programs traditionally have used very-low-calorie diets (VLCDs), which provide fewer than 3360 kJ/d^2 (800 kcal per day) and include large amounts of protein (70 to 100 g per day) to preserve lean body mass [23]. VLCDs typically induce losses of at least 3 lb per week (1.4 kg/wk) for the first few months. Adverse effects include gallstones, cold intolerance, hair loss, and constipation [23].

These symptoms are typically mild and easily managed. These diets are considered safe for selected patients under medical supervision [23]. The largest medically supervised proprietary programs are Health Management Resources, OPTIFAST, and Medifast.

The authors' search, which included lists of studies provided by all three companies, revealed several published evaluations of these programs and/or of their meal replacement plans. Only studies in which both the diet and lifestyle counseling program were provided by the company (as contrasted to studies in which a company's meal replacement products were combined with an investigator's own behavioral protocol) are reviewed here.

Health Management Resources (HMR)

Program components

HMR offers three treatment options for weight loss, all of which include meal replacements. The first is a VLCD that provides a range of medical supervision, depending upon patients' initial weight and health complications (see Table 2). Patients typically consume 2100 to 3150 kJ (500 to 750 kcal) per day during the period of rapid weight loss. The second plan, which is designed to induce more moderate weight loss, combines the use of meal replacements with conventional foods. This "Healthy Solutions" program provides approximately 5040 kJ (1200 kcal) per day. The third and newest option is a telephone-based program, also designed to induce more moderate weight loss. Losses of 3 to 6 lbs (1.4 to 2.7 kg) a week are expected with the VLCD program and 1 to 2 lbs (0.5 to 0.9 kg) a week with the more moderate plans. Most HMR clients participate in the VLCD program.

Participants in both the VLCD and the moderately-restricted plan attend 90-minute weekly lifestyle modification classes that emphasize accountability (eg, by record keeping and attending classes). Physical activity is encouraged, especially walking, and information is provided on the number of calories expended by different amounts and types of activity. The lifestyle modification curriculum lasts 18 to 20 weeks. Patients who do not reach their goal weight may attend extra classes (and continue the meal replacements) until they do so. The VLCD program is divided into three phases: (1) rapid weight loss (approximately 13 weeks); (2) transition (approximately 6 to 8 weeks); and (3) maintenance (variable duration). Participants in the VLCD program reportedly attend treatment for an average of 18 to 20 weeks, while those in the moderate weight loss plan participate for 13 weeks [24]. HMR encourages monthly weight maintenance visits after participants reach goal weight. The telephone-based program offers a less intensive lifestyle modification program, delivered over 6 weeks.

Costs

Health Management Resources is estimated to cost $1800 to $2000 for 12 weeks' treatment. This includes fees for the initial history and physical examination, cost of meal replacements, and fees for physician visits, laboratory tests, and classes. Follow-up costs are not included in this estimate (see Table 3).

Outcomes

There have been numerous reports of the safety and efficacy of the HMR VLCD program, [25–34], but no reports of HMR's moderate weight loss plans. Five studies evaluated the HMR program as it was provided to the public [25,27,28,34,35]. The first study was a randomized trial of 40 obese patients with type 2 diabetes. Participants received one of two 3360 kJ (800 kcal) diets. The first provided only HMR liquid meal replacements, and the second offered meal replacements with one meal per day of conventional foods. Both groups received the standard HMR protocol of intensive lifestyle modification. Weight losses in the two groups were 15.3% and 14.1% after 12 weeks, and attrition at this time was 0% and 2.5%, respectively. Thirty-six people (92% of the original sample) participated in a 1-year follow-up, at which time they maintained a loss of 8.4%. Results by group were not given separately [35].

The other four evaluations of HMR were all single-site case series. In the longest study of HMR, a retrospective case series evaluating 154 of 426 consecutive enrollees, who completed a 12-week core program and lost at least 10 kg during treatment, were asked to participate in a follow-up study [28]. Of these 154, 112 provided follow-up weights at least 2 years after the end of treatment (with 70% of weights assessed on-site and 30% by self-report). These 112 patients lost 29.7 kg (27.5%) in 5 months of treatment. Seventy-six of these individuals completed a 3-year evaluation, at which time they maintained a 7.4 kg (6.9%) loss. At a 5-year follow-up, 15 participants had a mean loss of 5.9 kg (5.5%), and at 7 years, 32 patients had a loss of 5.3 kg (4.9%) [28]. A second study evaluated 100 consecutive enrollees (71 women, 29 men), of whom 69 completed 17 or more weeks of treatment [27]. Women lost 19.2 kg (20.0%), and men lost 18.6 kg (16%). Three-year weight losses (assessed by telephone) were 7.3 kg (7.6%) and 7.2 kg (6.2%), respectively, among the 58 participants with follow-up data. A third study assessed 80 consecutive enrollees; 69 completed the program and lost a mean of 35.1 kg (27.3%) [25]. These individuals were provided an intensive weight loss maintenance program. Forty-six patients participated in a 2-year follow-up (either on-site or by telephone), at which time they maintained a loss of 16.8 kg (13.1%). A fourth study assessed 138 consecutive enrollees, of whom 102 participated in a 2- to 3-year telephone follow-up. The percentage of enrollees completing treatment was not given. These 73 women and 29 men lost a mean of 24.7 kg (24.8%) and 33.5 kg (28.9%), respectively, during 22 weeks of treatment. At follow-up, women maintained a loss of 9.7 kg (9.7%), and men maintained a loss of 15 kg (12.9%) [34].

OPTIFAST

Program components

The primary components of the OPTIFAST program consist of meal replacements, physician monitoring, and group lifestyle modification (see Table 2). The meal replacements include shakes, snack bars, and soups. Patients today typically consume a low-calorie liquid diet of 3360 to 4032 kJ (800 to 960 kcal) per day during the period of rapid weight loss. Most published OPTIFAST studies, however, used a VLCD of 1764 kJ (420 kcal) per day. The physician performs an initial history, physical exam, electrocardiogram, and laboratory tests, and monitors obesity-related health complications (see Table 2) [36].

The treatment program includes three phases; the overall structure is similar to that of HMR. During a 12- to 16-week full meal replacement phase, patients consume only OPTIFAST. Then, in a 4- to 6-week transition phase, conventional table foods gradually are reintroduced [36]. During the first two phases, patients attend weekly lifestyle modification classes (of approximately 60 minutes) conducted by behaviorists, dietitians, or exercise specialists. These individuals are retained by the physician. During the third phase, patients are encouraged to attend monthly visits (indefinitely) to prevent weight regain [36].

Costs

OPTIFAST is estimated to cost $1800 to $2000 for 12 weeks of treatment. This includes fees for an initial history and physical examination, costs of meal replacements, and costs for the lifestyle modification classes and follow-up physician visits. It does not include laboratory tests, EKGs, or follow-up visits after the first two phases of treatment (see Table 3).

Outcomes

There have been numerous studies of the OPTIFAST Program [37–47], five of which evaluated the program as it is offered to the public [37–41]. The strongest study was a prospective multi-center case series of 517 consecutive enrollees. Two hundred eighty five participants (55%) finished the 26-week program [37]. Women who completed treatment lost 22.1 kg (21%), and men lost 32.2 kg (25%). Women and men who dropped out lost 14.3 kg and 20.0 kg, respectively. In a 1-year (on-site) follow-up, 118 treatment completers participated out of 160 who were invited. These 118 individuals maintained 15.3 kg of an original 24.8 kg loss [37]. A second multi-center evaluation surveyed 929 participants who completed at least 3 weeks of treatment [38]. The study reported a loss of 16.7 kg (19%) in women and 26.9 kg (20.0%) in men, achieved over 16 weeks. The percentage of patients who completed the program was not given. A 1-year (telephone) follow-up of 704 women and men (76% of persons completing 3 weeks treatment) who participated in a maintenance program, revealed losses of 12.6 kg (14.3%) and 19.9 kg (14.8%) of initial weight, respectively.

Three studies of OPTIFAST included follow-up evaluations of at least 2 years, with weights assessed by telephone or mail [39–41]. One study evaluated 306 consecutive enrollees at a single OPTIFAST program and obtained 2-year follow-up data on a subset of 255 of these individuals [39]. These 255 individuals lost 21.4 kg (19.6%) during 24 weeks of treatment; 112 (44%) of the 255 completed treatment. At 2 years, these 255 patients reported a mean loss of 6.5 kg (5.6%) [39]. A second study, this one multi-center, provided follow-up data on 621 of 1283 patients who completed a 26-week program [40]. Among the 621 participants, end-of-treatment losses for women were 23.7 kg (22.6%), and for men, they were 34.3 kg (25.5%). At 2-year follow up, mean losses had declined to 9.6 kg (9.1%) and 17.6 kg (13.1%), respectively. A total of 337 participants participated in a 5-year assessment, at which time women reported a loss of 5.5 kg (5.1%), and men reported a loss of 10.3 kg (7.3%), respectively. A third study, also multi-center, sent a mail questionnaire to 325 individuals who completed an 18-week or 26-week OPTIFAST program [41]. A total of 192 persons responded to the questionnaire. These individuals lost 22 kg (21%) during treatment and maintained a 3 kg loss (2.9%) at 3-year follow-up [41].

Medifast

Program components

The main component of Medifast is a meal plan that provides 1890 or more kJ (450 kcal) per day (see Table 2) [48]. Unlike OPTIFAST and HMR, Medifast is sold directly to the public, and to participating providers. Dieters are instructed to use the meal replacements as a sole source of nutrition (ie, the complete plan) or as a supplement to one meal a day (of lean meat and low-carbohydrate vegetables) (ie, the modified plan) [48]. Participants are told to expect a loss of 3 to 7 lb (1.4 to 3.2 kg) a week with the complete plan and 2 to 4 lb (0.9 to 1.8 kg) a week with the modified plan [48]. Medifast states that its VLCD plans require medical monitoring to reduce the risk of health complications [48]. The company retains a network of physician referrals to provide medical monitoring but does not require documentation of physician care for dieters to order the product. Thus, Medifast is not provided consistently to consumers in accordance with guidance suggested by several expert panels, including the National Task Force on the Prevention and Treatment of Obesity [23]. Serious complications, including death, have been reported in obese individuals who consumed VLCDs in the absence of medical supervision [49]. Additionally, provision of a concurrent lifestyle modification program (as is mandatory with OPTIFAST and HMR) is at the discretion of the physician providing the medical monitoring. Participants in Take Shape For Life, a subsidiary of Medifast, also receive support from a health advisor trained by the company [50]. All Medifast clients can obtain free telephone consultation from company representatives and, when necessary, with the

company's registered nurses. Medifast recommends that the meal replacement program last approximately 16 weeks, with a period of 3 to 6
weeks for resuming consumption of conventional foods (see Table 2).

Costs

The cost of 12 weeks of treatment with Medifast is approximately $840.
This includes only the cost of meal replacements (see Table 3).

Outcomes

The authors were unable to identify any evaluations of the Medifast
program. The company's Web site reports abstracts of two studies, but
neither of these has been published.

Summary of medically monitored programs

Results of HMR- and OPTIFAST-sponsored studies suggest that
persons who complete a comprehensive low-calorie or very-low-calorie
diet program will lose approximately 15% to 25% of initial weight during 4
to 6 months of treatment. They can expect to maintain an approximate loss
of 8% to 9% at 1 year after treatment, 7% at 3 years, and 5% at 4 years
[26,27,35,37,39]. The values cited represent a best-case estimate, however.
They do not include individuals who dropped out of treatment or declined
a follow-up assessment. Weight losses in these studies were not adjusted for
drop-outs, as has been recommended [47]. Finally, the use of self-reported
weights in several studies is likely to have overestimated program efficacy.

A complete evaluation of HMR and OPTIFAST would require
a randomized trial that assigned participants to a (very) low-calorie meal
replacement program or to a comparison condition, such as a balanced 5040
to 6300 kJ (1200 to 1500 kcal) per day diet of conventional foods. Because of
the large initial weight losses and substantial reductions maintained (by
some patients) several years after treatment, some investigators have argued
in favor of VLCDs [51,52]. Multiple randomized trials from academic
centers that compared VLCDs and conventional diets (of 5040 to 6300 kJ
(1200 to 1500 kcal) per day), however, found equivalent weight losses for the
two approaches 1 or more years after treatment [53–61]. This was
a consequence of greater weight regain in people who received the VLCD.
Thus, the National Heart Lung and Blood Institute expert panel did not
recommend the use of VLCDs over less expensive conventional reducing
diets.

In general, VLCD plans would be a more attractive option if the large
weight losses could be maintained better. Results of the study by Anderson
et al suggest that patients who complete (very) low-calorie plans should
participate in a long-term maintenance program [26]. The results of randomized trials, however, show a more modest effect of weight maintenance programs [62–64]. During maintenance, patients also may wish

to replace one meal and one snack per day with a shake or bar. This practice appeared to facilitate an 8% reduction in initial weight for up to 4 years in a trial conducted in Germany [65,66]. Sibutramine also has been shown to facilitate the maintenance of weight loss achieved with a VLCD [67].

Health Management Resources and OPTIFAST are both expensive (ie, $1800 to $2000 for 3 months of treatment). This high cost limits access among patient populations with high rates of obesity, especially minorities, in whom the prevalence of obesity is as great as 50% [2]. Economic analyses of HMR and OPTIFAST would be useful. Medifast is significantly less expensive (approximately $720 for 3 months) than HMR or OPTIFAST, but only because the company fails to require medical supervision or behavior modification. The authors reiterate that mandatory medical supervision is critical to the safe use of VLCDs.

Internet-based commercial weight loss programs

Internet-based programs are the latest entry into the commercial weight loss field. This article discusses eDiets.com, the only Internet commercial program that has been evaluated by a randomized clinical trial. There are many Internet-based programs, including Nutrisystem.com, WebMD, Dietwatch.com, Caloriescount.com, Weight Watchers online, a-personaldietitian.com, mddiets.com, and others. Clinicians who want more information about Internet programs may consult Shape Up America, a nonprofit weight management organization that provides a list of online programs (www.shapeup.org).

eDiets.com

Program components

eDiets.com prescribes an individualized hypocaloric diet, designed to induce a loss of up to 2 lb (0.9 kg) per week, in conjunction with online counseling (see Table 2) [68]. Participants choose from 13 different diets, based on their nutritional preferences. The company provides clients with shopping lists for the diet selected. Participants purchase and prepare all of their own meals. eDiets.com promotes itself as a virtual dietitian program because of the variety of diet options and detailed individual advice given to clients. The company provides additional services with the membership package, including weekly online chats and personalized e-mail counseling from experts.

Costs

eDiets.com charges $65 for 13 weeks' participation in the program (see Table 3).

Outcomes

eDiets.com has not sponsored any evaluations of its program. Womble et al, however, compared (in a randomized trial) the efficacy of eDiets.com (as available on the Internet from February 2001 to September 2002) with treatment using a behavioral weight loss manual (ie, LEARN Program for Weight Management 2000) [70]. During the 1-year study, the 23 participants in each group had five 20-minute visits with a psychologist to review their progress. Participants also attended 11 brief assessment visits at which weight was measured. Participants in eDiets.com lost 0.7 kg (0.9%) and 0.8 kg (1.1%) at weeks 16 and 52, respectively. Corresponding losses for patients in the weight-loss manual group were 3.0 kg (3.6%) and 3.3 kg (4.0%). Using a last-observation-carried-forward analysis, differences in weight loss were statistically significant ($p < 0.05$) at both time points. Attrition was 34% at both week 16 and week 52 and did not differ significantly between groups.

Summary of internet-based programs

Currently, there is minimal evidence to recommend the use of commercial Internet interventions. Results of the study by Womble et al [69] are likely to be a best-case scenario concerning the efficacy of eDiets.com (as provided in 2001 to 2002). This is because participants were provided frequent on-site assessment visits and multiple meetings with a psychologist, neither of which is offered to eDiets.com subscribers. Larger controlled evaluations are needed to assess the efficacy of eDiets.com and other Internet-based commercial weight loss programs.

The results of two randomized trials from noncommercial Internet programs suggest that participants should keep daily records of their food intake and physical activity, as they do when attending a behavioral weight loss clinic [12,70]. Participants who recorded their food intake and physical activity and who received regular e-mail feedback on their performance lost over twice as much weight (ie, approximately 4.5 kg versus 2 kg) as participants who received information alone (on proper eating and activity habits) [71]. It is not known whether these results can be reproduced in commercial programs.

Organized self-help programs

Organized self-help programs differ from commercial programs in two principal ways. They are nonprofit and, thus, charge no or nominal fees, and they are led by locally selected volunteers. Self-help programs are conducted by laypersons, all of whom have struggled with a weight or eating problem. Self-help is based on the theory that people who have experienced the same condition (ie, obesity or overeating) may be more empathic and supportive.

Take Off Pounds Sensibly (TOPS)

Program components

Group meetings provide social support, weigh-ins, and the TOPS curriculum on diet, physical activity, and behavior change (see Table 2) [72]. A 5040, 6300, or 7560 kJ (1200, 1500, or 1800 kcal) per day diet of conventional foods typically is recommended [72]. It is based on an exchange plan, similar to the American Diabetes Association diet and to the Weight Watchers points system. Members who need additional guidance are encouraged to consult with their personal health care provider. Participants are not required to select a weight loss goal.

Costs

TOPS charges $20/year, and local chapters charge 50 cents or $1 per week to support their costs. Thus, 12 weeks of treatment would cost $26 to $32, including the annual fee (see Table 3).

Outcomes

According to the TOPS' Website, members lost 1,325,977 pounds, or 5.8 lbs (2.6 kg) per member in 2002 [72]. These numbers were derived from weigh-ins at weekly meetings. There are no recent reports on the efficacy of the TOPS program. Nearly 30 years ago, however, Levitz and Stunkard [73] evaluated 16 chapters of TOPS that were assigned to one of four conditions: (1) behavior modification conducted by a professional therapist; (2) behavior modification provided by a TOPS leader; (3) nutrition education conducted by a TOPS leader; or (4) the TOPS program, as provided in 1974. At 1 year, attrition rates were 38%, 41%, 55%, and 67%, respectively. Only individuals in the first group maintained a significant weight loss at 1-year follow-up (ie, 3.2% of initial weight) [73]. The results of this study reportedly contributed to TOPS' decision to incorporate behavior modification in its program [10].

Overeaters Anonymous

Program components

The OA philosophy holds that obesity is the result of compulsive eating, which, in turn, is thought to be the consequence of anger, sadness, loneliness, and other untoward emotions [74]. Participants frequently report that they are addicted to food. Overeaters Anonymous (OA) seeks to guide participants to physical, emotional, and spiritual recovery [74]. The program's philosophy and 12-step approach are similar to those of the older Alcoholics Anonymous. Supportive group meetings and a one-to-one sponsor relationship with an established member are the central features of OA (see Table 2). New members are encouraged to call their sponsor daily to discuss weight loss efforts [75]. Participants are also encouraged to stop using food as a solution to their difficulties and to work on the problems themselves, which may involve a lack of self-acceptance or intimacy with others [74]. OA does not prescribe specific diet or exercise plans. Instead, participants develop their own plan. They are encouraged to attend group meetings long-term to facilitate their continuing recovery.

Costs

Overeaters Anonymous relies entirely on member donations to support its program. There are no mandatory fees (see Table 3).

Outcomes

The authors' search revealed no studies of the efficacy of OA for weight loss.

Summary of organized self-help programs

There is little scientific evidence to recommend the use of organized self-help programs. Rigorous efficacy studies are unlikely to occur, given these programs' limited financial resources. It seems reasonable to encourage the use of programs such as TOPS or OA, however, given that they pose minimal financial or physical risks. Based on one author's (TAW) experience reviewing patients' dieting histories, the authors believe that a significant minority of patients will lose at least 5% of initial weight by attending TOPS or OA. TOPS appears to be similar to Weight Watchers, in that the program prescribes a hypocaloric diet and incorporates group support with weekly weigh-ins. Conversely, OA seems to be most appropriate for patients who seek intensive emotional support to facilitate weight loss. Because each OA chapter apparently has its own character, patients should sample several groups to find the best fit. Clinicians can help patients by familiarizing themselves with TOPS or OA chapters in their communities.

Summary

Weight Watchers is the only commercial weight loss program whose efficacy has been demonstrated in a randomized trial. Patients who regularly attend the program will lose approximately 5% of initial weight, which in conjunction with increased physical activity, may be sufficient to prevent or improve obesity-related health complications. Weight Watchers is moderately priced, but it is probably too costly for many patients in need of treatment. Thus, TOPS and OA are important options for weight control, despite their lack of supporting evidence. There is not sufficient evidence to support any commercial Internet programs.

Multiple studies of HMR and OPTIFAST, one of which was a randomized trial, suggest that these programs induce losses of approximately 15% to 25%

of initial weight in patients who complete treatment. As mentioned, medically supervised programs are expensive and were not recommended by the National Heart, Lung, and Blood Institute expert panel when compared with regimens that induce more modest initial weight loss [2]. A medically supervised program may be appropriate in selected patients with a BMI of at least 30 kg/m^2 who have not responded to less aggressive treatments for weight loss. More effective methods are needed to maintain the large weight losses achieved with medically supervised programs.

Supporting patients weight loss efforts

Psychiatrists and other healthcare providers may refer to the practical guide developed by the National Heart, Lung, and Blood Institute/North American Society for the Study of Obesity panel to help determine which patients have the greatest need for weight loss [1]. They can assist patients who are participating in commercial or self-help programs by regularly reviewing changes in weight, in obesity-related conditions, and in eating and activity habits [28]. The provider should praise patients' success, including not only for weight loss but for the prevention of weight gain and for positive lifestyle changes that may facilitate weight loss or maintenance. With these steps, psychiatrists and other mental health professionals can contribute to efforts to control obesity.

References

[1] National Heart Lung and Blood Institute (NHLBI) and North American Society for the Study of Obesity (NAASO). Practical guide to the identification, evaluation, and treatment of overweight and obesity in adults. Bethesda (MD): National Institute of Health; 2000.

[2] National Heart Lung and Blood Institute (NHLBI). Clinical guidelines on the identification, evaluation, and treatment of overweight and obesity in adults–the evidence report. National Institutes of Health. Obes Res 1998;51S–209S.

[3] Knowler WC, Barrett-Connor E, Fowler SE, et al. Reduction in the incidence of type 2 diabetes with lifestyle intervention or metformin. N Engl J Med 2002;346:393–403.

[4] World Health Organization. Obesity: preventing and managing the global epidemic. Geneva (Switzerland): World Health Organization; 1998.

[5] Institute of Medicine. Weighing the options: Criteria for evaluating weight management programs. Washington (DC): Government Printing Office; 1995.

[6] Tuomilehto J, Lindstrom J, Eriksson JG, et al. Prevention of type 2 diabetes mellitus by changes in lifestyle among subjects with impaired glucose tolerance. N Engl J Med 2001;344: 1343–50.

[7] Frank A. Futility and avoidance. Medical professionals in the treatment of obesity. JAMA 1993;269:2132–3.

[8] Tsai AG, Wadden TA. An evaluation of major commercial weight loss programs in the United States. Ann Intern Med, in press.

[9] Cleland R, Graybill D, Hubbard V, et al. Commercial weight loss products and programs: what consumers stand to gain and lose. A public conference on the information consumers need to evaluate weight loss products and programs. Crit Rev Food Sci Nutr 2001;41:45–70.

[10] Womble L, Wang S, Wadden T. Commercial and self-help weight loss programs. In: Wadden T, Stunkard A, editors. Handbook of obesity treatment. New York: Guilford Press; 2002. p. 395–415.

[11] Weight Watchers. About us, plan and products, flex points, FAQs. Available at: www.weightwatchers.com. Accessed October 2003.

[12] Tate DF, Jackvony EH, Wing RR. Effects of Internet behavioral counseling on weight loss in adults at risk for type 2 diabetes: a randomized trial. JAMA 2003;289:1833–6.

[13] Heshka S, Anderson JW, Atkinson RL, et al. Weight loss with self-help compared with a structured commercial program: a randomized trial. JAMA 2003;289:1792–8.

[14] Djuric Z, DiLaura NM, Jenkins I, et al. Combining weight-loss counseling with the Weight Watchers plan for obese breast cancer survivors. Obes Res 2002;10:657–65.

[15] Rippe JM, Price JM, Hess SA, et al. Improved psychological well-being, quality of life, and health practices in moderately overweight women participating in a 12-week structured weight loss program. Obes Res 1998;6:208–18.

[16] Christakis G, Miller-Kovach K. Maintenance of weight goal among Weight Watchers lifetime members. Nutr Today 1996;31:29–31.

[17] Lowe M, Miller-Kovach K, Phelan S. Weight-loss maintenance in overweight individuals one to five years following successful completion of a commercial weight loss program. Int J Obes 2001;25:325–31.

[18] Jenny Craig. Jenny Craig weight loss programs. www.jennycraig.com/programs; accessed October 2003.

[19] Wolfe BL. Long-term maintenance following attainment of goal weight: a preliminary investigation. Addict Behav 1992;17:469–77.

[20] LA Weight Loss. A record of success. www.laweightloss.com; accessed October 2003.

[21] Wadden TA, Berkowitz RI, Sarwer DB, et al. Benefits of lifestyle modification in the pharmacologic treatment of obesity: a randomized trial. Arch Intern Med 2001;161:218–27.

[22] Volkmar FR, Stunkard AJ, Woolston J, et al. High attrition rates in commercial weight reduction programs. Arch Intern Med 1981;141:426–8.

[23] National Task Force on the Prevention and Treatment of Obesity. Very low-calorie diets. JAMA 1993;270:967–74.

[24] Health Management Resources. About us. Available at: www.yourbetterhealth.com. Accessed October 2003.

[25] Anderson JW, Brinkman VL, Hamilton CC. Weight loss and 2-year follow-up for 80 morbidly obese patients treated with intensive very-low-calorie diet and an education program. Am J Clin Nutr 1992;56:244S–6S.

[26] Anderson J, Brinkman-Kaplan V, Lee H, et al. Relationship of weight loss to cardiovascular risk factors in morbidly obese individuals. J Am Coll Nutr 1994;13:256–61.

[27] Anderson J, Hamilton C, Crown-Weber E, et al. Safety and effectiveness of a multidisciplinary very-low-calorie-diet program for selected obese individuals. J Am Diet Assoc 1991; 91:1582–4.

[28] Anderson J, Vichitbandra S, Qian W, et al. Long-term weight maintenance after an intensive weight-loss program. J Am Coll Nutr 1999;18:620–7.

[29] Bryner R, Ullrich I, Sauers J, et al. Effects of resistance vs. aerobic training combined with an 800 calorie liquid diet on lean body mass and resting metabolic rate. J Am Coll Nutr 1999;18: 115–21.

[30] Collins R, Anderson J. Medication cost savings associated with weight loss for obese noninsulin-dependent diabetic men and women. Prev Med 1995;24:369–75.

[31] Donnelly J, Jacobsen D, Jakicic J, et al. Very low calorie diet with concurrent versus delayed and sequential exercise. Int J Obes 1994;18:469–75.

[32] Donnelly J, Jacobsen D, Whatley J. Influence of degree of obesity on loss of fat-free mass during very-low-energy diets. Am J Clin Nutr 1994;60:874–8.

[33] Daly A. Successful long-term maintenance of substantial weight loss: one program's experience. J Am Diet Assoc 2000;100:1456.

[34] Hartman W, Stroud M, Sweet D, et al. Long-term maintenance of weight loss following supplemented fasting. Int J Eat Disord 1993;14:87–93.

[35] Anderson JW, Brinkman-Kaplan V, Hamilton CC, et al. Food-containing hypocaloric diets are as effective as liquid-supplement diets for obese individuals with NIDDM. Diabetes Care 1994;17:602–4.

[36] OPTIFAST. Why choose OPTIFAST. Available at: www.optifast.com. Accessed October 2003.

[37] Wadden TA, Foster GD, Letizia KA, et al. A multi-center evaluation of a proprietary weight reduction program for the treatment of marked obesity. Arch Intern Med 1992; 152:961–6.

[38] Kanders B, Blackburn G, Lavin P, et al. Weight loss outcome and health benefits associated with the OPTIFAST program in the treatment of obesity. Int J Obes 1989;13:131S–4S.

[39] Flynn T, Walsh M. Thirty-month evaluation of a popular very-low-calorie-diet program. Arch Fam Med 1993;2:1042–8.

[40] Wadden TA, Frey DL. A multi-center evaluation of a proprietary weight loss program for the treatment of marked obesity: a five-year follow-up. Int J Eat Disord 1997;22: 203–12.

[41] Grodstein F, Levine R, Troy L, et al. Three-year follow-up of participants in a commercial weight loss program: can you keep it off? Arch Intern Med 1996;156:1302–6.

[42] Barrows K, Snook J. Effect of a high-protein, very low-calorie diet on resting metabolism, thyroid hormones, and energy expenditure of obese middle-aged women. Am J Clin Nutr 1987;45:391–8.

[43] Doherty J, Wadden T, Zuk L, et al. Long-term evaluation of cardiac function in obese patients treated with a very low-calorie diet: a controlled clinical study of patients without underlying cardiac disease. Am J Clin Nutr 1991;53:854–8.

[44] Genuth SM, Castro JH, Vertes V. Weight reduction in obesity by outpatient semistarvation. JAMA 1974;230:987–91.

[45] Kirschner M, Schneider G, Ertel N, et al. An eight-year experience with a very-low-calorie formula diet for control of major obesity. Int J Obes 1988;12:69–80.

[46] Vertes V, Genuth SM, Hazelton IM. Supplemented fasting as a large-scale outpatient program. JAMA 1977;238:2151–3.

[47] Beliard D, Kirschenbaum DS, Fitzgibbon ML. Evaluation of an intensive weight control program using a priori criteria to determine outcome. Int J Obes Relat Metab Disord 1992; 16:505–17.

[48] Medifast. About us. Available at: www.medifast.net. Accessed October 2003.

[49] Wadden TA, Stunkard AJ, Brownell KD, et al. The Cambridge diet. More mayhem? JAMA 1983;250:2833–4.

[50] Take Shape for Life. Our company. Available at: www.makemethinner.com. Accessed October 2003.

[51] Anderson JW, Konz EC, Frederich RC, et al. Long-term weight-loss maintenance: a meta-analysis of US studies. Am J Clin Nutr 2001;74:579–84.

[52] Astrup A, Rossner S. Lessons from obesity management programmes: greater initial weight loss improves long-term maintenance. Obes Rev 2000;1:17–9.

[53] Ryttig KR, Flaten H, Rossner S. Long-term effects of a very low calorie diet (Nutrilett) in obesity treatment. A prospective, randomized, comparison between VLCD and a hypo-caloric diet plus behavior modification and their combination. Int J Obes Relat Metab Disord 1997;21:574–9.

[54] Torgerson JS, Lissner L, Lindroos AK, et al. VLCD plus dietary and behavioural support versus support alone in the treatment of severe obesity. A randomised two-year clinical trial. Int J Obes Relat Metab Disord 1997;21:987–94.

[55] Wadden TA, Foster GD, Letizia KA. One-year behavioral treatment of obesity: comparison of moderate and severe caloric restriction and the effects of weight maintenance therapy. J Consult Clin Psychol 1994;62:165–71.

[56] Wadden TA, Sternberg JA, Letizia KA, et al. Treatment of obesity by very low calorie diet, behavior therapy, and their combination: a five-year perspective. Int J Obes 1989;13: 39S–46S.

[57] Wing RR, Blair E, Marcus M, et al. Year-long weight loss treatment for obese patients with type II diabetes: does including an intermittent very-low-calorie diet improve outcome? Am J Med 1994;97:354–62.

[58] Wing RR, Marcus MD, Salata R, et al. Effects of a very-low-calorie diet on long-term glycemic control in obese type 2 diabetic subjects. Arch Intern Med 1991;151:1334–40.

[59] Miura J, Arcu K, Tsukahara S, et al. The long-term effectiveness of combined therapy by behaviour modification and very-low-calorie diet: two year follow-up. Int J Obes 1989;13: 73S–7S.

[60] Pekkarinen T, Mustajoki P. Comparison of behaviour therapy with and without very-low-energy diet in the treatment of obesity. A 5-year outcome. Arch Intern Med 1997;157:1581–5.

[61] Saris WHM. Very-low-calorie diets and sustained weight loss. Obes Res 2001;9:295S–301S.

[62] Agras WS, Berkowitz RI, Arnow BA, et al. Maintenance following a very-low-calorie diet. J Consult Clin Psychol 1996;64:610–3.

[63] Wadden TA, Stunkard AJ. Controlled trial of very low calorie diet, behavior therapy, and their combination. J Consult Clin Psychol 1986;54:482–8.

[64] Wadden TA, Bartlett SJ, Foster GD, et al. Sertraline and relapse prevention training following treatment by very-low-calorie diet: a controlled clinical trial. Obes Res 1995;3: 549–57.

[65] Ditschuneit H, Flechtner-Mors M, Johnson T, et al. Metabolic and weight loss effects of long-term dietary intervention in obese subjects. Am J Clin Nutr 1999;69:198–204.

[66] Flechtner-Mors M, Ditschuneit HH, Johnson TD, et al. Metabolic and weight loss effects of long-term dietary intervention in obese patients: four-year results. Obes Res 2000;8:399–402.

[67] Apfelbaum M, Vague P, Ziegler O, et al. Long-term maintenance of weight loss after a very-low-calorie diet: a randomized blinded trial of the efficacy and tolerability of sibutramine. Am J Med 1999;106:179–84.

[68] eDiets.com. Company/what we do. Available at: www.ediets.com/company. Accessed October 2003.

[69] Womble LG, Wadden TA, McGuckin BG, et al. A randomized controlled trial of a commercial internet weight loss program. Obes Res 2004;12:1011–8.

[70] Brownell KD. The LEARN program for weight management 2000. Dallas (TX): American Health Publishing Company; 2000.

[71] Tate DF, Wing RR, Winett RA. Using Internet technology to deliver a behavioral weight loss program. JAMA 2001;285:1172–7.

[72] Take Off Pounds Sensibly. About TOPS/information. Available at: www.tops.org. Accessed October 2003.

[73] Levitz L, Stunkard A. A therapeutic solution for obesity: behavior modification and patient self-help. Am J Psychiatry 1974;131:423–7.

[74] Anonymous. Take it off and keep it off: based on the successful methods of Overeaters Anonymous. Chicago: Contemporary Books; 1989.

[75] Overeaters Anonymous. About OA. Available at: www.oa.org. Accessed October 2003.

ELSEVIER
SAUNDERS

PSYCHIATRIC
CLINICS
OF NORTH AMERICA

Psychiatr Clin N Am 28 (2005) 193–217

Drug Treatment of Obesity

George A. Bray, MD

Pennington Biomedical Research Center, Louisiana State University,
6400 Perkins Road, Baton Rouge, LA 70808, USA

A report from the Heart, Lung and Blood Institute of the National Institutes of Health (NIH) entitled Clinical Guidelines on the Identification, Evaluation, and Treatment of Overweight and Obesity in Adults—The Evidence Report [1] emphasizes the need for physicians to address obesity in their patients. This report sanctions the clinical use of weight loss drugs approved by the Food and Drug Administration (FDA) for long-term use as part of a concomitant lifestyle modification program. Appropriate patients include those who have been unsuccessful in previous weight loss attempts and whose body mass index (BMI) exceeds 27 kg/m²; those who have associated conditions such as diabetes, hypertension or dyslipidemia; or people whose BMI exceeds 30 kg/m². Still, for many physicians, treatment of obesity is not a routine part of their clinical practices, in part because of the stigma associated with medication usage.

Drug treatment for obesity has been tarnished by several problems [2]. Since the introduction of thyroid hormone to treat obesity in 1893, almost every drug that has been tried in obese patients has led to undesirable outcomes that have resulted in their termination. Thus, caution must be used in accepting any new drugs for treatment of obesity, unless the safety profile would make it acceptable for almost everyone.

An additional negative aspect to the use of drug treatment for obesity is the negative halo spread by the addictive properties of amphetamine [3]. Amphetamine stands for alpha-methyl-β-phenethylamine. It is indicated for narcolepsy and attention-deficit disorder, but it is also addictive. It reduces food intake, but it is not recommended for management of obesity. The addictiveness of amphetamine likely is related to its effects on dopaminergic neurotransmission. On the other hand, its anorectic effects appear to result from modulation of noradrenergic neurotransmission. Drugs such as phentermine, diethylpropion, fenfluramine, sibutramine,

---

E-mail address: brayga@pbrc.edu.

and the antidepressant venlafaxine are all β-phenethylamines. Phentermine and diethylpropion are sympathomimetic amines, like amphetamine, but differ from amphetamine in having little or no effect on dopamine release or reuptake at the synapse. Abuse of either phentermine or diethylpropion is rare [2]. Fenfluramine is also a β-phenethylamine, but it has no effect on reuptake or release of either norepinephrine or dopamine in the brain. Fenfluramine is a potent serotonin releaser, and it inhibits monoamine reuptake; its effect on dopamine is minimal, and it partially inhibits serotonin reuptake. There have been no reports of addiction to fenfluramine. Sibutramine has no evident abuse potential [4]. Thus, derivatives of β-phenethylamine have a range of pharmacologic effects and highly variable potential for abuse. If examined uncritically, however, they could all be lumped with amphetamine and carry its negative halo. It is thus misleading to use amphetamine-like in reference to appetite suppressant β-phenethylamine drugs except amphetamine and methamphetamine because of the negative linguistic images and inaccurate linguistic content.

A third issue surrounding drug treatment of obesity is the negative attitude that results when patients relapse after successful treatment. The perception arises that the drugs are ineffective, because weight regain occurs when drug treatment is stopped [5]. Cure for obesity is rare, and treatment thus is aimed at palliation. Clinicians do not expect to cure such diseases as hypertension or hypercholesterolemia with medications. Rather, they expect to palliate them. When the medications for any of these diseases are discontinued, clinicians expect the disease to recur. This means that medications only work when used. The same arguments go for medications used to treat overweight. It is a chronic, incurable disease for which drugs only work when used.

Reports of valvular heart disease associated with the use of fenfluramine, dexfenfluramine, and phentermine have provided the most recent ammunition for those who disapprove of treating obesity with medications [6–8]. This is an example of the law of unintended consequences. The reports of valvulopathy in patients treated with fenfluramine or dexfenfluramine were unexpected. Thankfully, the extent of the problem has not proven to be as great as first suspected [8]. It now is recognized that risk for valvulopathy associated with fenfluramine is associated with duration of exposure to the medication [8] and that the lesions are likely to remit off medication [9,10]. The finding, however, will add caution when any future drugs are marketed to treat obesity and will provide support for those who believe drug treatment of obesity is inappropriate and risky.

The final issue to address is the plateau of weight that occurs with all treatments for obesity [11–17]. At the beginning of treatment, a weight loss of less than 15% would be considered unsatisfactory by most obese patients [18]. This is a discrepancy in the amount of weight loss that is desired cosmetically and the amount of weight loss that will produce health benefits. Yet the reality is that none of the treatments, except gastric bypass [17], produces a consistent weight loss of greater than 15%. When weight loss plateaus at a level above their desired cosmetic goal, patients usually blame the treatment. The perceived loss of effectiveness often leads patients to terminate treatment, with the inevitable slow regain of the weight that had been lost.

In weighing the options regarding treatments for obesity, physicians must be cognizant of these barriers to success. It is against these limitations currently available medications will be reviewed.

Drugs that reduce food intake

Table 1 summarizes the effects of several drugs that are available in the United States to treat obesity [2,19].

Sympathomimetic drugs approved to treat obesity

Pharmacology

The sympathomimetic drugs are grouped together, because they can increase blood pressure (BP) and, in part, act like norepinephrine (NE). Drugs in this group work by several mechanisms, including the release of NE from synaptic granules (benzphetamine, phendimetrazine, phentermine, and diethylpropion), the blockade of NE reuptake (mazindol), or blockade of reuptake of NE and 5-HT (sibutramine).

These drugs are absorbed orally and reach peak blood concentrations within a short time. The half-life in blood is also short for all except the two pharmacologically active metabolites of sibutramine [2]. Although the two metabolites of sibutramine are active, this is not true for the metabolites of other drugs in this group. Liver metabolism inactivates a large fraction of these drugs before excretion. Adverse effects include dry mouth, constipation, and insomnia. Food intake is suppressed by delaying the onset of a meal or by producing early satiety. Sibutramine and mazindol have been shown to increase thermogenesis [20–24].

Table 1
Mechanisms that reduce food intake

System	Mechanism	Examples
Noradrenergic	α-1 Agonist, α-2 antagonist, β-2 agonist, stimulate NE release, block NE reuptake	Phenylpropanolamine, yohimbine, clenbuterol, phentermine, mazindol
Serotonergic	5-HT 1B or 1C Agonist, stimulate 5-HT release, block reuptake	Metergoline, fenfluramine, fluoxetine
Dopaminergic	D-2 Agonist	Apomorphine
Histaminergic	H-1 Antagonist	Chlorpheniramine

Efficacy

The criteria used by the FDA for the efficacy of appetite-suppressing drugs is the demonstration in randomized double-blind placebo-controlled clinical trials of statistically significant weight loss that is 5% below the placebo group [2]. A decrease in weight that is 10% below baseline and significantly greater than placebo is the major criterion for the European Committee on Proprietary Medicinal Products (CPMP). Clinical trials of sympathomimetic drugs done before 1975 were generally short-term, because it was widely believed that short-term treatment would cure obesity [2,25]. This was unfounded optimism, but because the trials were of short duration, and often cross-over in design, they provided few long-term data. This article will focus on longer-term trials lasting 24 weeks or more and only those trials in which there is an adequate control group.

Phentermine, diethylpropion, benzphetamine, and phendimetrazine

Only a few long-term clinical trials have been conducted on the first generation of sympathomimetic drugs [2,26–32]. The best and one of the longest of these clinical trials lasted 36 weeks and compared placebo treatment against continuous phentermine or intermittent phentermine [14]. Both continuous and intermittent phentermine therapy produced more weight loss than did placebo. In the drug-free periods the patients treated intermittently slowed their weight loss only to lose more rapidly when the drug was reinstituted.

Phentermine and diethylpropion are classified by the US Drug Enforcement Agency as schedule IV drugs, and benzphetamine and phendimetrazine are classified as schedule III drugs. This regulatory classification indicates the government's belief that they have the potential for abuse, although this potential appears to be very low. Phentermine and diethylpropion are only approved for a few weeks of use, which usually is interpreted as up to 12 weeks. Weight loss with phentermine and diethylpropion persists for the duration of treatment, suggesting that tolerance does not develop to these drugs. If tolerance were to develop, the drugs would be expected to lose their effectiveness or require increased amounts of drug for patients to maintain weight loss. This does not occur. Of the agents in this group, phentermine is prescribed most frequently in the United States, probably because it is inexpensive, since it is no longer protected by patents. Phentermine is not available in Europe. A recent review [33] recommends obtaining written informed consent if phentermine is prescribed for longer than 12 weeks, because this is off-label usage, and there are not sufficient published reports on the use of phentermine for long-term use.

Sibutramine

In contrast to the older sympathomimetic drugs, sibutramine has been evaluated extensively in several multi-center trials lasting 6 to 24 months

[11,34–46]. In a clinical trial lasting 8 weeks, sibutramine produced a dose-dependent weight loss with doses of 5 and 20 mg per day [47]. Several long-term, randomized, placebo-controlled, double-blind clinical trials have been conducted in men and women of all ethnic groups, with ages ranging from 18 to 65 years and with a BMI between 27 kg/m^2 and 40 kg/m^2. In a 6-month dose-ranging study of 1047 patients, 67% achieved a 5% weight loss, and 35% lost 10% or more [35]. There is a clear dose-response in this 24-week trial, and regain of weight occurred when the drug was stopped, indicating that the drug remained effective when used. Nearly two-thirds of the patients treated with sibutramine lost more than 5% of their body weight from baseline, and nearly one-third lost more than 10%. In an interesting study by virtue of the magnitude of weight lost, patients who initially lost weight eating a very low calorie diet were randomized to sibutramine 10 mg per day or placebo, and a behavioral program. Sibutramine produced additional weight loss (16% from baseline at 1 year), whereas the placebo-treated patients regained weight [36].

Several observations about sibutramine can be made from the Sibutramine Trial of Obesity Reduction and Maintenance (STORM Trial) [38], but the effects of sibutramine in aiding weight maintenance are persuasive. Seven centers participated in this trial, where patients initially were enrolled in an open-label fashion and treated with 10 mg per day of sibutramine for 6 months (Fig. 1). Those patients who lost more than 5% (77% of enrolled patients met this goal) were then randomized to sibutramine (two-thirds of patients) or placebo (one-third of patients). During the 18-month double-blind portion of the trial, the placebo-treated patients steadily regained weight, maintaining only 20% of their weight loss at the end of the trial. In contrast, the subjects treated with sibutramine maintained their weight for 12 months and then regained an average of 2 kg, thus maintaining 80% of their initial weight loss after 2 years [38]. In spite of the difference in weight at the end of the 18 months of controlled observation, the mean BP of the sibutramine-treated patients was still higher than in the patients treated with placebo, even though they had a weight difference of several kilograms.

Sibutramine given continuously for 1 year has been compared with placebo and sibutramine given intermittently [42]. In this study, patients who had lost 2% or 2 kg after 4 weeks of treatment with sibutramine dosed at 15 mg per day were randomized to placebo, continued sibutramine, or sibutramine prescribed intermittently (weeks 1 to 12, 19 to 30, and 37 to 48). Both sibutramine treatment regimens gave equivalent results and were significantly better than placebo. Stopping sibutramine results in small increases in weight, which is reversed when the medication is restarted.

Four clinical trials document sibutramine use in patients with diabetes. One is for 12 weeks [48] and the other three for 24 weeks [42–44]. In the 12-week trial, diabetic patients treated with sibutramine at 15 mg per day lost 2.4 kg (2.8%) compared with 0.1 kg (0.12%) in the placebo group [48]. In this study, hemoglobin A_{1C} fell 0.3% in the drug-treated group and

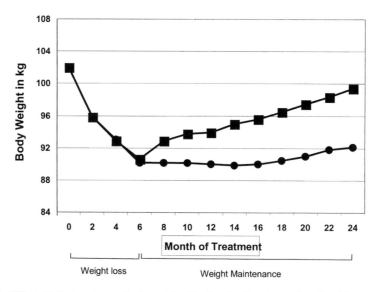

Fig. 1. Effect of sibutramine on body weight. During the first 6 months, all subjects were on sibutramine with adjustment in caloric intake at 3 months to maintain the rate of weight loss. At 5 months, patients were randomized to continue on sibutramine or placebo. Weight regain occurred in those on placebo, but only slightly on those remaining on sibutramine. Squares indicate placebo; circles indicate sibutramine. (*From* James WP, Astrup A, Finer N, et al. Effect of sibutramine on weight maintenance after weight loss: a randomised trial. STORM Study Group. Sibutramine Trial of Obesity Reduction and Maintenance. Lancet 2000;356(9248): 2119–25; with permission.)

remained stable in the placebo-treated group. In the study by Gokcel et al [44], 60 female patients who had poorly controlled glucose levels (HbA_{1c} greater than 8%) on maximal doses of sulfonylureas and metformin were randomly assigned to sibutramine at 10 mg twice daily or placebo. The weight loss at 24 weeks was 9.6 kg in sibutramine-treated patients and 0.9 kg in those on placebo. The improvements in glycemic control were equally striking. In sibutramine-treated patients, HbA_{1c} fell 2.73% compared with 0.53% with placebo. Insulin levels fell 5.67 µU/mL compared with 0.68 for placebo, and fasting glucose fell 124.9 mg/mL compared with 15.76 mg/mL for placebo. Although the weight loss in most of the studies of patients with diabetes does not appear as great as in nondiabetic patients, in all of the studies, the percentage of patients who achieved weight loss of at least 5% from baseline was significantly greater than placebo. In all studies, the degree of weight loss corresponds to the degree of improvement in glycemic control.

Two trials have been reported using sibutramine to treat hypertensive patients over 1 year [11,46], and two additional studies provide data on 12 weeks of treatment [49,50]. In all instances, the weight loss pattern favors sibutramine. Except for one study [50], however, mean weight loss, although favorable, was associated with mean BP increases. In a 3-month trial, all patients were receiving β-blockers with or without thiazides for their hypertension [49]. The sibutramine-treated patients lost 4.2 kg (4.5%) compared with a loss of 0.3 kg (0.3%) in the placebo-treated group. Mean supine and standing diastolic and systolic BP were not significantly different between drug-treated and placebo-treated patients. Heart rate, however, increased by 5.6 plus or minus 8.3 (M ± SD) beats per minute in sibutramine-treated patients as compared with an increase in heart rate of 2.2 plus or minus 6.4 (M ± SD) beats per minute in the placebo group. McMahon et al [11] conducted a 52-week trial in hypertensive patients whose BP was controlled with calcium channel blockers with or without β-blockers or thiazides. Sibutramine doses were increased from 5 to 20 mg per day during the first 6 weeks. Weight loss was significantly greater in sibutramine-treated patients, averaging 4.4 kg (4.7%) compared with 0.5 kg (0.7%) in the placebo-treated group. Diastolic BP decreased 1.3 mmHg in the placebo-treated group and increased by 2.0 mmHg in the sibutramine-treated group. The systolic BP increased 1.5 mmHg in the placebo-treated group and by 2.7 in the sibutramine-treated group. Heart rate was unchanged in the placebo-treated patients, and increased by 4.9 beats per minute in sibutramine-treated patients [11]. One small study in eight obese men demonstrated that an aerobic exercise program mitigated the adverse blood pressure effects of sibutramine [51].

Because the dose of sibutramine influences the amount of weight loss [34,35], the intensity of the behavioral component is also likely to have an effect. This is demonstrated in a study by Wadden [52]. With minimal behavioral intervention, the weight loss in that study was about 5 kg over 12 months. When group counseling to produce behavior modification was added to sibutramine, the weight loss increased to 10 kg, and when a structured meal plan using meal replacements was added to the medication and behavior plan, the weight loss increased further to 15 kg [52]. This indicates that the amount of weight loss observed during pharmacotherapy is caused in part by the intensity of the behavioral approach.

Sibutramine is available in 5-, 10-, and 15-mg pills; 10 mg per day as a single daily dose is the recommended starting level, with titration up or down based on response. Doses above 15 mg per day are not recommended by the FDA. The chance of achieving meaningful weight loss can be determined by the response to treatment in the first 4 weeks. In one large trial [35], of the patients who lost 2 kg in the first 4 weeks of treatment, 60% achieved a weight loss of more than 5%, compared with less than 10% of those who did not lose 2 kg in 4 weeks [35]. Except for BP, weight loss with sibutramine is associated with improvement in profiles of cardiovascular risk factors. Combining data from the 11 studies of sibutramine showed a weight-related reduction in triglyceride, total cholesterol, and low-density lipoprotein (LDL) cholesterol, and a weight loss-related rise in high-density lipoprotein (HDL) cholesterol that was related to the magnitude of the weight loss [53].

Safety

The adverse effect profile for sympathomimetic drugs is similar [2]. They produce insomnia, dry mouth, asthenia, and constipation. The sympathomimetic drugs phentermine, diethylpropion, benzphetamine, and phendimetrazine have very little abuse potential as assessed by the low rate of reinforcement when the drugs are self-injected intravenously to test animals [2]. In this same paradigm, neither phenylpropanolamine nor fenfluramine showed any reinforcing effects, and no clinical data show any abuse potential for either of these drugs. Sibutramine, likewise, has no abuse potential [4], but it is nonetheless a schedule IV drug.

Sympathomimetic drugs can increase BP. Phenylpropanolamine (PPA) is an α_1-adrenergic agonist, and at doses of 75 mg or more it can increase BP. Phenylpropanolamine has been associated with hemorrhagic stroke in women [54]. In December 2000, the FDA removed PPA from cold remedies and weight loss products because of the alleged relation to the development of hemorrhagic strokes [54]. Phenylpropanolamine also has a reported association with cardiomyopathy.

There are two issues to consider regarding BP management and sibutramine use. The first is the development of clinically significant BP elevations. Individual BP responses to sibutramine are variable. From the studies reviewed, withdrawals for clinically significant BP increase are usually 2% to 5% of trial participants. Higher doses tend to produce higher withdrawal rates [35]; thus, lower doses are preferred. The other issue with BP increases is the small mean increase of 2 to 4 mmHg in systolic and diastolic BP that occurs in sibutramine-treated patients versus controls. Weight loss usually is associated with improvement in risk factors for cardiovascular disease (blood pressure, lipids, measures of glycemic control). If sibutramine has mixed effects on risk factors, with improvement in some (lipids, glycemic control) but slight worsening of others, then the prescribing physician must use judgment in the decision to continue sibutramine.

Managing potential increases in blood pressure should be a part of the sibutramine treatment plan. Evaluation of blood pressure 2 to 4 weeks after starting sibutramine is recommended. The initial dose is usually 10 mg/day. About 5% of patients who take sibutramine will have unacceptable increases in blood pressure and for them, the medication should be stopped. If the blood pressure is less than 135/80 and there has been less than 10 mm Hg systolic and 5 mm diastolic rise from baseline, continued use of medication is acceptable. If patients have acceptable weight loss in the first month of treatment (four pounds in four weeks), the blood pressure response should then be a part of the decision to continue treatment.

Sibutramine should not be used in patients with a history of coronary artery disease, congestive heart failure, cardiac arrhythmias, or stroke. There should be a 2-week interval between termination of monoamine oxidase inhibitors (MAOIs) and beginning sibutramine and sibutramine should not be used with selective serotonin reuptake inhibitors (SSRIs). Because sibutramine is metabolized by the cytochrome P_{450} enzyme system (isozyme CYP3A4) when drugs like erythromycin and ketoconazole are taken, there may be competition for this enzymatic pathway and prolonged metabolism can result.

Sympathomimetic drugs not approved to treat obesity

Bupropion

Bupropion is a drug approved for treatment of depression, which produces weight loss [55]. It is a relative of diethylpropion, an approved drug for treating obesity. It probably acts through modulating the action of norepinephrine [55]. A 6-month randomized, double-blind, placebo-controlled trial [55] with a 6-month blinded extension where all patients received active medication has compared two doses of bupropion against placebo (Fig. 2). Both doses of medication produced significantly more weight loss than placebo.

During the 6-month extension, the weight loss largely was maintained. Bupropion has not been given approval by the FDA for weight loss.

Serotonergic drugs (none are approved to treat obesity)

No drugs working by this mechanism are approved by the FDA to treat obesity. Serotonergic drugs that act on specific serotonin receptors (5-HT_{1B} or 5-HT_{2C}) reduce food intake and specifically reduce fat intake. Several drugs that influence serotonin release (fenfluramine and dexfenfluramine) or

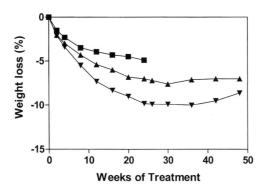

Fig. 2. Effect of bupropion on body weight. During the first 6 months, bupropion and placebo were administered in a double-blind, randomized, placebo-controlled trial. During the second 6 months, the remaining placebo-treated patients were rerandomized to either 300 or 400 mg/d of bupropion. Squares indicate placebo; triangles (facing up) indicate SR300, and triangles (facing down) indicate SR400. (*From* Anderson JW, Greenway FL, Fujioka K, et al. Bupropion SR significantly enhances weight loss: a 24-week double-blind, placebo-controlled, dose-ranging trial with placebo group randomized to bupropion SR during 24-week extension. Obes Res 2002;10:633–41; with permission.)

serotonin reuptake (fluoxetine and sertraline) have been used in obese patients. The clinical trial data are reviewed in detail elsewhere [2,56].

Other drugs in clinical trial

Topiramate

Topiramate is a neurotherapeutic agent approved for treatment of epilepsy, either as monotherapy, or in combination with other antiepileptic drugs. Topiramate is a carbonic anhydrase inhibitor that also affects the γ-aminobutyric acid (GABA$_A$) receptor. In uncontrolled clinical studies, the drug was noted to cause weight loss [57]. Data from a 6-month placebo-controlled, double-blind, randomized, dose-ranging clinical trial has been published [58] (Fig. 3), and several of studies from the terminated 2-year trials have been presented in abstract form. In the dose-ranging study, topiramate was titrated to final doses of 64, 96, 192 and 384 mg per day. All four doses produced significantly greater weight loss than placebo. The weight loss was similar with the two lower doses and with the two higher doses. Higher doses were associated with an increasing number of neurological adverse effects. In a 60-week trial, the lower dose of 96 mg per day produced nearly 9% weight loss. Higher doses of 192 and 256 mg per day produced even more weight loss of 12% to 13% [58]. These effects exceed those of any other monotherapy. In a trial where topiramate was introduced after an 8-week period of weight loss on a low calorie diet that produced an average of 10% weight loss, placebo treatment maintained therapeutic weight loss for 44 weeks, whereas doses of 96 and 192 mg per

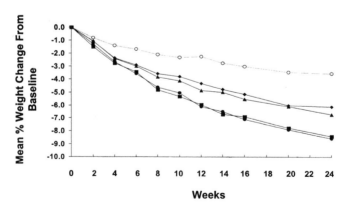

Fig. 3. Effect of topiramate on weight loss. The two lower doses (64 and 96 mg/d) produced comparable weight loss that was significantly greater than placebo. The two higher doses were also comparable, but also greater than placebo in this 6-month randomized, placebo-controlled trial. White ovals indicate placebo (n = 48); diamonds indicate TPM (64 mg/d, n = 57). Squares indicate TPM (192 mg/d, n = 50), and black ovals indicate TPM (384 mg/d n = 44). (*From* Bray GA, Hollander P, Klein S, et al. A 6-month randomized, placebo-controlled, dose-ranging trial of topiramate for weight loss in obesity. Obes Res 2003;11(6):722–33; with permission.)

day of topiramate produced further weight loss of 16% to 18%. Topiramate lowered blood pressure, but not lipids.

Rimonabant

Endocannabinoids may be involved in the leptin pathway, which regulates food intake. Rimonabant is a cannabinoid antagonist binding to the CB1A receptor [59]. It has been evaluated in year-long trials as an antiobesity drug and as a drug to reduce smoking. Doses of 5 and 20 mg per day were tested in both sets of trials. During the 52 weeks of treatment, 20 mg per day of rimonabant produced a 9 kg weight loss compared with 4 kg with 5 mg and 2 kg with placebo (Fig. 4). The therapeutic effect reached a maximum by 36 weeks, and the therapeutic effect was unaltered at 52 weeks. Of those treated with 20 mg per day, 72.9% of those on treatment lost more that 5%, and 44.3% lost more than 10% of initial weight at 1 year. HDL cholesterol increased more than 20%, and triglycerides decreased by more than 15% with the higher dose of rimonabant. Glucose and insulin also were reduced, and the number of patients with metabolic syndrome as defined by the Adult Treatment Panel III of the National Cholesterol Education Program fell from 52.9% at baseline to 25.8% at 1 year in patients treated with the 20 mg per day dose of rimonabant. Rimonabant also reduced BP in association with the weight loss. In the antismoking study, weight gain was 3.0 kg in the placebo group, compared with 0.7 kg in those treated with rimonabant at 20 mg per day. This reduced weight gain was associated with a 36.2% abstinence rate, compared with a 20.6% abstinence rate in the placebo group during the last 4 weeks of the 10-week treatment period.

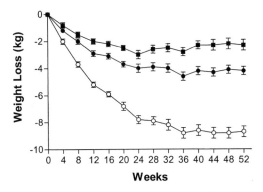

Fig. 4. Effect of rimonabant on weight loss. In this 52-week trial, subjects received placebo or one of two doses of rimonabant. Weight loss had plateaued by 36 weeks. Squares indicate placebo; black circles indicate rimonabant (5 mg), and white circles indicate rimonabant (20 mg). (*From* Press release, February 16, 2004; with permission.)

Zonisamide

Zonisamide is a neurotherapeutic drug that is approved as treatment for epilepsy. One 16-week randomized, placebo-controlled, clinical trial has been reported with this drug [60]. Weight loss was significantly greater in the zonisamide group than in the placebo treated group (Fig. 5).

Peptides that reduce food intake and are in early stages of drug development

Leptin

Leptin is a peptide produced almost exclusively in adipose tissue. Absence of leptin produces massive obesity in mice (ob/ob) and in people [61], and treatment with this peptide decreases food intake in the ob/ob mouse and the leptin-deficient person [62]. The diabetes mouse (db/db) and the fatty rat, which have genetic defects in the leptin receptor, are also obese, but they do not respond to leptin. Leptin levels in the blood are correlated highly with body fat levels, yet obesity persists, suggesting that there may be leptin resistance. A dose-ranging clinical trial with leptin has been reported [63]. In lean subjects treated for 4 weeks and in obese subjects treated for 24 weeks, there was a modest loss of weight with doses ranging from 0.01 to 0.3 mg/kg. The adverse effects of local irritation at the site of injection limit the use of this preparation. A long-acting leptin preparation may provide an improved way to use this drug [64].

Ciliary neurotrophic factor (axokine)

Axokine is pegylated ciliary neurotrophic factor (p-CNTF). It acts through the same janus–kinase signal for transduction and translation (JAK-STAT) system through which leptin acts. p-CNTF reduces food

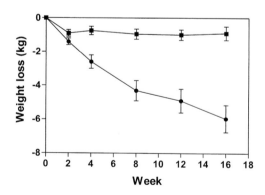

Fig. 5. Effect of zonisamide on weight loss. In this 16-week trial, zonisamide (squares), an anticonvulsant, produced significantly more weight loss than placebo (circles). (*From* Gadde KM, Franciscy DM, Wagner HR II, et al. Zonisamide for weight loss in obese adults: a randomized controlled trial. JAMA 2003;289:1820–5; with permission.)

intake in animals that lack leptin or the leptin receptors [65,66]. In a clinical trial for amyotrophic lateral sclerosis, the drug was noted to reduce weight, and a 3-month dose-ranging study was conducted that demonstrated a significantly greater dose-related weight loss in drug-treated patients [67]. In a dose-ranging clinical trial, p-CNTF produced a significant therapeutic response, with weight loss of 3% to 5%. Following termination of the drug, weight loss appeared to be maintained better in the patients who received p-CNTF than in the placebo-treated group. The first half of a 2-year randomized, placebo-controlled trial was reported in April 2003. About 70% of the p-CNTF-treated patients developed antibodies to the drug. Weight loss of about 5% occurred before the development of antibodies, but once antibodies appeared, the drug appeared to lose its effectiveness on reducing body weight.

Neuropeptide-Y

Neuropeptide-Y (NPY) is one of the most potent stimulators of food intake, and it appears to act through NPY Y-5 or Y-1 receptors [2]. Antagonists to these receptors might block NPY and thus decrease feeding. Several pharmaceutical companies are attempting to identify antagonists to NPY receptors [19].

Melanin-concentrating hormone

Melanin-concentrating hormone is found primarily in the lateral hypothalamic areas of the brain [68]. When injected into the brain, it reduces food intake. In transgenic mice that do not express melanin-concentrating hormone, there is modest weight gain. Conversely, when mice are prepared that overexpress this peptide, they become thinner. Thus, agonists to this peptide provide interesting potential agents for future evaluation.

Cholecystokinin

Cholecystokinin (CCK) reduces food intake in people and in experimental animals [2]. This effect does not require an intact hypothalamic feeding control system, but it does appear to require an intact vagus nerve. Peptide analogs have been developed and tested experimentally, but clinical data have not been published. A second strategy to modify CCK activity is to reduce the degradation of CCK. This approach also is being evaluated.

Glucagon and glucagon-like peptide-1

Pancreatic glucagon produces a dose-related decrease in food intake [2]. A fragment of glucagon (amino acids 6-29) called glucagon-like peptide-1 (GLP-1) reduced food intake when given either peripherally [69] or injected into the brain. Exendin, an analog of GLP-1, has been used in people, because infusion of GLP-1 in people reduces food intake [70].

Pramlintide

Pramlintide, an analog of amylin, is in clinical trial for diabetes. There is modest weight loss in these clinical trials, and more trials are planned.

Drugs that alter metabolism

Orlistat

Pharmacology

Orlistat is a potent selective inhibitor of pancreatic lipase that reduces intestinal digestion of fat. The drug has a dose-dependent effect on fecal fat loss, increasing it to about 30% of ingested fat on a diet that has 30% of energy as fat [71]. Orlistat has little effect in subjects eating a low-fat diet, as might be anticipated from the mechanism by which this drug works [71].

Efficacy

Several long-term clinical trials with orlistat lasting 6 months to 2 years have been published [12,72–82]. In all of the 2-year trials [74], patients received a hypocaloric diet calculated to be 2100 kJ per day below the patient's requirements. During the second year, the diet was calculated to maintain weight. By the end of year 1, the placebo-treated patients lost between 4% and 6% of their initial body weight, and the drug-treated patients lost between 8% and 10%. In one study, the patients were rerandomized at the end of year 1. Those switched from orlistat to placebo gained weight from 10% to 6.0% below baseline. Those switched from placebo to orlistat lost from 6% to 8.1%, which was essentially identical to the 7.9% in the patients treated with orlistat for the full two years. In a second 2-year study, 892 patients were randomized [75]. One group remained on placebo throughout the 2 years (N = 97 completers), and a second group remained on orlistat at 120 mg three times a day for 2 years (N = 109 completers). At the end of 1 year, two-thirds of the group treated with orlistat for 1 year were switched to orlistat at 60 mg three times a day (N = 102 completers), and the others were switched to placebo (N = 95 completers) [75]. After 1 year, the weight loss was 8.67 kg in the orlistat-treated group and 5.81 kg in the placebo group ($P < 0.001$). During the second year, those switched to placebo after 1 year reached the same weight as those treated with placebo for 2 years (4.5% in those with placebo for 2 years and 4.2% in those switched from orlistat to placebo during year 2). In a third 2-year study, 783 patients enrolled in a trial where, for 2 years, they remained in the placebo group or one of two orlistat-treated groups at 60 or 120 mg three times a day [77]. After 1 year with a weight loss diet, completers in the placebo group lost 7.0 kg, which was significantly less than the 9.6 kg lost by completers treated with orlistat 60 mg three times daily or 9.8 kg in completers treated with orlistat 120 mg three times daily. During the second year, when the diet was liberalized to a weight maintenance diet, all three groups regained some weight. At the end of 2 years, completers in the placebo group were 4.3 kg below baseline. The completers treated with orlistat 60 mg three times daily were 6.8 kg below baseline, and the completers treated with orlistat 120 mg three times daily were 7.6 kg below baseline. Another 2-year trial that has been published was performed on 796 subjects in a general practice setting [77]. After 1 year of treatment with orlistat at 120 mg per day, completers (N = 117) had lost 8.8 kg compared with −4.3 kg in the placebo group (N = 91). During the second year, when the diet was liberalized to maintain body weight, both groups regained some weight. At the end of 2 years, the orlistat group receiving 120 mg three times daily were 5.2 kg below their baseline weight compared with 1.5 kg below baseline for the group treated with placebo (Fig. 6).

Weight maintenance with orlistat was evaluated in a 1-year study [76]. Patients were enrolled who lost more than 8% of their body weight over 6 months eating a 4180 kJ per day diet. The 729 patients were divided into one of four groups randomized to receive either placebo or 30, 60, or 120 mg of orlistat three times a day for 12 months. At the end of 1 year, the placebo-treated patients had regained 56% of their body weight, compared with 32.4% in the group treated with orlistat at 120 mg three times a day. The other two doses of orlistat were not statistically different from placebo in preventing the regain of weight.

Effects of orlistat on lipids and lipoproteins

The modest weight reduction observed with orlistat treatment may have a beneficial effect on lipids and lipoproteins [19]. Orlistat seems to have an independent effect on LDL cholesterol. From a meta-analysis [83] of the

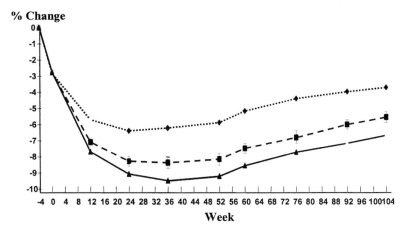

Fig. 6. Effect of orlistat on weight loss over 2 years, comparing 60 mg (squares) three times daily against 120 mg (triangles) three times daily. Diamonds indicate placebo. (*Data from* the pooled experience of Hoffmann La Roche; used with permission of Dr. J. Hauptman.)

data relating orlistat to lipids, orlistat-treated subjects had almost twice as much reduction in LDL cholesterol as their placebo-treated counterparts for the same weight loss category reached after 1 year.

One study is representative of the effects of orlistat on weight loss and on cardiovascular risk factors, particularly serum lipids, in obese patients with hypercholesterolemia [84]. The main findings were that orlistat promoted clinically significant weight loss and reduced LDL cholesterol in obese patients with elevated cholesterol levels more than could be attributed to weight loss alone. The ObelHyx study demonstrates an additional 10% LDL cholesterol lowering in obese subjects with baseline elevated LDL cholesterol levels compared with placebo [85]. These data indicate that the difference in mean percentage change in LDL cholesterol between orlistat and placebo is roughly 10% to 12% in all studies, whether this difference is computed as change from the start of the single-blind placebo dietary run-in or from the start of double-blind treatment. LDL cholesterol levels continued to decline after the start of double-blind treatment in orlistat-treated subjects in all trials, but that LDL cholesterol either remained largely unchanged or increased during double-blind therapy in placebo-treated recipients, despite further weight loss. This independent cholesterol-lowering effect probably reflects a reduction in intestinal absorption of cholesterol. Because lipase inhibition by orlistat prevents the absorption of approximately 30% of dietary fat, the prescribed diet of 30% of energy from fat would thus become in effect 20% to 24% when associated with orlistat treatment. It has been hypothesized that inhibition of gastrointestinal (GI) lipase activity may lead to retention of cholesterol in the gut through a reduction in the amount of fatty acids and monoglycerides absorbed from the gut, or may lead to sequestration of cholesterol within a more persistent oil phase in the intestine. Partial inhibition of intestinal fat and cholesterol absorption probably leads to decreased hepatic cholesterol and saturated fatty acid concentration, upregulation of hepatic LDL receptors, and decreased LDL cholesterol levels. The decrease in LDL cholesterol observed in the study with hypercholesterolemic subjects [83] is comparable to the 14% LDL cholesterol reduction that was achieved previously with a plant stanol ester-containing margarine but of a lesser magnitude than the LDL cholesterol lowering effects that commonly are observed with fibrate or statin drugs [86,87].

Effects of orlistat on glucose tolerance and diabetes

The orlistat-treated subjects in trials lasting for at least 1 year were analyzed by Heymsfield et al [88], who found that orlistat reduced the conversion of impaired glucose tolerance (IGT) to diabetes and that the transition from normal to impaired glucose tolerance also was reduced in subjects treated with orlistat for 1 year. In orlistat-treated subjects, the conversion from normal glucose tolerance to diabetes occurred in 6.6% of patients, whereas approximately 11% of placebo-treated patients had a similar worsening of glucose tolerance. Conversion from IGT to diabetes was less frequent in orlistat-treated patients than in placebo-treated obese subjects, by 3.0% and 7.6%, respectively [88]. Although these data are based on a retrospective analysis of 1-year trials in which data on glucose tolerance were available, they show that modest weight reduction with pharmacotherapy may lead to an important risk reduction for the development of type 2 diabetes.

One study [81] randomized 550 insulin-treated patients to receive either placebo or orlistat at 120 mg three times a day for 1 year. Weight loss in the orlistat-treated group was 3.9% plus or minus 0.3% compared with 1.3% plus or minus 0.3% in the placebo-treated group. Hemoglobin A1c (HbA$_{1c}$) was reduced 0.62% in the orlistat-treated group, but only 0.27% in the placebo group. The required dose of insulin decreased more in the orlistat group, as did plasma cholesterol [81].

In a study of patients with diabetes [80], orlistat improved metabolic control with a reduction of up to 0.53% in HbA$_{1c}$ and a decrease in the concomitant ongoing antidiabetic therapy, despite limited weight loss. Independent effects of orlistat on lipids also were shown in this study [80]. Orlistat also has an acute effect on postprandial lipemia in overweight patients with type 2 diabetes [89]. By lowering remnant-like particle cholesterol and free fatty acids in the postprandial period, orlistat may contribute to a reduction in atherogenic risk [90].

The longest clinical trial with orlistat is the Xenical Diabetes Outcome Study (XENDOS) [91]. In this 4-year randomized, placebo-controlled clinical trial, 1640 patients were assigned to receive orlistat at 120 mg three times daily plus lifestyle intervention, and 1637 were assigned to receive matching placebos plus lifestyle intervention. The study enrolled Swedish patients with a BMI of at least 30 kg/m^2 with normal or impaired glucose tolerance (21%). More than 52% of the orlistat- and 34% of the placebo-treated patients continued to adhere to the clinical protocol. The patients receiving orlistat were 6.9 kg below their baseline weight by the end of year 4 compared with 4.1 kg below baseline for the placebo-treated group (p < 0.001). Cumulative incidence of diabetes was 9.0% in the placebo group and 6.2% in the orlistat group, a 37% reduction in relative risk. Thus, it is clear that long-term clinical trials of antiobesity drugs can be implemented.

In an analysis of orlistat's effect on patients with syndrome X, Reaven et al [92] subdivided patients who participated in previously reported studies into those in the highest and lowest quintile for triglycerides and HDL cholesterol. Those with high triglycerides and low HDL were labeled syndrome X or metabolic syndrome, and those with the lowest triglycerides and highest HDL were the nonsyndrome X controls. In this analysis, there were almost no males in the nonsyndrome X group compared with an equal gender breakdown in the syndrome X group. The other differences between these two groups were the slightly higher systolic and diastolic blood pressure in those with syndrome X and the nearly two-fold higher level of fasting insulin. The only difference besides weight loss between placebo and orlistat-treated patients was the drop in LDL cholesterol. The syndrome X subgroups, however, showed a significantly greater decrease in triglycerides and insulin than those without syndrome X. HDL cholesterol rose more in the syndrome X subgroup, but LDL cholesterol showed a smaller decrease than in the nonsyndrome X group.

An analysis of quality of life in patients treated with orlistat showed improvements over the placebo group in spite of the concerns about GI symptoms. In addition, orlistat-treated patients showed a significant decrease in serum cholesterol and LDL cholesterol that is greater than can be explained by the weight loss alone.

Safety

Orlistat is not absorbed to any significant degree, and its adverse effects are related to the blockade of triglyceride digestion in the intestine [71]. Fecal fat loss and related GI symptoms are common initially, but these subside as patients learn to use the drug [74,75]. During treatment, small but significant decreases in fat-soluble vitamins can occur, although these almost always remain within the normal range [93]. A few patients, however, may need supplementation with fat-soluble vitamins that can be lost in the stools. Because it is impossible to tell a priori which patients need vitamins, the author routinely provides a multi-vitamin with instructions to take it before bedtime. Absorption of other drugs does not seem to be affected by orlistat significantly.

Combining orlistat and sibutramine

Because orlistat works peripherally to reduce triglyceride digestion in the GI track, and sibutramine works on noradrenergic and serotonergic reuptake mechanisms in the brain, their mechanisms do not overlap, and combining them might provide additive weight loss. To test this possibility, Wadden et al [94] randomly assigned patients to orlistat or placebo following a year of treatment with sibutramine, as depicted in Fig. 7. During the additional 4 months of treatment, there was no further weight loss, This result was a disappointment, but additional studies are needed before firm conclusions can be made about combining therapies.

Drugs that increase energy expenditure

Ephedrine and caffeine

Pharmacology

Ephedrine is a derivative of phenylpropanolamine used to relax bronchial smooth muscles in patients with asthma. It also stimulates thermogenesis in

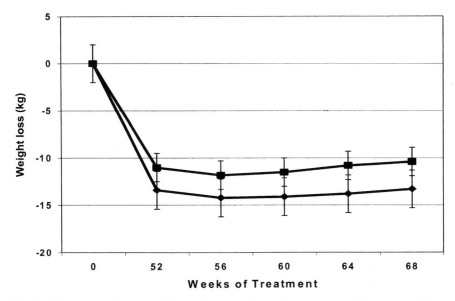

Fig. 7. Effect on weight loss of adding orlistat to patients who have received sibutramine during the previous year. Squares indicate sibutramine plus placebo; diamonds indicate sibutramine plus orlistat. (*From* Wadden TA, Berkowitz RI, Womble LG, et al. Effects of sibutramine plus orlistat in obese women following 1 year of treatment by sibutramine alone: a placebo-controlled trial. Obes Res 2000;8(6):431–7; with permission.)

people [95–98]. Caffeine is a xanthine that inhibits adenosine receptors and phosphodiesterase. In experimental animals, the combination of ephedrine and caffeine reduces body weight, probably through stimulation of thermogenesis and a reduction in food intake [2].

Efficacy

One long-term placebo-controlled clinical trial enrolled 180 patients treated with ephedrine, caffeine, or the combination of ephedrine and caffeine [97]. Patients treated with the combination of ephedrine and caffeine lost more weight than did patients treated with ephedrine alone, caffeine alone, or placebo (Fig. 8). In a 6-month open-label extension, subjects who completed the initial trial were offered additional treatment with ephedrine and caffeine. Nearly two thirds of the group opted for this treatment and were able to maintain their initial weight loss for the next 6 months. No other long-term data are available using ephedrine and caffeine. During controlled metabolic studies, patients treated with ephedrine and caffeine lost less lean tissue than did those in the placebo-treated group. Using the changes in body composition from these studies, Astrup et al have estimated the contribution of thermogenesis and food intake to the weight loss [97]. They concluded that 60% to 75% of the weight loss was caused by a decrease in food intake, and 25% to 40% was caused by the thermogenic effects of ephedrine and caffeine.

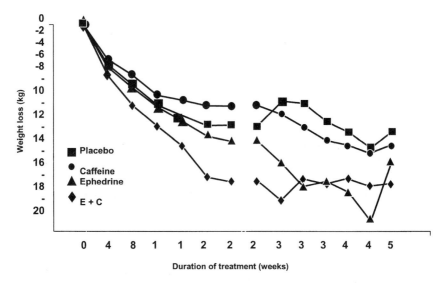

Fig. 8. Effect of ephedrine and caffeine on weight loss and maintenance for 1 year. Squares indicate placebo; circles indicate caffeine. Triangles indicate ephedrine, and diamonds indicate both caffeine and ephedrine.

Safety

Although caffeine and ephedrine have a long record of clinical use separately, neither drug alone nor the combination is approved for treating obesity.

β-Adrenergic receptor agonists in early stages of drug development

The sympathetic nervous system has a tonic role in maintaining energy expenditure and BP. Blockade of the thermogenic part of this system will reduce the thermic response to a meal. Norepinephrine, the neurotransmitter of the sympathetic nervous system, also may decrease food intake by acting on β_2- or β_3-adrenergic receptors. Several synthetic β_3-agonists have been developed against rodent β_3-receptors, but the clinical responses have been disappointing [2]. After cloning of the human β_3-receptor, a new round of compounds is being synthesized that will be tried in obese human subjects.

One clinical trial of a third generation of β_3 drugs has been reported in an abstract; it showed no significant effect on thermogenesis in people when studied in a metabolic chamber after treatment for 28 days [99]. Other drugs are being tested.

Summary

Only two drugs are approved for long-term treatment of obesity. Sibutramine inhibits the reuptake of serotonin and norepinephrine. In clinical trials, it produces a dose-dependent 5% to 10% decrease in body weight. Adverse effects include dry mouth, insomnia, asthenia, and constipation. In addition, in clinical trials, sibutramine produces a small mean increase in BP and pulse that mandates attention to BP monitoring on follow-up visits. Sibutramine is contraindicated in some individuals with heart disease.

Orlistat is the other drug approved for long-term use in treating obesity. It works by blocking pancreatic lipase and thus increasing the fecal loss of triglyceride. One valuable consequence of this mechanism of action is the reduction of serum cholesterol that averages about 5% more than can be accounted for by weight loss alone. In clinical trials, it produces a 5% to 10% loss of weight. Adverse effects are caused entirely by undigested fat in the intestine (steatorrhea) that can lead to increased frequency and change in the character of stools. It also can lower fat-soluble vitamin levels. The ingestion of a vitamin supplement before bedtime is a reasonable treatment strategy when orlistat is prescribed. All medications currently available for obesity management should be used as adjuncts to dietary and physical activity approaches to weight management. Patients who meet prescribing guidelines (BMI of at least 30 kg/m^2 or at least 27 kg/m^2 with a comorbid condition) and who are motivated to undertake concurrent lifestyle changes may receive health benefits from the additional weight loss that accompanies medication use.

References

[1] National Institutes of Health. National Heart, Lung, and Blood Institute. Clinical guidelines on the identification, evaluation, and treatment of overweight and obesity in adults—the Evidence report. Obes Res 1998;6(Suppl 2):51S–210S.

[2] Bray GA, Greenway FL. Current and potential drugs for treatment of obesity [review]. Endocr Rev 1999;20:805–75.

[3] Weintraub M, Bray GA. Drug treatment of obesity [review]. Med Clin North Am 1989;73: 237–49.

[4] Cole JO, Levin A, Beake B, et al. Sibutramine: a new weight loss agent without evidence of the abuse potential associated with amphetamines. J Clin Psychopharmacol 1998;18(3): 231–6.

[5] Bray GA. Obesity—a time-bomb to be defused. Lancet 1998;352:160–1.

[6] Connolly HM, Crary JL, McGoon MD, et al. Valvular heart disease associated with fenfluramine-phentermine. N Engl J Med 1997;337:581–8.

[7] Ryan DH, Bray GA, Helmcke F, et al. Serial echocardiographic and clinical evaluation of valvular regurgitation before, during, and after treatment with fenfluramine or dexfenfluramine and mazindol or phentermine. Obes Res 1999;7:313–22.

[8] Jick H. Heart valve disorders and appetite-suppressant drugs. JAMA 2000;283:1738–40.

[9] Hensrud DD, Connolly HM, Grogan M, et al. Echocardiographic improvement over time after cessation of use of fenfluramine and phentermine. Mayo Clin Proc 1999;74:1191–7.

[10] Mast ST, Jollis JG, Ryan T, et al. The progression of fenfluramine-associated valvular heart disease assessed by echocardiography. Ann Intern Med 2001;134:261–6.

[11] McMahon FG, Fujioka K, Singh BN, et al. Efficacy and safety of sibutramine in obese white and African-American patients with hypertension. Arch Intern Med 2000;160:2185–91.

[12] Finer N, James WP, Kopelman PG, et al. One-year treatment of obesity: a randomized, double-blind, placebo-controlled, multi-centre study of orlistat, a gastrointestinal lipase inhibitor. Int J Obes Relat Metab Disord 2000;24:306–13.

[13] Flechtner-Mors M, Ditschuneit HH, Johnson TD, et al. Metabolic and weight loss effects of long-term dietary intervention in obese patients: four-year results. Obes Res 2000;8:399–402.

[14] Munro JF, MacCuish AC, Wilson EM, et al. Comparison of continuous and intermittent anorectic therapy in obesity. BMJ 1968;1:352–4.

[15] Greenway FL, Ryan Greenway FL, Ryan DH, et al. Pharmaceutical cost savings of treating obesity with weight loss medications. Obes Res 1999;7:523–31.

[16] Astrup A, Breum L, Tourbro S, et al. The effect and satiety of an ephedrine/caffeine compound compared to ephedrine, caffeine and placebo in obese subjects on an energy restricted diet. A double-blind trial. Int J Obes 1992;16:260–77.

[17] Sjostrom CD, Lissner L, Wedel H, et al. Reduction in incidence of diabetes, hypertension and lipid disturbances after intentional weight loss induced by bariatric surgery: the SOS Intervention Study. Obes Res 1999;7:477–84.

[18] Foster GD, Wadden TA, Vogt RA, et al. What is a reasonable weight loss? Patients' expectations and evaluations of obesity treatment outcomes. J Consult Clin Psychol 1997;65: 79–85.

[19] Bray GA, Tartaglia LA. Medicinal strategies in the treatment of obesity [review]. Nature 2000;404(6778):672–7.

[20] National on the Task Force Prevention and Treatment of Obesity. Long-term pharmacotherapy in the management of obesity [review]. JAMA 1996;276:1907–15.

[21] Astrup A, Hansen DL, Lundsgaard C, et al. Sibutramine and energy balance. Int J Obes Relat Metab Disord 1998;22(Suppl 1):S30–42.

[22] Hansen DL, Toubro S, Stock MJ, et al. Thermogenic effects of sibutramine in humans. Am J Clin Nutr 1998;68:1180–6.

[23] Sykas SL, Danforth E Jr, Lien EL. Anorectic drugs which stimulate thermogenesis. Life Sci 1983;33:1269–75.

[24] Lupien JR, Bray GB. Effect of mazindol, d-amphetamine and diethylpropion on purine nucleotide binding to brown adipose tissue. Pharmacol Biochem Behav 1986;25:733–8.

[25] Scoville B. Review of amphetamine-like drugs by the Food and Drug Administration: clinical data and value judgments. In: Bray GA. (ed.). Obesity in perspective. Washington (DC): Department of Health Education and Welfare; 1975. p. 441–3.

[26] Bray GA. Evaluation of drugs for treating obesity [review]. Obes Res 1995;3(Suppl 4): 425S–34S.

[27] Silverstone JJ, Solomon T. The long-term management of obesity in general practice. Br J Clin Pract 1965;19:395–8.

[28] McKay RHG. Long-term use of diethylpropion in obesity. Curr Med Res Opin 1973;1: 489–93.

[29] Langlois KJ, Forbes JA, Bell GW, et al. A double-blind clinical evaluation of the safety and efficacy of phentermine hydrochloride (Fastin) in the treatment of exogenous obesity. Curr Ther Res 1974;16:289–96.

[30] Gershberg H, Kane R, Hulse M, et al. Effects of diet and an anorectic drug (phentermine resin) in obese diabetics. Current Therapeutic Research 1977;22:814–20.

[31] Campbell CJ, Bhalla IP, Steel JM, et al. A controlled trial of phentermine in obese diabetic patients. Practitioner 1977;218:851–5.

[32] Williams RA, Foulsham BM. Weight reduction in osteoarthritis using phentermine. Practitioner 1981;225:231–2.

[33] Yanovski SZ, Yanovski JA. Drug obesity. N Engl J Med 2002;346:591–602.

[34] Bray GA, Ryan DH, Gordon D, et al. A double-blind randomized placebo-controlled trial of sibutramine. Obes Res 1996;4:263–70.

[35] Bray GA, Blackburn GL, Ferguson JM, et al. Sibutramine produces dose-related weight loss. Obes Res 1999;7:189–98.

[36] Apfelbaum M, Vague P, Ziegler O, et al. Long-term maintenance of weight loss after a very-low-calorie diet: a randomized blinded trial of the efficacy and tolerability of sibutramine. Am J Med 1999;106:179–84.

[37] Fanghanel G, Cortinas L, Sanchez-Reyes L, et al. A clinical trial of the use of sibutramine for the treatment of patients suffering essential obesity. Int J Obes 2000;24:144–50.

[38] James WPT, Astrup A, Finer N, et al. Effect of sibutramine on weight maintenance after weight loss: a randomized trial. Lancet 2000;356:2119–25.

[39] Cuellar GEM, Ruiz AM, Monsalve MCR, et al. Six-month treatment of obesity with sibutramine 15 mg—a double-blind, placebo-controlled monocenter clinical trial in a Hispanic population. Obes Res 2000;8(1):71–82.

[40] Smith IG, Goulder MA. Randomized placebo-controlled trial of long-term treatment with sibutramine in mild-to-moderate obesity. J Fam Pract 2001;50(6):505–12.

[41] Dujovne CA, Zavoral JH, Rowe E, et al. Effects of sibutramine on body weight and serum lipids: a double-blind, randomized, placebo-controlled study in 322 overweight and obese patients with dyslipidemia. Am Heart J 2001;142(3):489–97.

[42] Wirth A, Krause J. Long-term weight loss with sibutramine. JAMA 2001;286(11):1331–9.

[43] Fujioka K, Seaton TB, Rowe E, et al, and the Sibutramine/Diabetes Clinical Study Group. Weight loss with sibutramine improves glycemic control and other metabolic parameters in obese type 2 diabetes mellitus. Diabetes Obes Metab 2000;2:1–13.

[44] Gockel A, Karakose H, Ertorer EM, et al. Effects of sibutramine in obese female subjects with type 2 diabetes and poor blood glucose control. Diabetes Care 2001;24:1957–60.

[45] Serrano-Rios M, Melchionda N, Moreno-Carretero E. Spanish Investigators. Role of sibutramine in the treatment of obese type 2 diabetic patients receiving sulphonylurea therapy. Diabet Med 2002;19(2):119–24.

[46] McMahon FG, Weinstein SP, Rowe E, et al. Sibutramine is safe and effective for weight loss in obese patients whose hypertension is well controlled with angiotensin-converting enzyme inhibitors. J Hum Hypertens 2002;16:5–11.

[47] Weintraub M, Rubio A, Golik A, et al. Sibutramine in weight control: a dose-ranging, efficacy study. Clin Pharmacol Ther 1991;50:330–7.

[48] Finer N, Bloom SR, Frost GS, et al. Sibutramine is effective for weight loss and diabetic control in obesity with type 2 diabetes: a randomised, double-blind placebo-controlled study. Diabetes Obes Metab 2000;2:105–12.

[49] Hazenberg BP. Randomized, double-blind, placebo-controlled, multi-center study of sibutramine in obese hypertensive patients. Cardiology 2000;94:152–8.

[50] Sramek JJ, Seiowitz MT, Weinstein SP, et al. Efficacy and safety of sibutramine for weight loss in obese patients with hypertension well controlled by β-adrenergic blocking agents: a placebo-controlled, double-blind, randomized trial. Am J Hypertens 2002;16:13–9.

[51] Berube-Parent S, Prud-homme D, St-Pierre S, et al. Obesity treatment with a progressive clinical tri-therapy combining sibutramine and a supervised diet-exercise intervention. Int J Obes Relat Metab Disord 2001;25(8):1144–53.

[52] Wadden RA, Berkowitz RI, Sarwer DB, et al. Benefits of lifestyle modification in the pharmacologic treatment of obesity: a randomized trial. Arch Intern Med 2001;161:218–27.

[53] Van Gaal LF, Wauters M, De Leeuw IH. The beneficial effects of modest weight loss on cardiovascular risk factors. Int J Obes 1997;21(Suppl 1):S5–9.

[54] Kernan WN, Viscoli CM, Brass LM, et al. Phenylpropanolamine and the risk of hemorrhagic stroke. N Engl J Med 2000;343(25):1826–32.

[55] Anderson JW, Greenway FL, Fujioka K, et al. Bupropion SR significantly enhances weight loss: a 24-week double-blind, placebo-controlled trial with placebo group randomized to bupropion SR during 24-week extension. Obes Res 2002;10:633–41.

[56] Haddock CK, Poston WSC, Dill PL, et al. Pharmacotherapy for obesity: a quantitative analysis of four decades of published randomized clinical trials. Int J Obes 2002;26:262–73.

[57] Reife R, Pledger G, Wu S. Topiramate as add-on therapy: pooled analysis of randomized controlled trials in adults. Epilepsia 2000;41(Suppl 1):S66–71.

[58] Bray GA, Klein S, Levy B, et al. Topiramate produces dose-related weight loss in obese patients [abstract]. Diabetes 2002;51(Suppl 2):A420–1.

[59] Rissanen A, Wilding J, Van Gaal L, et al. The effect of topiramate on body weight and blood pressure in obese subjects: a long-term, randomized, placebo-controlled trial. Presented at 18th International Diabetes Federation Congress. August 2003.

[60] Gadde KM, Franciscy DM, Wagner HR II, et al. Zonisamide for weight loss in obese adults: a randomized, controlled trial. JAMA 2003;289:1820–5.

[61] DiMarzo V, Goparaju SK, Wang L, et al. Leptin-regulated endocannabinoids are involved in maintaining food intake. Nature 2001;410(6830):822–5.

[62] Montague CT, Farooqi IS, Whitehead JP, et al. Congenital leptin deficiency is associated with severe early-onset obesity in humans. Nature 1997;387:903–8.

[63] Farooqi IS, Jebb SA, Langmack G, et al. Effects of recombinant leptin therapy in a child with congenital leptin deficiency. N Engl J Med 1999;341:879–84.

[64] Heymsfield SB, Greenberg AS, Fujioka K, et al. Recombinant leptin for weight loss in obese and lean adults: a randomized, controlled, dose-escalation trial. JAMA 1999;282:1568–75.

[65] Huckshorn CJ, Saris WH, Westerterp-Plantenga M, et al. Weekly subcutaneous pegylated recombinant native human leptin (PEG-OB) administration in obese men. J Clin Endocrinol Metab 2000;85:4003–9.

[66] Guler HP, Ettinger TW, Littlejohn SL, et al. Axokine causes significant weight loss in severely and morbidly obese subjects [abstract]. Int J Obes 2001;25(Suppl 1):S111.

[67] Lambert PD, Anderson KD, Sleeman MW, et al. Ciliary neurotrophic factor activates leptin-like pathways and reduces body fat, without cachexia or rebound weight gain, even in leptin-resistant obesity. Proc Natl Acad Sci U S A 2001;98:4652–7.

[68] Ludwig DS, Tritos NA, Mastaitis JW, et al. Melanin-concentrating hormone overexpression in transgenic mice leads to obesity and insulin resistance. J Clin Invest 2001;107:379–86.

[69] Flint A, Raben A, Astrup A, et al. Glucagon-like peptide 1 promotes satiety and suppresses energy intake in humans. J Clin Invest 1998;101:515–20.

[70] Al-Barazanji KA, Arch JR, Buckingham RE, et al. Central exendin-4 infusion reduces body weight without altering plasma leptin in (fa/fa) Zucker rats. Obes Res 2000;8:317–23.

[71] Hauptman J. Orlistat: selective inhibition of caloric absorption can affect long-term body weight. Endocrine 2000;13(2):201–6.

[72] James WP, Avenell A, Broom J, et al. A one-year trial to assess the value of orlistat in the management of obesity. Int J Obes Relat Metab Disord 1997;21(Suppl 3):S24–30.

[73] Van Gaal LF, Broom JI, Enzi G, et al. Efficacy and tolerability of orlistat in the treatment of obesity—a 6-month dose-ranging study. Eur J Clin Pharmacol 1998;54:125–32.

[74] Sjostrom L, Rissanen A, Andersen T, et al. Randomised placebo-controlled trial of orlistat for weight loss and prevention of weight regain in obese patients. European Multi-centre Orlistat Study Group. Lancet 1998;352:167–72.

[75] Davidson MH, Hauptman J, DiGirolamo M, et al. Long-term weight control and risk factor reduction in obese subjects treated with orlistat, a lipase inhibitor. JAMA 1999;281:235–42.

[76] Hill JO, Hauptmann J, Anderson JW, et al. Orlistat, a lipase inhibitor, for weight maintenance after conventional dieting: a 1-year study. Am J Clin Nutr 1999;69:1108–16.

[77] Hauptmann J, Lucas C, Boldrin MN, et al. Orlistat in the long-term treatment of obesity in primary care settings. Arch Fam Med 2000;9:160–7.

[78] Rossner S, Sjostrom L, Noack R, et al. Weight loss, weight maintenance, and improved cardiovascular risk factors after 2 years treatment with orlistat for obesity. Obes Res 2000;8:49–61.

[79] Lindgarde F, on behalf of the Orlistat Swedish Multi-morbidity Study Group. The effect of orlistat on body weight and coronary heart disease risk profile in obese patients: the Swedish Multi-morbidity study. J Intern Med 2000;248:245–54.

[80] Hollander P, Elbein SC, Hirsch IB, et al. Role of orlistat in the treatment of obese patients with type 2 diabetes. Diabetes Care 1998;21:1288–94.

[81] Kelley D, Bray G, Pi-Sunyer FX, et al. Clinical efficacy of orlistat therapy in overweight and obese patients with insulin-treated type 2 diabetes mellitus: a one-year, randomized, controlled trial. Diabetes Care 2002;25:1033–41.

[82] Miles JM, Leiter L, Hollander P, et al. Effect of orlistat in overweight and obese patients with type 2 diabetes treated with metformin. Diabetes Care 2002;25(7):1123–8.

[83] Zavoral JH. Treatment with orlistat reduces cardiovascular risk in obese patients. J Hypertens 1998;16:2013–7.

[84] Muls E, Kolanowski J, Scheen A, et al. The effects of orlistat on weight and on serum lipids in obese patients with hypercholesterolemia: a randomized, double-blind, placebo-controlled, multicenter study. Int J Obes Relat Metab Disord 2001;25:1713–21.

[85] Tonstad S, Pometta D, Erkelens DW, et al. The effects of gastrointestinal lipase inhibitor, orlistat, on serum lipids and lipoproteins in patients with primary hyperlipidaemia. Eur J Clin Pharmacol 1994;46:405–10.

[86] Linton MF, Fazio S. Re-emergence of fibrates in the management of dyslipidemia and cardiovascular risk. Curr Atheroscler Rep 2000;2:29–35.

[87] Maron DJ, Fazio S, Linton MF. Current perspectives on statins. Circulation 2000;101:207–13.

[88] Heymsfield SB, Segal KR, Hauptman J, et al. Effects of weight loss with orlistat on glucose tolerance and progression to type 2 diabetes in obese adults. Arch Intern Med 2000;160:1321–6.

[89] Tan MH. Current treatment of insulin resistance in type 2 diabetes mellitus. Int J Clin Pract Suppl 2000;113:54–62.

[90] Ceriello A. The postprandial state and cardiovascular disease: relevance to diabetes mellitus. Diabetes Metab Res Rev 2000;16:125–32.

[91] Torgerson JS, Hauptman J, Boldrin MN, et al. XENical in the prevention of diabetes in obese subjects (XENDOS) study: a randomized study of orlistat as an adjunct to lifestyle changes for the prevention of type 2 diabetes in obese patients. Diabetes Care 2004;27:155–61.

[92] Reaven G, Segal K, Hauptman J, et al. Effect of orlistat-assisted weight loss in decreasing coronary heart disease risk in patients with syndrome X. Am J Cardiol 2001;87:827–31.

[93] Drent ML, van der Veen EA. First clinical studies with orlistat: a short review. Obes Res 1995;3:S623–5.

[94] Wadden TA, Berkowitz RI, Womble LG, et al. Effects of sibutramine plus orlistat in obese women following 1 year of treatment by sibutramine alone: a placebo-controlled trial. Obes Res 2000;8(6):431–7.

[95] Bray GA. Drug treatment of obesity [review]. Endocrine and Metabolic Disorders 2001;2:403–18.

[96] Astrup A, Bulow J, Madsen J, et al. Contribution of BAT and skeletal muscle to thermogenesis induced by ephedrine in man. Am J Physiol 1985;248:E507–15.

[97] Astrup A, Breum L, Toubro S. Pharmacological and clinical studies of ephedrine and other thermogenic agonists [review]. Obes Res 1995;3(Suppl 4):537S–40S.

[98] Astrup A, Breum L, Toubro S, et al. Ephedrine and weight loss. Int J Obes Relat Metab Disord 1992;16(9):715.

[99] Larsen TM, Toubro S, van Baak MA, et al. No thermogenic effect after 28 days treatment with L-796,568, a novel beta-3-adrenoceptor, in obese men. Obes Res 2000;8(Suppl 1):44S.

ELSEVIER
SAUNDERS

PSYCHIATRIC
CLINICS
OF NORTH AMERICA

Psychiatr Clin N Am 28 (2005) 219–234

Surgical Treatment of Obesity

John R. Pender, MD, Walter J. Pories, MD, FACS*

Department of Surgery, Brody School of Medicine, East Carolina University, Brody Medical Science Building, 2E-67 Greenville, NC 27858, USA

Imagine, for a moment, that the United States was involved in an epidemic that spread so quickly that within 15 years, it affected 23 million people and accounted for seven times the mortality of vehicle accidents. And imagine that this disease was associated with an increase in the most costly illnesses, including diabetes, heart failure, arthritis, and cancer. Then finally consider that effective treatment was available, in fact several forms of that treatment, and that only 0.5% of those afflicted had access to it.

That is the challenge confronting bariatric surgery today.

This article will familiarize the reader with the types of weight reduction surgery practiced today and explain the risks and benefits of each.

Morbid obesity: the indication for surgical intervention

Morbid obesity is properly named. It is the most severe form of the disease and associated with the highest mortality and morbidity. The term morbid is applied when the body mass index (kg/m^2) exceeds 35. The 1991 National Institutes of Health (NIH) Consensus Conference on the Surgery of Obesity underscored the importance of this threshold with its declaration that diets, exercise, behavioral modification, and drugs are not effective in the morbidly obese. Based on that conclusion and a review of the therapies available at that time, the panelists concluded that gastrointestinal (GI) surgery may be the next step for people who remain severely obese after trying nonsurgical approaches, or for people who have an obesity-related disease. Candidates for surgery have:

- BMI of 40 or more.
- A life-threatening obesity-related health problem such as diabetes, severe sleep apnea, or heart disease, and a BMI of 35 or more.

---

* Corresponding author.

E-mail address: poriesw@mail.ecu.edu (W.J. Pories).

0193-953X/05/$ - see front matter. Published by Elsevier Inc. All rights reserved.
doi:10.1016/j.psc.2004.09.007 **psych.theclinics.com**

- Obesity-related physical problems that interfere with employment, walking, or family function.

The panelists also recommended limiting age to those older than 18 years of age and recommended two operations, the vertical banded gastroplasty and the gastric bypass as the preferred procedures.

These guidelines proved to be invaluable but are now out of date. Surgery appears to have a place in the treatment of morbidly obese children and adolescents, and bariatric surgery has evolved with additional operations and the introduction of laparoscopic techniques [1].

Indications and evaluation

Obesity surgery is not without complications, including death and permanent disability. For this reason, preoperative screening is extensive at most centers. The authors favor a slow approach. Several months usually pass from the time the patient first is seen until the day of the surgery. The delay allows a trial of dieting, often an indicator of the patient's willingness to participate in follow-up. In addition, the authors require extensive education and adherence to every class, clinic appointment, and support group. Patients must be motivated and well-informed concerning the surgery's risks, benefits, and alternatives. Well-informed and highly motivated patients have better results.

The authors adhere to the 1991 National Institute of Diabetes and Digestive and Kidney Diseases guidelines regarding BMI as an indicator for bariatric surgery (ie, if the patients present with a BMI at least 35 with comorbidities or a BMI at least 40 without these diseases). There is a need to explore this issue. Should a woman with a BMI of 32 with type 2 diabetes be denied surgery until she gains additional weight?

Similarly, there has been much discussion recently about the role of surgery in the most worrisome area of the obesity epidemic: children whose BMIs are greater than 40. These children are at increased risk of morbidity and early mortality. Research in this area is needed.

Bariatric surgery

Bariatric surgery began with the observation that loss of a significant portion of the small bowel led to long-term weight loss. This led to the development of the first malabsorptive operation, the intestinal bypass, a procedure that met the goal of weight reduction but with a high cost of complications. Stimulated by the challenge, but deeply concerned about the effects of that draconian procedure, Mason developed the two basic approaches that represent the foundation of bariatric surgery: the restrictive and the malabsorptive procedures.

Roux en Y gastric bypass

There are several types of procedures for weight reduction. The Roux en Y gastric bypass (RYGB), however, is the gold standard to which all procedures are compared in the United States. The favorable risk to benefit ratio of the RYGB and the ability to perform it laparoscopically are what make it the gold standard of obesity procedures in the United States. Although historically it is not the first procedure to be performed, it is the result of modifications of other procedures that led to the development of what is the most common operation for weight loss performed in America today. It combines restrictive and malabsorptive procedures. It is helpful, therefore, to describe this procedure first, and compare it with the others.

Roux en Y gastric bypass is restrictive in that the stomach is stapled in a manner that reduces its size to around 15 cc. It is malabsorptive in that a large portion of the small intestines is bypassed. The success of weight loss with the procedure depends on the size of the gastric pouch and the length of the bypassed intestine. Originally performed open, this procedure now is performed laparoscopically at most major bariatric centers. At East Carolina University, this is the procedure for morbid obesity.

A 15 cc balloon is placed by anesthesia into the patient's stomach and inflated. This sizes the pouch, which then is divided from the distal stomach by staples. The jejunum is divided 50 cm from the end of the duodenum. This creates two limbs of intestine. One protrudes from the duodenum (proximal to the division) containing all the digestive juices of the pancreas and biliary tree (the biliopancreatic limb). The other limb (distal to the division) will connect to the stomach as a gastrojejunostomy (the alimentary limb).

A side-to-side anastomosis is performed 100 cm distal to this division, connecting the biliopancreatic limb to the alimentary limb. The 100 cm alimentary limb then is brought up to the stomach pouch, and the stapled gastrojejunostomy is preformed. This creates a 1 cm outlet from the pouch. The result is a Y-shaped configuration in which the two limbs of the Y are the biliopancreatic and alimentary limbs that join together to for a common channel that runs to the ileocecal valve. Because the digestive juices of the biliopancreatic limb are separated from the food bolus in the alimentary limb for about 100 cm, there is malabsorption in this section of intestine. The operation is restrictive, in that the stomach is now 15 cc in size and has a 1 cm outlet. The operations last about 1 to 2 hours, and hospitalization lasts 2 to 3 days generally (Fig. 1).

Postoperatively, the patient undergoes a limited contrast study of the anastomosis on postoperative day 1. This study is used to rule out an anastomotic leak and confirm patency before advancing the diet. For the first few days, the patient's diet consists of 30 cc of a liquid nutritional supplement three times a day and water. The patient is discharged on full liquids until his or her 2-week postoperative visit. Over the next 6 weeks, the

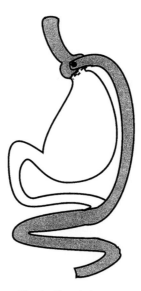

Fig. 1. Gastric bypass.

diet slowly is increased to soft foods with meats such as fish. By the end of 3 months, the patient is able to eat a well-balanced diet, but in limited amounts (secondary to the small pouch size and limited out flow).

These patients generally do not eat sweets or other caloric-dense foods because of the associated dumping syndrome that is experienced post-prandially. Patients who have a gastroenteric anastomosis experience bloating, nausea, weakness, and tachycardia about 30 minutes after ingesting a caloric-dense carbohydrate meal. Patients must be counseled on their diet initially so as to avoid the adverse effects of emesis and dumping syndrome that are associated with overeating and sweets. This is a good deterrent from sweets. Dietary supplementation consists of multi-vitamins and B-12 injections once a month. Laboratory values reflecting liver function, electrolytes, and nutritional status are checked periodically. The patient is seen every month for the first 6 months and then every 6 months. The doctor–patient relationship between the postoperative bariatric patient and the surgeon is for life.

The authors' series of 608 RYGB patients followed for a 14-year period demonstrated a 68% excess weight loss after the first year. At 14 years, most patients maintained a 50% excess weight loss. In a 1995 study weight loss with the RYGB in 608 patients followed over 14 years [2]. Other studies have shown the effectiveness of gastric bypass on hypertension in morbidly obese persons [3,4]. Since this 1995 study, modifications to the RYGB consisting of smaller pouch size and a longer (150 cm) bypass limb for the super obese have resulted in greater weight loss that is maintained. As weight loss increases, however, so does the rate of malabsorption problems.

A careful balance between operative procedure and postoperative manage-ment is essential for successful weight loss that is free of malabsorptive complications.

The mortality and morbidity rates for RYGB vary significantly with centers and surgeons, probably according to patient selection, surgeons' experience, and risk. Wittgrove (unpublished data, 2003) recently reported one death in 2500 patients. Most big centers with significant high-risk patients report mortality rates of 0.5% to 1.5% and morbidity rates of 8.5% to 14%, respectively [2,5–7]. Early complications include pulmonary embolism, wound infection, anastomotic leak, and abscess. Late complica-tions include B12 deficiency, anemia, incisional hernia, staple line failure, and marginal ulcers at the gastrojejunostomy site [2,8].

Malabsorptive procedures

In 1954, Kremen et al first reported the jejunal–ileal bypass (JI) [9]. This procedure resulted in excellent weight loss through bypassing most of the small bowel (as opposed to only 100 cm with the RYGBP). The procedure, although popular for around 20 years, has been abandoned. Through dividing the proximal jejunum and creating an anastomosis at the terminal ileum, the patient's ingested meals quickly passed through the alimentary tract without much absorption. Although good for weight loss, this pro-cedure resulted in profound long-term nutritional complications. Patients suffered dehydration with electrolyte abnormalities that further caused hyperoxaluria, renal stones, liver failure, and skin lesions. The patients' experienced severe diarrhea and gas bloat syndrome also. This procedure was abandoned by 1980, and almost all required revision.

Malabsorptive/restrictive procedures

Biliopancreatic diversion (with and without duodenal switch)

Around the same time that the JI bypass was being abandoned, Scopinaro et al were developing their version of a malabsorptive procedure. Marceau and Hess modified this procedure with the addition of a duodenal switch in the 1990s. Recently, it also has made the transition from open to laparoscopic surgery. The biliopancreatic diversion (BPD) involves creating a 200 to 500 cc gastric pouch (restrictive) with closure of the duodenal stump by dividing the first portion of the duodenum from the pylorus. A gastrojejunostomy then is created, and the biliopancreatic limb anastomosis is created 50 cm proximal to the ileocecal valve.

With the duodenal switch, the 50 cm common channel is lengthened to 100 cm. A sleeve resection of the stomach is performed (instead of a partial gastrectomy). The duodenum is divided just above the second portion of the duodenum, and an end-to-end duodenoileostomy is performed. A 250 cm alimentary limb is created in both procedures, with an ileoileal anastomosis proximal to the ileocecal valve. The digestive juices of the pancreas and the biliary system travel down the biliopancreatic limb, where these juices finally mix with the alimentary limb that is carrying the food and gastric juices. This procedure is restrictive (sleeve resection of stomach) and malabsorptive (only 100 cm of intestine where digestive juices and food travel together) (Fig. 2).

Marceau reports an operative mortality rate of 1.9% and a morbidity of 16.3%. A third of the deaths were caused by pulmonary emboli. Complications include gastric retention, abdominal abscess, pancreatitis, fistula, and wound infection [10]. The long-term complication rate reported by Scopinaro for the BPD was less than 5%. These included anemia, stomal ulcers, bone demineralization, neurologic complications peripheral neuropathy and Wernicke encephalopathy), and protein malabsorption [11].

Weight loss after BPD has been reported as high as 75% for Scopinaro's 21-year series of 2241 patients. Postoperative supplementation with iron, folate, B12, calcium, vitamin D, thiamine, and H2-blockers is essential. If protein malabsorption is severe, intravenous amino acids may be administered. BPD patients do not experience dumping syndrome; therefore they can maintain their weight by eating high caloric foods. For the first year however, food in the ileum curbs the patient's appetite. Bowel movements are increased to three to four often foul-smelling, soft stools a day. Flatulence also is increased. Metronidazole and neomycin can help manage these adverse effects [11]. The addition of a duodenal switch reduces some of these also. Duodenal switch also demonstrated initial excess weight loss superior to that of BPD alone (61% versus 73%) [10].

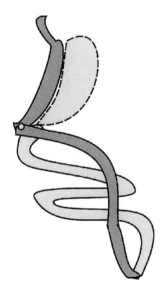

Fig. 2. Duodenal switch.

Restrictive procedures

Restrictive procedures produce weight loss through the creation of a small gastric pouch and a limited gastric outlet. This limitation in volume and the delay in emptying require compliance with a diet to maximize weight loss. Restrictive procedures do not affect digestion or absorption. Although effective, they do not achieve as much weight loss as seen following the malabsorptive procedures. These procedures are simpler in that they have few or no staple lines, and they have lower morbidity and mortality. They also do not generally require vitamin and mineral supplementation.

Mason and Ito, in response to the complications of the intestinal bypass, developed the gastric bypass in 1963 [12]. Whereas the jejunoileal bypass interfered with the digestion and absorption of food, the gastric bypass interfered with the intake of food. A modification to this initial procedure has developed into the vertical banded gastroplasty (VBG) and the Roux en Y gastric bypass (RYGB).

Vertical banded gastroplasty

Mason's continued modifications to his initial procedure led to the development of the vertical banded gastroplasty in 1980. The procedure is based on the creation of a 15 to 30 cc pouch that is vertically oriented. A 32 F tube is placed down the esophagus and held against the lesser curvature of the stomach to aid in sizing the stomach pouch. An end-to-end stapler then is used to create a window next to the tube on the opposite side of the lesser curvature. This window is reinforced by a piece of mesh that is wrapped about the lesser curvature and through the window. This mesh maintains the restrictive outlet. Above the window, a linear stapler is fired along side of the tube (dividing or partitioning the stomach), completing the pouch (Fig. 3).

The extent of weight loss is variable. Sugarman compared the weight loss of sweet eaters with nonsweet eaters who had undergone the VBG procedure. At 1 year, sweet eaters had only lost 36% of their excess weight, while nonsweet eaters lost 57% of their excess weight [5]. As the study group was studied longer, however, some nonsweet eaters became sweet eaters. Several patients found themselves eating more sweets than they had before surgery to maintain the same caloric intake [5]. Because the procedure is purely restrictive, patients can maintain their weight by consuming high caloric foods that pass easily through the 32 F outlet. Milkshakes, sodas, candy, and other high caloric liquid carbohydrates readily pass through the VBG pouch, delivering a daily caloric intake of presurgery proportions.

Roux en Y gastric bypass has an added benefit over VBG in that most sweet eaters learn not to like high caloric carbohydrates because of the dumping syndrome they experience. Purely restrictive procedures such as the VBG do not provide this deterrent.

Because VBG is purely a restrictive procedure, the nutritional deficiencies of the malabsorptive procedures are seen only rarely. Some feel that the

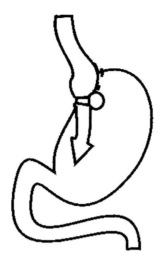

Fig. 3. Vertical banded gastroplasty.

VBG procedure reduces gastroesophageal reflux disease directly because of the procedure's similarity to the antireflux Collis gastroplasty [6]. Others have found the procedure to cause severe reflux even in those who did not suffer from reflux preoperatively [13].

Other complications seen in long-term follow-up include persistent vomiting, solid food intolerance, stomal stenosis, staple line disruption/leak, ulcer formation, band erosion, and incisional hernia. All of these can be seen in late follow-up of RYGB patients also. There is some debate as to which procedure has a higher complication rate, but most studies report a lower short-term morbidity and mortality rate for VBG than for RYGB [5–7,13].

For weight loss, most papers report a percentage of excess weight loss (EWL) equal to or less than RYGBP [5–7,13]. In a prospective trial comparing VBG with RYGB, less than 50% of the VBG patients lost greater than 50% of their excess weight during the first year. Nearly 100% of the RYGB patients lost greater than 50% of their excess weight, however. This study reported a 20% conversion of VBG to RYGB because of complications or poor weight loss [7]. In the long term, the comparison between the two operations fades. Few US surgeons now perform VBG, preferring RYGB.

Adjustable band

Kuzmak introduced a silicone band that can be placed about the stomach in 1986. Gastric banding, especially adjustable banding, has become popular in Australia and Europe, where it has probably become the gold standard of obesity surgery (Fig. 4). It is popular, because it is less invasive and permits a more gradual weight loss. Estimated weight loss with banding is reported at 2 years to be between 52% and 65% [14]. Banding also has less morbidity

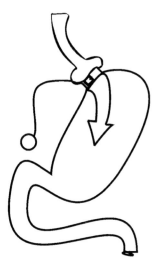

Fig. 4. Adjustable gastric band.

and mortality than the other procedures. The Australian Safety and Efficacy Register of New International Procedures-Surgical (ASERNIP-S) reported only three (0.05%) deaths in 5827 cases. These data compare well to the 25 (0.3%) deaths in the ASERNIP-S review of 7232 RYGB cases [7]. Early morbidity associated with the gastric band includes infection, stomach prolapse through the band, and delayed emptying through the band. Late complications include malfunctioning of the tubing requiring replacement/ repair, obstruction of the stomach outlet (prolapse), and erosion/perfora- tion [14]. International studies have reported an overall morbidity for laparoscopic adjustable banding of 11.3%, 25.7% for RYGBP, and 23.6% for VBG.

Weight loss with the band depends heavily upon follow-up. The band is inserted when the stomach is empty, and on the first postoperative visit, it is adjusted based on the patient's weight loss and satiety. Every 1 to 2 months, the patient must return for adjustment until a steady state is reached. Even then the physician must keep in close contact with the patient for the life of the band.

Proponents of the band also assert that it is not permanent and can be removed easily [15]. It certainly can be removed, and the operation can be reversed. Upon reversal however, patients almost invariably regain their weight. In addition, the normal anatomy is not fully restored. Many patients develop significant adhesions that make conversion to RYGB difficult.

Although some international authors report comparable weight loss data between banding and RYGBP, US reports indicate that the bypass patients lose significantly more weight, and the weight loss is more durable.

The benefits of weight loss with band are the same as any weight loss: remission of some diabetes, improvement in insulin levels, and resolution of sleep apnea. The difference is that should the band be removed, or if it fails, the patient will regain weight, and comorbid conditions will return. But the weight loss is without the morbidity of the malabsorption associated with the RYGB. Band patients do not need as close monitoring of their nutritional status. Studies have demonstrated a 64% remission of diabetes after laparoscopic banding [16]. This is compared with the 82.9% remission rate in an RYGB diabetes study [2].

In the United States, there is debate concerning use of this band. Early Food and Drug Administration (FDA) trials did not produce the same results as international studies [40]. The FDA trial A demonstrated an inferior percent EWL at 2 years of 38%. The complication rates were much higher also. After surgery, 50% of the patients experienced nausea and vomiting; 34% experienced reflux, and 14% experienced obstruction of the stomach outlet (prolapse) [17]. The discrepancy is probably a mix between experience, technique, and subjects in the study model in the United States. In Australia, O'Brien demonstrated an impressive learning curve. His first few bands took up to 4 hours, but the last 50 (in a study of 302 patients) took an hour on average. Also, there was a decrease in the complication rate from 15 prolapses with the first 50 patients to zero prolapses with the last 100 [18]. But there could also be differences in the populations compared. The obese American probably has easier access to high caloric foods than the obese Australian or European. Sugerman has demonstrated that sweet eaters can maintain their weight after having the purely restrictive VBG [7].

There are continued trials in the United States using the band, and some centers have had good results. Modifications have been made to the band and to the technique in placing the band that has reduced the morbidity and improved the weight loss [17]. The approach is gaining popularity in the United States. With time and experience, it is likely that the operation will be used widely as indications and procedural details become more defined.

Laparoscopy

The advent of laparoscopy has revolutionized many areas of surgery. Its use in obesity surgery has been developed over the past 10 years for all of the procedures described. And with the elimination of a large incision, the rate of incisional hernias has been reduced from about 25% to about 2%, according to early reports. Pulmonary function postoperatively returns to baseline much quicker, eliminating some perioperative morbidity. Patients are able to return to activities of daily living sooner than with open surgery [18,19]. Laparoscopy decreases hernia rates, but there is still a potential of herniation through port sites or undiagnosed/repaired umbilical hernia. Studies have found that a midline incision on an obese individual is more likely to result in a hernia than in a patient on chronic steroids for ulcerative colitis who undergoes a midline laparotomy [20,21].

The effects of surgery on associated comorbid conditions

The metabolic syndrome or syndrome X has been documented [22]. This describes the increased resistance to insulin, hyperinsulinemia, dyslipidemia, essential hypertension, noninsulin-dependent diabetes (NIDDM), and an increased risk of cardiovascular disease [22,23]. Additionally, severity of this syndrome has been found to be associated with the distribution of fat (intra-abdominally rather than subcutaneously). Intra-abdominal fat cells correlate are associated with higher glucose and insulin levels [24].

Respiratory disease

Intermittent obstruction of the pharynx results in episodes of apnea during sleep. This occurs frequently in the obese because of reduced tone in the pharyngeal muscles and redundant soft tissue. Obstructive sleep apnea (OSA) results in daytime drowsiness, morning headaches, and cognitive dysfunction. Obesity hypoventilation syndrome is associated with hyper-carbia and hypoxemia while awake. This syndrome is the result of decreased lung volumes, and it also can cause right heart failure. Surgery for obesity is associated with significant improvements in lung volumes, arterial blood gases, and sleep apnea [25].

Type 2 diabetes mellitus

The most serious comorbidity of morbid obesity is diabetes. One third of the patients meet the criteria of the American Diabetic Association for type 2 diabetes; another third have impaired glucose tolerance (IGT) or prediabetes. The most worrisome part of this problem is that morbidly obese children are being seen in increasing number with diabetic glucose tolerance curves.

The RYGB is not just a weight loss procedure that reverses the comorbid conditions of hypertension and NIDDM. In the authors' study of 608 patients undergoing RYGB, 82.9% had remission of their NIDDM, and 98.7% had improvements in their glucose control, insulin levels, and glycosylated hemoglobin [2] (Fig. 5). Studies have demonstrated improvements in diabetes with restrictive surgeries (VBG and adjustable banding,) but not to the extent of the improvements with RYGB [16,26]. The return to euglycemia and normal insulin levels occurs within days after RYGB. Thus, the improvements in glucose control are not just because of weight loss. The actual mechanisms for the remarkable improvement remain unexplained. Those patients who improved but did not attain full remission were older and had the diabetes longer than those who demonstrated full success, suggesting that the presence of diabetes in morbid obesity should be an indication for early surgery [2,3].

Gastroesophageal reflux

There is an increase in the prevalence of gastroesophageal reflux disease in the obese. It is estimated that between 37% and 72% of obese patients

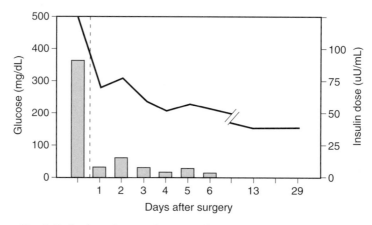

Fig. 5. Reduction of serum glucose and insulin dose after gastric bypass.

suffer from this condition. Increased abdominal pressure is believed to overcome the lower esophageal resting pressure, resulting in reflux [13,27].

Hypertension

Several theories have been developed to explain the increased prevalence of high blood pressure in the obese, including sodium reabsorption and increased catecholamine sensitivity as a result of the metabolic syndrome. Other theories are based on increased abdominal pressure and its effects on the renin-angiotensin-aldosterone system. Sodium retention, increased blood pressure, and proteinuria are seen in the severely obese [23,28,29]. In 45 patients followed for 39 months after RYGB, 70% had resolution or improvement in their hypertension [3].

Idiopathic intracranial hypertension

Headaches, visual disturbances, pulsatile tinnitus, cranial nerve dysfunction, and increased cerebrospinal fluid (CSF) pressure affect the patient with idiopathic intracranial hypertension. Also called pseudo tumor cerebri (PTC), this syndrome is most commonly seen in obese females. In a study of eight patients with PTC before obesity surgery, 100% of the patients had resolution of their symptoms and a decrease in their CSF pressures after obesity surgery [30,31].

Hormone imbalance and cancer

Infertility, irregular menses, and hirsutism are seen commonly in the obese female. Elevated levels of estradiol and dehydroepiandrosterone sulfate (DHEAS) and increases in sex-hormone-binding globulin (SHBG) have been measured in preoperative obese patients [32]. This occurs in the obese, because androgens are converted into estrogens in the white fat tissue, and this correlates with the degree of adiposity in women. Men tend to have normal levels of testosterone. Reports of higher mortality rates from breast, ovarian, endometrial, and prostate cancers also have been reported [32,33].

Psychosocial

"Disdain for the obese is one of the last widely permitted prejudices in the United States" [34]. Obese patients report an overwhelming discrimination and prejudice toward themselves because of their weight [35]. Although there is no single personality type to characterize the obese patient, these patients do demonstrate higher levels of axis I disorders [36,37]. Specifically, these patients have higher rates of depression, eating disorders, and anxiety disorders than people in the general population [38–39].

Quality of life (QOL) is compromised in this patient population. Disparagement of the body image and recurrent health problems impede their QOL. They frequently avoid situations in which they may be stigmatized, and they suffer from lower rates of employment, marriage, and sexual relations.

Surgically induced weight loss improves QOL. Psychiatric, health, and economic status have been demonstrated to improve after obesity surgery. Morbidly obese patients report an improvement after surgery in their social relationships, sexual relationships, marriage, employment, and self-esteem [37].

Other comorbid conditions

Improvement in other comorbidities after RYGB and the other bariatric operations may be related to factors other than weight loss alone, although the reduction in adipose tissue probably plays a major role. Incretins, inflammatory cytokines from adipose tissues, increased use of glucose by muscle, and differences in satiety signals may be factors also. All of the following comorbid conditions can be reduced and eliminated permanently by most obesity-reducing surgeries.

Increased abdominal pressure has been deemed the cause of several other comorbid conditions, including pressure on the urinary tract that results in high rates of urgency and incontinence. Weight loss results in almost universal resolution of these problems [40]. Poor venous return from the lower extremities secondary to increased abdominal pressure causes venous stasis ulcer in the obese. With adequate weight loss, these ulcers can resolve [41].

Musculoskeletal problems plague the morbidly obese, with an estimated 50% rate of some degree of disability, including sharp limitations of activity, with dependence on canes and wheel chairs in a significant number. The morbidly obese suffer from pain in weight-bearing joints, and from ruptured or compressed vertebral discs. Obesity is a contraindication for repair of most of these orthopedic issues.

Increased rates of diabetes, wound infections, subcutaneous injections of insulin, ventral hernia, and poor blood flow to the pannus have been blamed on the development of pannicular abscess [42]. Obviously, losing weight will reduce or remove the pannus and the risk of this serious and sometimes fatal complication of obesity. Surgical panniculectomy can be an additional procedure after obesity-reduction surgery.

Obesity also has been demonstrated as an important prognostic indicator in severe surgical diseases, including pancreatitis and diveriticular disease. Obesity was demonstrated to be an important prognostic factor in acute pancreatitis. Increased retroperitoneal fat was suggested to be the reason for the increase in severity of pancreatitis in the obese [43]. Diveriticular disease has also been demonstrated to require surgery and is more common in young obese patients [44].

Regardless of the method of weight loss, these comorbid conditions can be reduced. Diet programs and pharmacotherapy, however, have demonstrated poor long-term success rates in weight reduction [45]. Surgery produces permanent changes.

Summary

Bariatric surgery is a demanding discipline that requires well-trained surgeons and a hospital and staff prepared to care for these patients with skill and compassion. The best centers manage large volumes of patients with rigorous evaluations, precise care plans, and involvement of specialists at every level, providing behavioral support and great attention to detail. Morbidly obese patients present major challenges in terms of their bulk, their special needs, the requirement for equipment capable of dealing with these individuals, and the recognition that they have little resistance to infection. The American Society for Bariatric Surgery and the Surgical Review Corporation have delineated the requirements for a bariatric surgery center of excellence. Medical centers preparing to enter this field are advised to consult these sources.

References

[1] VanItallie TB. Health implications of overweight and obesity in the United States. Ann Intern Med 1985;103:983–8.
[2] Pories WJ, Swanson MS, MacDonald KG, et al. Who would have thought it? An operation proves to be the most effective therapy for adult-onset diabetes mellitus. Ann Surg 1995;222: 339–50.
[3] Carson JL, Ruddy ME, Duff AE, et al. The effect of gastric bypass surgery on hypertension in morbidly obese patients. Arch Intern Med 1994;54:193–9.
[4] Foley EF, Benotti PN, Borlase BC, et al. Impact of gastric restrictive surgery on hypertension in the morbidly obese. Am J Surg 1992;163:294–7.
[5] Sugerman HJ, Starkey JV, Birkenhauer R. A randomized prospective trial of gastric bypass versus vertical banded gastroplasty for morbid obesity and their effects on sweets versus nonsweets eaters. Ann Surg 1987;205:613–24.

[6] Sugerman HJ, Kellum JM, DeMaria EJ, et al. Conversion of failed or complicated vertical banded gastroplasty to gastric bypass in morbid obesity. Am J Surg 1996;171:263–9.

[7] Brolin RE, Robertson LB, Kenler HA, et al. Weight loss and dietary intake after vertical banded gastroplasty and Roux-en-y gastric bypass. Ann Surg 1994;220:782–90.

[8] Mason EE, Printen KG, Barron P, et al. Risk reduction in gastric operations for obesity. Ann Surg 1979;190:158–65.

[9] Kremen AJ, Linner LH, Nelson CH. An experimental evaluation of the nutritional importance of proximal and distal small intestine. Ann Surg 1954;140:439–44.

[10] Marceau P, Hould FS, Simand S, et al. Biliopancreatic diversion with duodenal switch. World J Surg 1998;22:947–54.

[11] Scopinaro N, Adami GF, Marinari GM, et al. Biliopancreatic diversion. World J Surg 1998; 22:936–46.

[12] Mason EE, Ito C. Gastric bypass in obesity. Surg Clin North Am 1967;47:1345–51.

[13] Kim CH, Sarr MG. Severe reflux esophagitis after vertical banded gastroplasty for treatment of morbid obesity. Mayo Clin Proc 1992;67:33–5.

[14] O'Brien PE, Dixon JB. Weight loss and early and late complications—the international experience. Am J Surg 2002;184:42S–5S.

[15] Favretti F, O'Brien PE, Dixon JB. Patient management after LAP-BAND placement. Am J Surg 2002;184:38S–41S.

[16] Dixon JB, O'Brien PE. Health outcomes of severely obese type 2 diabetic subjects 1 year after laparoscopic adjustable gastric banding. Diabetes Care 2002;25:358–62.

[17] Ren CJ, Horgan S, Ponce J. US experience with the LAP-BAND system. Am J Surg 2002; 184:46S–50S.

[18] O'Brien PE, Brown WA, McMurrick PJ, et al. Prospective study of a laparoscopically placed, adjustable gastric band in the treatment of morbid obesity. Br J Surg 1999;85:113–8.

[19] Higa KD, Boone KB, et al. Laparoscopic Roux-en-Y gastric bypass for morbid obesity: technique and preliminary results of our first 400 patients. Arch Surg 2000;135:1029–34.

[20] Ngyen NT, Lee SL, Goldman C, et al. Comparison of pulmonary function and postoperative pain after laparoscopic versus open gastric bypass: a randomized trial. J Am Coll Surg 2001; 192:4469–77.

[21] Sugerman HJ, Kellum JM, Reines HD, et al. Greater risk of incisional hernia with morbidly obese than steroid-dependent patients and low recurrence with prefascial polypropylene mesh. Am J Surg 1996;171:80–4.

[22] Björntorp P. Abdominal obesity and the metabolic syndrome. Ann Med 1992;24:465–8.

[23] Gillum RF. The association of body fat distribution with hypertension, hypertensive heart disease, coronary heart disease, diabetes and cardiovascular risk factors in men and women aged 18–79 years. J Chronic Dis 1987;40:421–8.

[24] Kissebah AH, Vydelingum N, Murray R, et al. Relation of body fat distribution to metabolic complications of obesity. J Clin Endocrinol Metab 1982;54:254–7.

[25] Sugerman HJ, Fairman RP, Sood RK, et al. Long-term effects of gastric surgery for treating respiratory insufficiency of obesity. Am J Clin Nutr 1992;55:597S–601S.

[26] Kellum JM, Kuemmerle JF, O'Dorisio TM, et al. Gastrointestinal hormone responses to meals before and after gastric bypass and vertical band gastroplasty. Ann Surg 1990;211: 764–71.

[27] Kahrilas PJ. Gastroesophageal reflux disease. JAMA 1996;276:983–8.

[28] Bloomfield GL, Blocher CR, Fahkry IF, et al. Elevated intra-abdominal pressure upregulates the renin-angiotensin-aldosterone system. J Trauma 1996;40:193A.

[29] Sugerman HJ, Wolfe LG, Sica DA, et al. Diabetes and hypertension in severe obesity and effects of gastric bypass-induced weight loss. Ann Surg 2003;237:751–8.

[30] Sugerman HJ, Felton WL, Salvant JB, et al. Effects of surgically induced weight loss on idiopathic intracranial hypertension on morbid obesity. Neurology 1995;45:1655–9.

[31] Sugerman HJ, Felton WL, Sismanis A, et al. Gastric surgery for pseudotumor cerebri associated with severe obesity. Ann Surg 1999;229:634.

[32] Deitel M, To TB, Stone E, et al. Sex hormonal changes accompanying loss of massive excess weight. Gastroenterol Clin North Am 1987;16:511–5.

[33] Garfinkel L. Overweight and cancer. Ann Intern Med 1985;103:1034–6.

[34] Buchwald H, Ikramuddin S. Introduction. Am J Surg 2002;184:1S–3S.

[35] Rand CSW, Macgregor AMC. Morbid obese patients' perceptions of social discrimination before and after surgery for obesity. South Med J 1990;83:1390–5.

[36] Stunkard AJ, Wadden TA. Psychological aspects of severe obesity. Am J Clin Nutr 1992;55: 524S–32S.

[37] Herertz S, Kielmann R, Wolf AM, et al. Does obesity surgery improve psychosocial functioning? A systematic review. Int J Obes Relat Metab Disord 2003;27:1300–14.

[38] Sarlio-Lähteenkorva S, Stunkard A, Rissanen A. Psychosocial factors and quality of life in obesity. Int J Obes Relat Metab Disord 1995;19(Suppl 6):S1–5.

[39] Onyike CU, Crum RM, Lee HB, et al. Is obesity associated with major depression? Results from the Third National Health and Nutrition Examination survey. Am J Epidemiol 2003; 158:1139–47.

[40] Bump RC, Sugerman HJ, Fantl JA, et al. Obesity and lower urinary tract function in women: Effect of surgically induced weight loss. Am J Obstet Gynecol 1992;167:392–9.

[41] Sugerman HJ, Sugerman EL, Wolfe L, et al. Risks and benefits of gastric bypass in morbidly obese patients with severe venous stasis disease. Ann Surg 2001;234:41–6.

[42] Nauta RJ. A radical approach to bacterial panniculitis of the abdominal wall in the morbidly obese. Surgery 1990;107:134–9.

[43] Funnell IC, Bornman PC, Weakley SP, et al. Obesity: an important prognostic factor in acute pancreatitis. Br J Surg 1993;80:484–6.

[44] Schauer PR, Ramos R, Ghiatas AA, et al. Virulent diverticular disease in young obese men. Am J Surg 1992;164:443–8.

[45] Ayyad C, Anderson T. Long term efficacy of dietary treatment of obesity: review of studies published 1931–1999. Obes Rev 2000;1(2):113–9.

ELSEVIER
SAUNDERS

PSYCHIATRIC
CLINICS
OF NORTH AMERICA

Psychiatr Clin N Am 28 (2005) 235–252

Public Policy and Obesity: The Need to Marry Science with Advocacy

Shirley S. Wang, MS, Kelly D. Brownell, PhD*

*Department of Psychology, Yale University, 2 Hillhouse Avenue, Box 208205
New Haven, CT 06520-8250, USA*

Obesity rates have skyrocketed. Nearly half a billion people worldwide are considered overweight or obese [1], and twice as many American adults are overweight than not [2]. Being obese is associated with serious health problems, including cardiovascular disease and diabetes [1–3]. The economic costs of obesity are also great; the direct costs account for approximately 7% of health care costs in the United States [4], and indirect costs caused by obesity-related sick leave and disability account for 10% of lost worker productivity [5].

Although obesity is a major public health issue [6–11], prevention has received little attention. The focus of obesity treatment and research still centers on individual responsibility and individual-level changes, and there is no coherent national strategy to reduce prevalence. Indeed, the US government has stood in the way of global progress on the issue [13–15].

This article addresses the causes of obesity. Biased by misattributions of cause, the nation has sidestepped the need for changes in the environment and instead has focused on the individual, typically by assigning blame to individuals and calling for personal responsibility. The article discusses medical versus public health models as they relate to obesity issue, and ends by proposing changes in public policy the authors believe may help advance the field.

Causes of obesity

Responsibility for obesity has been ascribed mainly to the individual with the problem. For the general public, the misbehavior of overweight individuals is considered the cause of their obesity. This sentiment also

---

* Corresponding author.
E-mail address: kelly.brownell@yale.edu (K.D. Brownell).

doi:10.1016/j.psc.2004.09.001   *psych.theclinics.com*

pervades the health professions, which is why the primary approach in health agencies like the National Institutes of Health (NIH) is to focus on treatment rather than prevention, hoping that people can be persuaded (eg, with lifestyle interventions, drugs, or surgery) to make better choices. Agencies such as the US Department of Agriculture and the Department of Health and Human Services also have focused on the individual, hoping that imploring people to eat better and to exercise more will reverse the situation.

Individual responsibility is woven indelibly into the nation's emphasis on the treatment of obesity. Behavioral treatment teaches overweight individuals to change eating and exercise habits without addressing the environment that fosters the behavior, and medications are targeted at mechanisms such as hunger and satiety, thought to be deficient in overweight individuals. Diet advertisements on television and in magazines suggest repeatedly that the individual must take charge, and that the right pill, device, or book will enable them to do so. Individuals, therefore, are blamed if they fail to lose weight. These individuals are stigmatized as being weak or unable to exhibit self-control, and are sometimes discriminated against in a variety of domains [15–17].

At least 36 guidelines about healthy weight have been issued from federal agencies and private organizations since 1952 [18]. As Nestle and Jacobson point out, however, most of these guidelines are geared toward individuals, and very few discuss the social conditions that contribute to the condition. They note that one report in 1977 spoke of the social and environmental influences on obesity; this report also proposed a long list of possible federal, community, and private actions to change the food and physical activity environment [11]. Little came of this report, however, which Nestle and Jacobson suggest may be because of the sheer number of suggestions, their broadness and lack of priority, and no talk of feasibility with funding.

With the ever-increasing number of overweight individuals in the United States and abroad, it is imperative to examine environmental contributors to obesity, and how these factors might be altered in a way that improves public health. Rates of obesity have increased year after year. It is not possible to ascribe these changes to biology or to declining levels of personal responsibility. The most important question is how changes in the environment have undermined personal responsibility so profoundly.

Evidence that environment matters

Laboratory experiments demonstrate that animals are adept at regulating a very steady body weight until they are placed in a situation in which palatable, high-fat, high-sugar food is consistently accessible to them. Under these conditions, laboratory animals overeat and become far heavier than their normal body weight [19], even when nutritionally balanced food is available.

In people, cross-country and migration studies provide support for the impact of environment on body weight. Migration evidence suggests that when individuals move from countries with less obesity to countries with more, weight gain is common.

The Pima Indians of the southwestern United States are notable for the high prevalence of obesity and obesity-related diseases, such as glucose intolerance and diabetes [20–22]. In 1994, Ravussin et al investigated whether the prevalence of obesity in the Pimas might be related to lifestyle factors, rather than genetics alone, by comparing a population of Pima ancestry in northwestern Mexico separated several hundred years ago from the American Pimas, to the Pima Indians now living in Arizona [21]. Those in Mexico lived a more traditional lifestyle with a diet comprised of less animal fat, more complex carbohydrates, and more physical activity than the lifestyle of the American Pimas.

The data showed that the Pimas living in Mexico had a mean body mass index (BMI) of 24.9 kg/m^2, which was significantly lower than that of the American Pimas, who had a mean BMI of 33.4 kg/m^2, well within the obese range. The Mexican Pimas had significantly lower cholesterol levels and diabetes than the American Pimas. This study is a compelling demonstration that environment plays a critical role in body weight, even if individuals have a genetic predisposition toward obesity.

This association between industrialization and body weight has been demonstrated in several populations. People of African (Benin) descent in the United States are heavier than those in less-industrialized West Africa, while people living in the Caribbean are in between [23]. Rates of obesity among Mexican Americans are far higher than among people in Latin America or Haiti [24]. Peruvian residents in South America have lower total cholesterol, blood pressure, and BMI in men, and higher rates of physical activity in women compared with Peruvian immigrants in California [25]. Even within the same country, lifestyle is related to body weight. South Indians in urban settings are heavier than those in rural settings [26].

To place genetics and environment in context, it appears that other than with rare genetic syndromes, obesity is unlikely to occur in the absence of an unhealthy environment. An individual's genetics may set the boundaries for upper and lower weights, and appear to make some individuals more vulnerable than others to environmental changes, but with two thirds of the population overweight, it appears that genetic susceptibility occurs in most people. It is difficult to ignore the relationship between living in the particular environments and having a heavier body weight. The environment is causing the obesity crisis.

Environmental contributors to obesity

Food environment

The current food environment so effectively promotes heavy consumption of foods high in sugar, fat, and calories that it is not an overstatement to call it toxic. The economic balance sheet of the main determinants of eating—taste, accessibility, convenience, promotion, and cost—encourages unhealthy eating [7,27–29]. Nutrition is not the foremost concern when the average person makes most food choices [28]. Because unhealthy foods tend to be high in fat, salt, and sugar, and hence taste better than healthy alternatives, calorie intake is high for reasons of palatability [29].

Unhealthy foods can be found virtually anywhere in the current environment, not only at fast food and other restaurants, convenience stores, and vending machines, but at gas stations, museums, bookstores, and hospitals. Healthier foods, especially fresh fruits and vegetables, are generally less accessible. In some neighborhoods, particularly lower-income areas, full-service grocery stores with a wide selection of produce may not exist. In addition, preparation of many healthful foods requires more time and knowledge than eating out or obtaining less healthy but conveniently prepared foods.

The prevalence of eating out increased 89% from 1972 to 1995, and in 1998, 46% of US adults ate at some establishment away from home each day [8]. Outside-the-home foods also have more calories than at-home foods; people consume almost 200 more calories per day eating the same food outside the home rather than at home [8]. Also, the portion sizes at restaurant-type establishments can be massive. The calories in one order of the largest size fries at a typical fast-food restaurant will encompass nearly 30% of the recommended calorie levels for an entire day [12]. Sodas, which began in 8-ounce bottles, now commonly are found in 12- and 20-ounce containers, more than double their original size.

The advertisement and promotion of unhealthy foods overwhelms that for healthy foods, with massive advertising targeting children. In a given year, children view an average of 10,000 food commercials, with 95% of those advertising candy, fast food, sodas, sugared cereals, and other unhealthy foods [7]. Coca-Cola spent $277 million on advertising in 1997; McDonalds spent $571.7 million, and Burger King spent $407.5 million in 1998 [8]. In contrast, recent milk promotion campaigns were limited to less than $30 million, and the NIH spent a mere $1 million on its "5-A-Day" fruit and vegetable campaign [8].

The food industry claims that advertisements affect only brand choice, say whether a child wants Lucky Charms or Fruity Pebbles, but not overall desire for classes of foods such as soft drinks or sugared cereals. This is an indefensible claim, as it defies common sense and science [6,12,30,31]. The billions of dollars devoted to promoting unhealthy foods have done more than persuade people, particularly children, to just like one brand over another.

Also, the cost of healthy foods may be perceived to be greater than that of unhealthy foods. People are encouraged to supersize a meal at fast-food restaurants (more food for what seems a bargain), but no similar incentives exist for say oranges, spinach, or carrots. In addition, the perishable nature of many more healthful foods may raise concerns about wasting food.

Environment for physical activity

At the same time that Americans are consuming more energy, they also are expending less energy throughout the day at work and during leisure time [8]. The Surgeon General recommends 30 minutes of moderate activity 5 days per week, yet more than 25% of Americans report being completely sedentary [32]. More people have sedentary jobs than ever before, and energy-saving devices decrease the demand of physical work also [7,8,18,33]. In addition, commuting and taking short trips by vehicle has increased, whereas walking and biking to work have decreased. Forty years ago, half of all US children walked to school; now an estimated 10% of children walk to school [34]. Outside of work, television is by far the most popular leisure activity for Americans [8]. Seventy-six percent of Americans owned more than one television set in 2000; just 20 years ago only 50% of households had even one set. The increasing presence of computers also may contribute to increases in sedentary activities among adults and children. Modern conveniences like air-conditioning also make it more appealing to stay inside than be active outside [8]. Schools are cutting physical education from their curricula because of budget cuts [18]. Indeed, the opportunity for physical activity in day-to-day activities has decreased dramatically. It is, thus, increasingly important to increase physical activity.

Environmental structures appear to be critical in inhibiting or promoting physical activity. Most of those who report exercising say that they do so on neighborhood streets [35]. Saelens et al [36] found that residents in high-walkability neighborhoods exercise more than people in low-walkability neighborhoods and have lower rates of obesity. Neighborhood character-istics that are associated with physical activity include the presence of sidewalks, streetlights, access to trails, and enjoyable scenery [35,37]. These structures, however, often are not taken into account in neighborhood design. The suburbanization of many metropolitan areas has made it difficult for people to walk or bike to do errands, because the distances between places are usually too great. Yet even when commercial areas are nearby, poor neighborhood planning may inhibit such activity, such as lack of sidewalks, cross walks at intersections, or safe ways to cross heavy traffic.

An added social concern is that exercise opportunities appear to vary by the socioeconomic status (SES) of neighborhoods. Higher SES neighbor-hood residents appear to have more structures for exercise. While pay-for-exercise facilities, like fitness clubs, ironically do not differ by SES, low- and medium-SES neighborhoods have fewer free exercise resources, such as biking trails and parks, than high-SES neighborhoods [38]. Also, the perceived safety of neighborhoods tends to vary by SES, which limits outdoor physical activity.

When efforts are made to change the environment, lifestyles change. St. Louis University built 17 walking trails in communities in Missouri to provide safe and convenient places to exercise and found that 42% of residents reported using the trails. In addition, 60% of trail users said that they are more physically active than before the trails were built [38]. Interventions need not take place on such a large scale, however. Several studies have shown that simply putting up a sign about stair use increases their use in the short-term [39,40].

Increasing energy intake and decreasing energy expenditure leads to imbalance in the energy balance equation. Although individuals have the ability to make choices, it is difficult to make healthy choices and to succeed when the environment is stacked against them. As Kumanyika stated, "The question of how easy or feasible it is to make the right choices is usually not asked" [10].

Medical versus public health perspective on obesity

Traditionally, obesity has been conceptualized from the medical or disease model perspective. This model views obesity as a disease (or even personal failing) that affects some vulnerable individuals, which then needs to be eradicated in those who are stricken. This philosophy was apparent in earlier attempts to treat the condition, in which overweight or obese individuals were expected to shed all excess weight and return to their ideal weight. Treatment is oriented toward the individual using traditional medical approaches such as medication, surgery, or suggestions for lifestyle change.

Such an approach emphasizes individual rather than population causes and leads to treatment of individuals rather than efforts to reduce prevalence, and does not lend itself to prevention. This bias is noteworthy with obesity, since treatment is difficult and of questionable effectiveness. Even with the most effective behavioral and pharmacological treatments, patients typically lose 8% to 12% of initial body weight, but often regain much or all of their lost weight [41].

Even for those who succeed in maintaining large weight losses, the effort is considerable and unyielding. The National Weight Control Registry, which is comprised of people who report successfully maintaining weight losses of 30 pounds or more for 1 year or more, finds that successful maintainers exercise with moderate intensity for about 1 hour each day and consume 1400 calories per day [42], which is substantially more exercise and fewer calories than the average American. These maintainers also appear vigilant about monitoring their weight. Forty-four percent of Registry members weigh themselves at least once per day, and another 31% report doing so once a week. Thus, even if individuals are able to lose weight initially, keeping the weight off requires consistent energy.

Prevention of obesity, on the other hand, may be easier than treatment, and more important for the population as a whole. From a public health perspective, small improvements among many individuals make more of a population-wide impact than large improvements in a few individuals. One way to reach a greater number of individuals is to target the environmental contributors to obesity.

Medical and public health models have their place. Obese individuals have a serious medical condition to face, and deserve effective, compassionate help. Although this sounds trite, the pervasive bias and stigma directed at overweight persons has inhibited compassionate care in important ways [15–17]. Beliefs that obese people are defective and bring the condition on themselves affects funding for treatment research, quality of medical care, and the social experiences of people who struggle with weight.

Treatment, therefore, can be conceptualized as needed care for the suffering, but not as a means of reducing prevalence. For every person successfully treated and therefore removed from the obese population, thousands more are entering it because of the toxic environment. Prevention, based in a public health model, must be the priority for reducing the impact of obesity on individuals and nations.

What must be done?

It is time to be courageous. Environmental changes will be key, and these must be brought about by changes in public policy. In some cases, policy changes might occur at state or national levels, but they also might involve local institutions such as schools (eg, banning soft drinks and snack foods) or community organizations (eg, sponsoring walking/bike trails).

A focus on prevention leads naturally to children. Rates of childhood obesity are skyrocketing, and overweight children are much more likely to become overweight adults [43,44]. The young may be the most vulnerable victims of the toxic environment, but they are also the group in which prevention strategies are likely to be most effective. Food preferences, brand loyalties, and connections of certain foods and classes of foods with cultural icons such as cartoon characters, sports stars, and music celebrities can have powerful influences on food intake. The food industry has exploited this key phase of development; diet has deteriorated, and children, like adults, are becoming less physically active. It is important that children be protected from negative influences and that childhood be a time when children are exposed to conditions that promote good health.

It is common, when speaking of prevention, for education about healthy eating and exercise to be considered the solution. Education may be necessary but not nearly sufficient to prevent obesity. The rudiments of healthy eating are well-known, and knowledge that exercise is beneficial is nearly universal, so assuming that knowledge can overcome such an unhealthy environment is wishful thinking [6,45].

There are multiple actions that could be taken to address the obesity issue from policy and legislative angles. These ultimately will be possible as changes occur in social changes, and a strong collective will exist for systemic changes (Box 1). For instance, improving the food and physical activity environments in schools could be brought about by national or state legislation, pressure from parent groups in particular schools, or inspired

Box 1. Summary of recommended actions

Thinking differently

Appreciate that a changing environment has caused the obesity epidemic, and that the environment is a logical place to intervene.

Recognize that personal resources (responsibility) can be overwhelmed when the environment is toxic, that culture already places heavy emphasis on personal responsibility, and that further emphasis likely will have limited impact on the obesity epidemic.

Move beyond the "no good foods or bad foods" stance into a public perspective that identifies types of the food people should consume less of or more of.

Recognize that treating obesity is difficult and can be costly; thus prevention must be a national priority.

Appreciate that investing in children will likely produce the first victories in the fight against poor diet and inactivity.

Pledge to the nation's children that they will be provided with a healthy environment.

Physical activity

Develop a national strategic plan to increase physical activity.

Earmark transportation funding to increase activity (eg, bike and walking paths, buses with bike racks, traffic calming).

Design activity-friendly communities.

Promote walking and biking to school and enhance physical education.

Offer incentives for physical activity and strive to decrease sedentary behavior.

Promote activity through work sites and physician practices.

Commercialization of childhood

Object to thinking of children as market objects.

Protest to companies that offer up their characters to sell unhealthy foods.

Encourage celebrities not to promote unhealthy food and to help promote healthy eating and physical activity.

Encourage entertainment executives to stop using product placements in programming aimed at children.

Level the playing field so that healthy foods are promoted at least as much as unhealthy foods.

Mandate equal time for pronutrition and activity messages to counter those for unhealthy foods.

Create a superfund to promote healthy eating, perhaps from assessments placed on food advertisements or small taxes on the sale of unhealthy foods.

Enforce the Children's Television Act.

Promote media literacy among children.

Food and soft drinks in schools

Show how healthy eating and activity are connected with academic performance.

Permit commercial television in schools only if it is free of advertising for unhealthy foods.

Rid children's books and educational materials of references to unhealthy foods and cease connection with brand-name food products.

If food is used as an academic incentive, use healthy foods.

Have nonfood or healthy food fundraisers.

Do not allow food company logos or advertisements on school property, including buses.

Improve school lunch programs and use the cafeteria as a learning laboratory.

Find alternatives to snack foods, soft drinks and fast foods in schools, with the goal of eliminating unhealthy foods entirely.

Support programs that teach children about nutrition and activity.

Make schools commercial-free zones and use zoning laws to prohibit establishments with unhealthy foods from operating near schools.

Have only healthy foods and beverages in vending machines. If this is impossible, use pricing to encourage purchase of healthy items.

Require schools to be open and clear about industry contacts and connections.

Challenge industry claims that they are helping education.

Portions

Help make the public, health professionals, and government leaders aware that larger portion sizes lead to greater eating, and that people do not appear to compensate for the additional calories at later meals.

Educate people on appropriate serving sizes.

Encourage food companies to show reasonable portions in advertisements and avoid suggestions about eating larger amounts.

(*continued on next page*)

Require food labeling at restaurants.
Require food packaging to have the number of servings in
a container accompany weight or volume figures on the front
of containers.

Economic issues
Help make the public aware of the economic forces that
contribute to obesity, noting how the imbalance of incentives
to eat unhealthy foods versus healthy foods by itself would
predict an epidemic for obesity.
Increase the awareness of social inequities (eg, conditions that
predispose the poor to obesity) and increase access to healthy
foods and opportunities to be active for those living in poverty.
Engage federal food programs as allies in the fight against
obesity.
Consider changing the price structure of food, first by lowering
the cost of healthy foods and perhaps increasing the cost of
unhealthy foods.
Think of food taxes, not as a means for punishing people for bad
choices but as a means for raising revenues for programs
aimed at improving the nation's diet.
Sensitize consumers to financial inducements to buy large
amounts of unhealthy foods.

Interacting with the food industry
Celebrate positive changes the industry makes in its products
and the support it provides for programs aimed at improving
diet and activity.
Make transparent the impact of the industry on national nutrition
policy.
Increase awareness of industry tactics in dealing with being
challenged; reinforce reasonable tactics and fight those that
will impede progress.
Challenge the industry for connections with tobacco and for
funding provided to shadow groups like the Center for
Consumer Freedom that fight efforts to curtail smoking or to
change practices of the food industry.
Encourage political leaders to be bold and innovative in
addressing the obesity crisis and to remove political barriers to
taking action.
Curb food commercialism in public and community institutions.
Promote activities known to help with body weight.
Mobilize parents to demand a healthy environment for their
children.

school officials. Social norms that place a higher priority on the health of children than income from selling unhealthy foods could precipitate any or all of these actions.

Establishing priorities leads to complicated but fascinating questions. Would it have more impact to restrict food advertising directed at children, improve the food environment in schools, educate the public on healthy eating, or tax unhealthy foods to subsidize healthier ones? Existing science in the obesity field will not answer questions of this nature. Information must be assembled from areas like marketing, tax policy, agricultural economics, trade policy, and more to develop a coherent plan. There has not been the will or resources to approach this task. This situation must change. Otherwise, one can foresee no appreciable impact on the prevalence of obesity; staggering health care costs will continue, and the opportunity to reduce premature morbidity and mortality will be missed.

Box 1 presents suggestions for change. The following section describes several areas in detail.

Legislative efforts

Legislation is one means for making the environment healthier. Efforts to create conditions that increase physical activity are likely to succeed with little resistance (except for reluctance for funding programs in general), because the food industry is in full support, as are business-friendly legislators. Changing the food environment may be at least as important, but will encounter strong pushback from the food industry.

At one point, legislation to change the food environment was inconceivable, as the food industry was immovable in terms of accepting responsibility or making positive changes. In 1994, for instance, Brownell wrote an opinion/editorial about the obesity epidemic in the *New York Times* [46]. This piece recommended changes in the food environment by decreasing children's exposure to food advertising and if needed, taxing foods of poor nutrition quality. The response at that time was negative and blistering, especially from the political right, and from groups funded by the food industry.

Now the situation is different. Legislation is no longer impossible. Partly because the food industry has reacted late to growing criticism, legislative action, particularly at the state level, is occurring as never before. What at one point seemed the most radical idea, taxing foods, is now part of public debate and is being considered as a legitimate action to combat obesity. With the door now open, it is imperative that policy research be done to define the most fruitful legislative approaches.

Encouraging legislative efforts have been made, including ones targeting children and directed at improving the nutrition environment in schools. Arkansas' Act 1220 was signed into law, instructing the state board of education to create a committee by the 2003–2004 school year, to make recommendations about foods, vending, food service training, physical education, and how revenue from such contracts should be used. In addition, the bill prohibits vending machines in elementary schools, demands that revenues from food contracts be published, and instructs schools to report each student's BMI to his or her parents [38].

The Arkansas act is illustrative as a beginning, but as with any initial effort, it has flaws that should be corrected. Prohibiting soft drink machines in elementary schools is good, but most machines are in middle and high schools. A survey in Kentucky found that 44% of elementary schools have soft drink machines, compared with 88% of middle schools and 97% of high schools [47]. Further, elementary schools probably have fewer machines per student, and the children are less likely than older children to have discretionary money. The authors are not privy to behind the scenes negotiations of the Arkansas bill, but they wonder whether the soft drink industry withdrew opposition in exchange for overlooking middle and high schools.

California passed a bill in 2001 that prohibits soft drink sales in middle schools during lunchtime, and has followed up with an additional bill that will ban all soda from middle schools by 2005. Massachusetts is considering House Bill 3519, which would ban the sale of low-nutrition foods and drinks during school hours in all schools. The New York State Assembly and Senate both approved a bill that would create a childhood obesity prevention program, a media campaign designed to target children and parents, and nutrition and physical activity programs in schools. Missouri and Montana passed similar bills on improving nutrition in schools [38].

Similar bills have been voted down or tabled in Connecticut, Virginia, New Mexico, and Kentucky, but such is the history of new legislation that challenges a powerful industry, as was clear with tobacco. The authors expect legislative efforts to grow in number and impact.

Legislation ultimately could address many issues, including schools, the price of food, advertising policy, and more. Thus far there is no coordinated effort to affect legislation or even a measure for understanding which legislative effects might be most helpful, most feasible, or both. There is a need for advances in this area.

The National Conference of State Legislatures' Health Policy Tracking Service provides monthly updates on legislative efforts related to child and adolescent nutrition and obesity (contact Lee.Dixon@netscan.org to subscribe). Searchable databases of state physical activity and nutrition legislation are provided by the National Conference of State Legislatures at http://www.ncsl.org/programs/health/pp/healthpromo.cfm or by the Centers for Disease Control and Prevention's Division of Nutrition and Physical Activity at http://apps.nccd.cdc.gov/DNPALeg/. Additional information on legislative and policy changes can be found at the Center for Science in the Public Interest at http://cspinet.org/nutritionpolicy/policy_ options.html.

The food industry

The food industry is motivated to stay active in policy discussions about obesity and has been invited by the federal administration to do so. This is a key strategic issue facing the country, namely how to involve the industry in nutrition policy. The nation must decide whether the industry is trustworthy. Whereas public sentiment becomes more skeptical of the industry, the federal administration behaves as if the industry is trustworthy, acted out in statements by the Secretary of Health and Human Services and the Surgeon General. Couched in phrases like "involving all stakeholders," industry is part of key decisions. History will tell whether this is wise, but the deadly history of tobacco offers lessons that should not be ignored. That industry distorted science, paid leading scientists who then took industry positions with the press, developed "safe" products like filtered cigarettes that were not safer at all, and more. There are eerie parallels with what is happening now with food.

In the last 2 years, major players in the food industry have made announcements about change. For instance, in 2002, McDonalds made the announcement that it would change the type of oil it uses to cook its fried items, reducing transfatty acids by 48% and saturated fats by 16%, while increasing polyunsaturated fat by 167%. McDonalds retracted this promise later. In contrast, Frito-Lay has eliminated trans fat from its products.

Kraft, America's largest food company, announced in 2003 that it would scale back on advertising some products to children, would pull out of schools, and would help in the fight against obesity by advertising more reasonable portion sizes [48]. McDonald's announced in 2004 that it would scale back supersizing, and the largest size of French fries would drop from 7 to 6 ounces (the original size of French fries was 2.5 ounces).

The authors believe that companies should be applauded for positive changes they make, but not be issued public relations or legal immunity for negative practices. McDonalds introducing a wider range of salads is good, perhaps. It is possible that weight-conscious parents will now feel more willing to take children to McDonalds, but without proper research, it is unknown whether this is the case. Giving McDonalds the benefit of the doubt and not inferring pernicious motives, one can celebrate salads. One cannot celebrate if the company uses a tiny fraction of its advertising budget to promote healthier options compared with its traditional fast food.

Case studies

There are other examples of policy and environmental changes that focus particularly on children. In 2002, the Los Angeles Unified School Board voted to ban sales of soft drinks in school vending machines and in the cafeteria. The board unanimously decided that the health issue of selling sugary, non-nutritive drinks was separate from the economic issue of how soft drink contracts provide extra funding to the school system. The existing contract stipulated that schools received a 36% commission on soft drink sales but only 15% commission on healthier drinks [49].

A major initiative for environmental change of physical activity is the "Safe Route to School Program," established by the Surface Transportation Policy Project coalition. This program aims to increase the safety for children when walking or biking to school, thus increasing their physical activity [34]. Support for this program is growing, and already specific examples of improvements can be cited. The Phoenix Department of Transportation has responded by increasing the safety at high pedestrian traffic areas by expanding sidewalks at traffic lights, adding crosswalks, and adding speed-reduction measures near schools. California passed a bill in 1999 that provides funding to improve the safety and design of the streets and sidewalks along routes to school [34].

There are many more examples of such victories [12]. These show that individuals, grass roots organizations, and advocacy groups can make a difference. The authors believe that these signal the beginning of a growing movement to change the food and activity environments.

Policy approaches

These examples are encouraging, but more public policy on environmental change is needed. Public policy can lead to widespread change systematically and immediately. There is a long-standing history in most countries of policy changes made for the good of public health [10,12]. For instance, the addition of fluoride to water was once a controversial innovation, but is now routine. More recently with smoking, there were outcries from the tobacco companies about a number of policies, but the public is not complaining that Joe Camel is gone from advertisements targeting children.

In addition, with obesity, it could be argued that the extraordinary prevalence rates are a result of letting people fend for themselves in this toxic environment. Clearly the environment is prevailing over individuals' choices. It is becoming apparent that individuals are overwhelmed and need help in overcoming the unhealthy environment that surrounds them.

Policy priorities and suggestions

The authors believe that policy priorities should center on prevention and children. Policies aimed at modifying the school environment should include improving the quality of the nutrition in the foods served, removing food company logos and advertisements from school property, finding alternative sources of funding for schools than from marketing unhealthy foods to children, and doing everything possible to increase physical activity [10,12]. The Child and Adolescent Trial for Cardiovascular Health (CATCH) provides support that policy changes work [50–52]. This 3-year study promoted healthy eating and physical activity in 5000 elementary school children. The schools lowered the amount of fat in their school lunches and increased physical education class time. Results showed that the children lowered the amount of fat that they consumed per day and increased their amount of physical activity each day also.

Advertising toward children also needs to be regulated better. This includes promoting healthy foods as much as unhealthy foods or stopping use of product placements in programming aimed at children [12].

Other policy approaches include subsidizing healthier foods [7], making physical activity more accessible and affordable [53], and levying small taxes on snack or other foods with the revenue earmarked for promoting healthy foods [54]. French et al have conducted several studies in the community to measure the impact of cost on consumption of healthy foods [27]. In one study conducted at work sites and schools, they [55] found that lowering the cost of lower fat snack foods by 10%, 25%, and 50% increased sales by 9%, 39% and 93%, respectively, compared with sales of the same snacks with their usual prices. They found that price reductions of fresh fruit and carrots yielded similar sales increases. Thus policy changes that decrease the price of healthy foods may have a substantial impact on consumption.

Taxing unhealthy foods is a more complicated policy change. Several concerns have been raised, including how to decide what foods to tax, the "slippery slope" of taxing one food item and expanding the list to include similar items, and the regressive nature of such taxes. Jacobson and Brownell [54] proposed a very small tax on snack foods, low enough that consumers would not object, with the revenue used to subsidize healthy food or to fund other projects to make the environment healthier.

Other policies geared toward prevention should focus on the physical environment. Communities can be built with healthy lifestyles in mind, by incorporating sidewalks and shared outdoor space (eg, parks and trails), building crosswalks at traffic intersections, and perhaps building bike lanes if the shared roads otherwise would be too dangerous for bikers.

Feasibility and funding

Funding to carry out policy suggestions is an appropriate concern. Ideally federal, state, community, and private organizations will recognize the critical importance of these initiatives and work together to fund them. Tax money also can be used to fund programs. In addition, it is important to examine the relative cost of various approaches.

For instance, West Virginia used snack taxes to fund health promotion programs encouraging consumers to switch from higher fat to lower fat milk. The 7-week campaign increased the market share of 1% or fat-free milk from 18% to 41%, and the cost of the television and radio campaign was only 22 cents per resident. More strikingly, as Jacobson and Brownell [54] state, "A campaign reaching about 200,000 people would cost about the same as one coronary-bypass operation." Similarly, a 20-week television-advertising campaign in Louisville, KY, that cost only 30 cents per person resulted in a 5% increase in produce sales in supermarkets area [38]. Thus, while funding is a very real issue, much can be done with relatively little, especially compared with the cost of treatment.

Summary

Obesity is an epidemic that likely will worsen if strong, broad-reaching changes are not made to the current environment. Although treatment of the individual traditionally has been the focus of the obesity field, prevention using a public health model will be essential for making progress. There are encouraging signs that nations are taking the obesity problem seriously, that there is growing recognition that prevention must be the priority, and that a full-scale effort must be made to protect children. One important area of research is to understand what makes local victories possible, say a school system banning soft drinks and snack foods, or a neighborhood creating ways for citizens to be more physically active, and then to help make such changes spread to other communities. Public policy changes long have been used to combat infectious and chronic diseases and will be vital in the attempt to reduce the toll of poor diet, physical inactivity, and obesity.

References

[1] Rossner S. Obesity: the disease of the twenty-first century. Int J Obes 2002;26:S2–4.
[2] Mokdad AH, Bowman BA, Ford ES, et al. The continuing epidemics of obesity and diabetes in the United States. JAMA 2001;286:1195–200.
[3] Visscher TLS, Seidel JC. The public health impact of obesity. Annu Rev Public Health 2001; 22:355–75.
[4] Colditz GA. Economic costs of obesity and inactivity. Med Sci Sports Exerc 1999;31:S663–7.
[5] Narbro K, Jonsson E, Larsson B, et al. Economic consequences of sick-leave and early retirement in obese Swedish women. Int J Obes 1996;20:895–903.
[6] Battle EK, Brownell KD. Confronting a rising tide of eating disorders and obesity: treatment vs. prevention and policy. Addictive Behav 1996;21:755–65.
[7] Brownell KD. Public health approaches to obesity and its management. Annu Rev Public Health 1986;7:521–33.
[8] French SA, Story M, Jeffery RW. Environmental influences on eating and physical activity. Annu Rev Public Health 2001;22:309–35.
[9] Jeffery RW. Public health approaches to the management of obesity. In: Brownell KD, Fairburn CG, editors. Eating disorders and obesity: a comprehensive handbook. New York: Guilford Press; 1995. p. 558–63.
[10] Kumanyika SK. Minisymposium on obesity: overview and some strategic considerations. Annu Rev Public Health 2001;22:293–308.
[11] Stunkard AJ. Obesity and the social environment: current status, future prospects. In: Bray GA, editor. Obesity in America. Washington, DC: Department of Health, Education, and Welfare; 1979. Publication #NIH. 79–359.

[12] Brownell KD, Horgen KB. Food fight: the inside story of the food industry, America's obesity crisis, and what we can do about it. New York: McGraw Hill; 2004.

[13] Brownell KD, Nestle M. The sweet and lowdown on sugar. New York Times. January 23, 2004; Opinion/editorial section: A23.

[14] Nestle M. Food politics: how the food industry influences nutrition and health. Berkeley (CA): University of California Press; 2002.

[15] DeJong W. Obesity as a characterological stigma: the issue of responsibility and judgments of task performance. Psychol Rep 1993;73:963–70.

[16] Puhl R, Brownell KD. Bias, discrimination, and obesity. Obes Res 2001;9:788–805.

[17] Puhl RM, Brownell KD. Bias, discrimination, and obesity. In: Bray GA, Bouchard C, editors. Handbook of obesity: clinical applications. 2nd edition. New York: Marcel Dekker; 2004. p. 69–74.

[18] Nestle M, Jacobson MF. Halting the obesity epidemic: a public health policy approach. Public Health Rep 2000;115:12–24.

[19] Gale SK, Van Itallie TB, Faust IM. Effects of palatable diets on body weight and adipose tissue cellularity in the adult obese female Zucker rat (fa/fa). Metabolism 1981;30:105–10.

[20] Lillioja S, Bogardus C. Obesity and insulin resistance: lessons learned from the Pima Indians. Diabetes Metab Rev 1988;4:517–40.

[21] Ravussin E, Valencia ME, Esparza J, et al. Effects of a traditional lifestyle on obesity in Pima Indians. Diabetes Care 1994;17:1067–74.

[22] Saad MF, Knowler WC, Pettitt DJ, et al. The natural history of impaired glucose tolerance in the Pima Indians. N Engl J Med 1988;319:1500–6.

[23] Wilks R, McFarlane-Anderson N, Bennett F, et al. Obesity in peoples of the African diaspora. Ciba Found Symp 1996;201:37–48.

[24] Martorell R, Khan LK, Hughes ML, et al. Obesity in Latin American women and children. J Nutr 1998;128:1464–73.

[25] Lizarzaburu JL, Palinkas LA. Immigration, acculturation, and risk factors for obesity and cardiovascular disease: a comparison between Latinos of Peruvian descent in Peru and in the United States. Ethn Dis 2002;12:342–52.

[26] McKeigue PM. Metabolic consequences of obesity and body fat pattern: lessons from migrant studies. Ciba Found Symp 1996;201:54–64.

[27] French SA. Pricing effects on food choices. J Nutr 2003;133:841S–3S.

[28] Glanz K, Basil M, Maibach E, et al. Why Americans eat what they do: taste, nutrition, cost, convenience, and weight control concerns as influences on food consumption. J Am Diet Assoc 1998;98:1118–28.

[29] Sorensen LB, Moller P, Flint A, et al. Effect of sensory perception of foods on appetite and food intake: a review of studies on humans. Int J Obes 2003;27:1152–66.

[30] Report by the Kaiser Family Foundation. The role of media in childhood obesity. Available at: http://www.kff.org/entmedia/7030.cfm. Accessed May 5, 2004.

[31] Report by the American Psychological Association Taskforce. Television advertising leads to unhealthy habits in children. Available at: http://www.apa.org/releases/childrenads_summary.pdf. Accessed May 5, 2004.

[32] Centers for Disease Control and Prevention. Physical activity trends—United States: 1998. MMWR Morb Mortal Wkly Rep 2001;50:166–9.

[33] Blair SN, Nichaman MZ. The public health problem of increasing prevalence rates of obesity and what should be done about it. Mayo Clinic Proc 2002;77:109–13.

[34] Surface Transportation Policy Project. The 2002 summary of safe routes to school programs in the United States. New York: Transportation Alternatives; 2002.

[35] Brownson RC, Baker EA, Housemann RA, et al. Environmental and policy determinants of physical activity in the United States. Am J Public Health 2001;91:1995–2003.

[36] Saelens BE, Sallis JF, Black JB, et al. Neighborhood-based differences in physical activity: an environment scale evaluation. Am J Public Health 2003;93:1552–8.

[37] Huston SL, Evenson KR, Bors P, et al. Neighborhood environment, access to places for activity, and leisure-time physical activity in a diverse North Carolina population. Am J Health Promot 2003;18:58–69.

[38] Estabrooks PA, Lee RE, Gyurcsik NC. Resources for physical activity participation: does availability and accessibility differ by neighborhood socioeconomic status? Ann Behav Med 2003;25:100–4.

[39] Andersen RE, Franckowiak SC, Snyder J, et al. Can inexpensive signs encourage the use of stairs? Results from a community intervention. Ann Intern Med 1998;129:363–9.

[40] Brownell KD, Stunkard AJ, Albaum JM. Evaluation and modification of exercise patterns in the natural environment. Am J Psychiatry 1980;137:1540–5.

[41] Wing RR. Behavioral weight control. In: Wadden TA, Stunkard AJ, editors. Handbook for obesity treatment. New York: Guilford Press; 2002. p. 301–16.

[42] Wing RR, Hill JO. Successful weight loss maintenance. Annu Rev Nutr 2001;21:323–41.

[43] Dietz WH. Overweight in childhood and adolescence. N Engl J Med 2004;350:855–7.

[44] Ebbeling CB, Lawlak DB, Ludwig DS. Childhood obesity: public health crisis, common sense cure. Lancet 2002;360:473–82.

[45] Jeffery RW. Public health strategies for obesity treatment and prevention. Am J Health Behav 2001;25:252–9.

[46] Brownell KD. Get slim with higher taxes (editorial). New York Times. December 15, 2004: A29.

[47] Study conducted between 12/1/02 and 1/18/02 on The Status of Vending Machines, Schools and Physical Activity in KY Schools. Conducted by the University of Kentucky Cooperative Extension, Lexington Fayette Country Health Department, and the Kentucky Dept. of Public Health. Available at: http://www.cspinet.org/nutritionpolicy/status_of_vending_machines_school.pdf. Accessed October 20, 2004.

[48] Higgins M. Kraft to go lean, starve appetite for obesity suits. The Washington Times. July 2, 2003, p. A01.

[49] California Leaders Encouraging Activity and Nutrition. What it took to ban soft drinks in the LAUSD. Lean Times. November 2002.

[50] Edmundson EP, Guy S, Feldman HA, et al. The effects of the child and adolescent trial for cardiovascular health upon psychosocial determinants of diet and physical activity behavior. Prev Med 1996;25:442–54.

[51] McKenzie TL, Nader PR, Strikmiller PK, et al. School physical education: effect of the child and adolescent trial for cardiovascular health. Prev Med 1996;25:423–31.

[52] Lytle LA, Stone EJ, Nichaman MZ, et al. Changes in nutrient intakes of elementary school children following a school-based intervention: results from the CATCH study. Prev Med 1996;25:465–77.

[53] Mitka M. Economist takes aim at big fat US lifestyle. JAMA 2003;289:33–4.

[54] Jacobson MF, Brownell KD. Small taxes on soft drinks and snack foods to promote health. Am J Public Health 2000;90:854–7.

[55] French SA, Jeffery RW, Story M, et al. Pricing and promotion effects on low-fat vending snack purchases: the CHIPS study. Am J Public Health 2001;91:112–7.

SPECIAL ARTICLES

ELSEVIER
SAUNDERS

PSYCHIATRIC
CLINICS
OF NORTH AMERICA

Psychiatr Clin N Am 28 (2005) 255–274

Neuroleptic-induced Movement Disorders: An Overview

Perminder S. Sachdev, MD, PhD, FRANZCP

School of Psychiatry, University of New South Wales, Sydney NSW 2052, Australia
Neuropsychiatric Institute, Prince of Wales Hospital, Barker Street,
Randwick NSW 2031, Australia

Movement disorders commonly are associated with many psychotropic drugs. Tricyclic antidepressants often cause a tremor in the hands and myoclonic jerks. In some patients, they result in agitation and restlessness, referred to as the jitteriness syndrome [1]. Occasional anecdotes of dyskinesia and dystonia have been reported with these drugs, but tardive dyskinesia typically is not associated with tricyclics, with the possible exception of amoxapine [2]. Movement disorders are reported somewhat more commonly with serotonin-specific reuptake inhibitors (SSRIs), including mild parkinsonian symptoms, dystonia, dyskinesia, and akathisia. There have been some reports of irreversible dyskinesia and dystonia with these drugs [3]. Lithium most commonly is associated with a peripheral tremor, which is usually a mild action tremor, but becomes coarse when toxic levels are reached. Lithium produces myoclonus less often, and is also known to exacerbate the parkinsonian adverse effects of neuroleptics. Stimulants are associated with stereotypes, dyskinesia, tremor, dystonia, and myoclonus. Anticonvulsants (eg, phenytoin or carbamazepine) are associated with dyskinesia, tremor, and tics, and in toxic doses will produce nystagmus, ataxia, and dysarthria. Anticholinergic drugs can exacerbate dyskinesias. Of course there many other drugs used in medicine that may cause disorders of movement, and the reader is referred to some recent publications on this topic [4–6].

The overwhelming concern of psychiatrists is with neuroleptic-induced movement disorders (NIMD). These may be categorized on the basis of the temporal relationship to neuroleptic use (acute and delayed or tardive) or their characteristics (hyperkinetic or hypokinetic, sometimes referred to as positive or negative). Acute NIMDs include acute dystonia, akathisia,

---

E-mail address: p.sachdev@unsw.edu.au

0193-953X(05)/$ - see front matter © 2005 Elsevier Inc. All rights reserved.
doi:10.1016/j.psc.2004.10.004

parkinsonism, and neuroleptic malignant syndrome. The typical tardive syndrome is tardive dyskinesia (TD), although several related syndromes have been described.

Acute neuroleptic-induced movement disorders

Acute dystonia

A dystonia is an involuntary movement in which the muscle action is sustained at the point of maximal contraction for at least a short period. The movements are typically slow, but rapid dystonia, referred to as myoclonic dystonia, has been described [7]. The disconnection between the agonist action and the reflex antagonist inhibition often results in a twisting distortion of the affected part, with sustained abnormal postures. The symptomatology is varied, with common manifestations being torticollis, retrocollis, tongue protrusion, opening or closing of the jaw, facial grimacing, limb torsion, opisthotonus, or rolling the eyes upwards, sometimes with deviation to the side (oculogyric crisis). The sudden occurrence of a muscle spasm is often very frightening to the patient, thereby presenting as a medical emergency, although it is in most cases not dangerous. The exception is the occasional occurrence of a laryngopharyngeal spasm that may compromise respiration and may even cause death. Dystonias, and in particular oculogyric crises, may be preceded by prodromal symptoms such as restlessness, anxiety, irritability, or an exacerbation of psychosis, which sometimes may be so severe that the movement disorder itself may be ignored by the patient and the clinician [8].

Although acute neuroleptic-induced dystonia is common, its incidence is determined greatly by the type of drug used, dosage, route of administration, and age of the individual. Although reported rates of acute dystonia vary from 2.3% [9] to over 90% [10], high-potency drugs such as haloperidol generally produce acute dystonia in 30% to 40% of cases. The rates are lower with atypical neuroleptics, and clozapine does not appear to produce acute dystonia. The incidence increases with dose, but this has an inverted U-shaped relationship. Most dystonias occur within 2 to 3 days of the initiation or significant increment in dose of neuroleptic, and parenteral administration increases the risk. They also may occur after the abrupt discontinuation of anticholinergic medication within the first few weeks of initiating neuroleptics. Children and young adults appear to have greater risk, and males develop it twice as often as females. Some coexisting conditions, such as hypocalcemia, hyperthyroidism, and hyperparathyroidism, or recent cocaine use have been reported as risk factors in several case series. The pathophysiology of acute dystonia is understood incompletely, with the focus having been on dopaminergic mechanisms. Arguments have been presented for acute dopamine antagonism (DA hypofunction hypothesis) and a compensatory increase in dopamine release leading to mismatch (DA hyperfunction hypothesis) [11].

Acute dystonia is generally easy to treat. In the acute situation, the parenteral administration of benztropine, benzhexol, biperiden, procyclidine or other anticholinergic drug, or the antihistaminic/anticholinergic diphenhydramine, is usually effective in 15 to 20 min, although a second treatment may be necessary after 30 min. If it is less severe, oral medication may be sufficient. This will need to be continued for a further 24 to 48 hours to avoid a recurrence. Prophylactic use of anticholinergic drugs to prevent dystonia is controversial, but in a high-risk patient, they may be used for 7 to 14 days when neuroleptics are first initiated, after which they can be discontinued slowly over a few days.

Acute neuroleptic-induced akathisia

The syndrome of akathisia (from Greek, literally unable to sit) has come to refer to the development of restlessness seen most commonly as an acute adverse effect of neuroleptics, although other drugs such as the selective serotonin reuptake inhibitors (SSRIs), calcium channel antagonists also may produce it. Additionally, it may develop as a tardive syndrome [12]. Most investigators agree that there are two aspects to akathisia: a subjective report of restlessness or inner tension, particularly referring to the legs, with a consequent inability to maintain a posture for several minutes; and the objective (or observational) manifestations of restlessness in the form of semipurposeful or purposeless movements of the limbs, a tendency to shift body position in the chair while sitting, or marching on the spot while standing [13]. There is disagreement about the relative importance of these two aspects [14,15], with emphasis on the subjective component (akathisia as a mental disorder) or the objective component (akathisia as a movement disorder) by different investigators. A combination of the two has been argued as being necessary for a definite diagnosis [15] (ie, akathisia as both mental and movement disorder). A less certain diagnosis (probable or possible) of akathisia sometimes may be made if either the subjective or the objective features, but not both, are present (Box 1). Even when fairly characteristic features of akathisia are present, and the clinical situation is appropriate for the diagnosis, a clinical decision often must be made to distinguish it from anxiety or agitation or restlessness caused by other causes.

The urge to move in akathisia may be unrelenting and may preoccupy the person's thinking. Mild cases often can be detected by asking patients if they have difficulty in checking out at supermarkets, cooking a meal while standing, or sitting to watch television. Lying down provides some relief for most patients, contrasting akathisia from restless legs syndrome. The sensations in the legs usually are localized deep inside, and paresthesia are uncommon. Akathisia first may become apparent when a patient refuses medication, and it has been recognized as an important cause of noncompliance in schizophrenic patients [16]. Some patients may experience

---

Box 1. Research diagnosis of drug-induced akathisia [12]

Prerequisites (necessary for all diagnoses)
A history of exposure to drugs known to cause akathisia
    (antypsychotics can cause all subtypes; nonantipsychotics can
    cause acute akathisia and chronic akathisia, acute onset)
Presence of characteristic subjective or objective features of
    akathisia
Absence of other known causes of akathisia (eg, restless legs
    syndrome, Parkinson's disease, subthalamic lesion) and
    absence of peripheral neuropathy, myelopathy, or myopathy

Diagnoses[a]
Acute akathisia (antipsychotic or non-antipsychotic
    drug-induced; if has a duration of at least 3 months,
    categories as chronic akathisia, acute-onset)
Tardive akathisia (if has a duration of at least 3 months,
    categorize as chronic akathisia, tardive onset)
Withdrawal akathisia (if has a duration of at least 3 months,
    categorize as chronic akathisia, withdrawal onset)
Chronic akathisia (acute, tardive or withdrawal onset; state if
    patient is not receiving antipsychotics)

---
[a] State if only subjective or objective features are present.

---

their internal distress in the form of apprehension, irritability, impatience, or general unease. Others may exhibit fear, anxiety, terror, anger or rage, vague somatic symptoms, an exacerbation of psychosis, or as sexual torment. There has been some recent debate on the relationship between akathisia and aggressive, self-destructive, or suicidal behavior, and case reports of violence [17] and suicidal behavior attributed to akathisia have been published [18].

Akathisia usually develops within a few days of the initiation or increment in dose or change to high-potency neuroleptic, with most cases developing in the first 2 weeks. With conventional neuroleptic drugs, rates reported vary from 8% to as high as 76% [19]. A conservative estimate is 20% to 30%, but this rate is significantly affected by treatment-related variables and other variables. The risk with atypical neuroleptics is lower but not absent, and the published evidence for this is inconsistent because of the problems of carryover effects and equivalent doses not always being used. The risk increases with higher drug doses, rapid increment of the dosage, and higher potency of the drug. The development of parkinsonism also increases the likelihood of akathisia developing, although the latter may occur first, or concurrently, with the parkinsonism. The role of sociodemographic factors and other treatment-related variables is modest. The presence of psychiatric disorder is not necessary for akathisia to develop, but certain organic brain disorders may increase the vulnerability. Although some evidence exists that iron deficiency may be a predisposing factor, this is far from established, and its role is likely to be minor. The literature on akathisia in childhood and adolescence is scant, although akathisia has been reported, especially in Tourette's disorder patients treated with neuroleptics [20].

Akathisia is difficult to treat, and its prevention or modification through the appropriate use of neuroleptics is the most important strategy. Drugs that are used to treat akathisia include anticholinergics, β-adrenergic antagonists, and benzodiazepines, although the effect of the latter is probably nonspecific. There is a suggestion that anticholinergics may be more effective in those who have associated parkinsonian symptoms. Sometimes a combination of an anticholinergic drug and a β-blocker may be necessary. The reader is referred to a recent article for a more detailed discussion of management [21].

Neuroleptic-induced parkinsonism

Sometimes referred to as pseudoparkinsonism, the symptoms of neuroleptic-induced parkinsonism are clinically indistinguishable from Parkinson's disease and comprise rigidity, bradykinesia, tremor at rest, and postural instability. Patients develop a poverty of spontaneous, generally automatic, movements. The face appears masked; there may be drooling of saliva. The posture is flexed, and speech becomes slow and lacking in intonation. The initial symptom may be a tremor or muscle stiffness, and reduce arm swing and increased muscle tone are obvious on examination. With the exception of seborrhea (and sialorrhea), autonomic symptoms are usually not present. The symptoms are usually bilateral but may be asymmetrical.

Parkinsonism develops later than dystonia or akathisia, although most people develop it in the first week of neuroleptic treatment or dose increment [9]. It is the adverse effect related most clearly to dopamine antagonism. It is therefore dose-related and more prevalent with high-potency drugs. Increasing age, and possibly female gender, are other risk factors [22]. Drugs with an intrinsic anticholinergic property have a lower propensity. The rate of dose increment is also important, suggesting the development of some tolerance with time. It is reversible with the cessation of the drug, although this may take many months, especially after the use of depot neuroleptics. In the elderly, however, persistence of parkinsonian symptoms occurs in a proportion; it was 11% at 1 year after neuroleptic cessation in one study [23].

The development of parkinsonism once was considered to be a necessary condition of antipsychotic drug action, until the introduction of so-called atypical neuroleptics, with clozapine as the flag-bearer. What makes a neuroleptic atypical is debated, but the essential characteristic of these drugs is the lack of parkinsonian adverse effects at therapeutic doses. There appears to be more than one mechanism by which this occurs: antagonism of dopamine (D2) and serotonin (S2) receptors, rapid dissociation from binding with dopamine receptors, relative specificity for limbic rather than striatal dopamine receptors, intrinsic anticholinergic action, and other mechanisms. This atypical character is lost if the dose is increased above a certain threshold (eg, greater than 6 mg/day in the case of risperidone). Recent neuroimaging studies have suggested that there may a window of dopamine D2 receptor blockade at which antipsychotic effect is induced without parkinsonian symptoms. This may be between 60% and 80% of receptors. With haloperidol, at the usual therapeutic dose, more than 90% of D2 receptors are blocked; with atypical drugs, this is about 70% to 80%, with clozapine being less than 60% to 70% [24,25].

The emergence of neuroleptic-induced parkinsonism is managed best by a modification of the antipsychotic regimen. If this cannot be achieved, anticholinergic drugs are the main intervention. There is no clear evidence that any one anticholinergic is superior to the others, although M1 selectivity is the property that would be desirable. Drugs are to be used only if parkinsonism is clearly manifest, and their prophylactic use is best avoided. L-dopa and directly acting dopamine agonists do not appear to be effective in neuroleptic-induced parkinsonism, although data on this question are limited. Amantadine may have a role, especially if anticholinergics are unsuccessful or not tolerated.

Neuroleptic malignant syndrome

Although uncommon, neuroleptic malignant syndrome (NMS) is the most serious adverse effect of neuroleptics, and it is potentially fatal. The principal features are hyperthermia, muscle rigidity, alteration in consciousness, and autonomic dysfunction [26,27]. Fever may be low-grade to higher than 42°C. Rigidity, which may be described as lead-pipe or cogwheel, is present in more than 90% of cases and may be so severe as to lead to rhabdomyolysis. Patients often are agitated, but they may become mute and catatonic. Confusion and delirium are common, and these in severe cases may progress to stupor or coma. Autonomic features commonly present are diaphoresis, pallor or flushing of the skin, tachycardia, lability of blood pressure, hypertension or hypotension, arrhythmia, tachypnea, dyspnea, and urinary incontinence. Movement disorders associated with NMS include bradykinesia, tremor, dystonia (blepharospasm, opisthotonus, oculogyric crises, trismus, chorea [including oro-buccal dyskinesia]), and myoclonus. Rarely, seizures, ataxia, nystagmus, and reflex changes may occur. The symptoms are acute in onset, and the full syndrome usually develops within 24 to 48 hours of the onset.

Laboratory findings are nonspecific but useful in supporting the diagnosis. The most important is a rise in creatine kinase (CK), which may vary from greater than 200 to several thousand IU/L. A rise in CK in the absence of clinical features of NMS is not enough to make a diagnosis. Two- to threefold rises in CK levels are not uncommon after neuroleptic administration, but rises above 1000 IU/L suggest caution, and such patients should be monitored for clinical signs of NMS. CK levels are useful in the follow-up of patients. Polymorphonuclear leukocytosis is another consistent finding. Less common findings are elevated liver cell enzymes, hypocalcemia, hypomagnesemia, hypoferremia, proteinuria, and myoglobinuria.

The diagnosis of NMS is a clinical one and relies on the exclusion of other causes of fever, rigidity, and altered sensorium, although the acute development of these symptoms in a patient on neuroleptics always should arouse the suspicion of NMS. It is not certain how many features are necessary for a diagnosis. Most sets of criteria for NMS need the presence of rigidity and fever for a definite diagnosis, but patients have been described who lacked one of more of the features. These may well be forme fruste of the syndrome, and a dimensional approach to NMS has been advocated by some authors [28]. All neuroleptic drugs, including clozapine, may cause NMS. The risk appears to be greatest in patients who are agitated and compromised medically through dehydration and malnutrition, especially if they are treated with large doses of parenterally administered neuroleptics over short periods to control their agitation [27,29]. Severely disturbed male manic patients often fit this description.

Neuroleptic malignant syndrome is not confined to psychiatric patients. Any patient treated with neuroleptics runs the risk of NMS. The reported incidence is variable, with rates varying from 0.1% to 2% [30,31]. This range may depend on the differences in the definition of the disorder and prescribing practices. Although most patients develop it at the time of initiation of neuroleptics, it may occur after a change in drug or dose, or in patients on stable medication because of an intercurrent illness or sometimes for no obvious cause. Parkinson's disease patients on dopaminergic drugs (L-dopa or directly acting dopamine agonists) can develop a NMS-like syndrome if the drug is stopped suddenly. A similar syndrome can develop in cocaine users. NMS resembles some other disorders, which must be considered in the differential diagnosis. Malignant hyperthermia (MH), a genetically determined, myopathic disorder can be differentiated by a history of exposure to inhalant anesthetics and depolarizing muscle relaxants rather than neuroleptics. Lethal catatonia resembles NMS in its presentation but occurs in the absence of exposure to neuroleptics.

Once it develops, NMS progresses rapidly and often leads to medical complications that may be respiratory (pneumonia or pulmonary embolism), cardiovascular (arrhythmia or cardiac arrest), renal (myoglobinuria, azotemia, and failure) or neurological (movement disorders or cognitive failure). Mortality was reported in 11% to 30% in earlier series, but this figure has decreased progressively with early detection and management. The pathogenesis of NMS is not understood fully, but a central dopamine shutdown is the most prevalent current theory [32].

When NMS is suspected, treatment should be prompt, with the immediate cessation of any neuroleptic medication, and the institution of supportive treatment for dehydration, fever, metabolic abnormalities, and any complications. Most mild cases do not need any other measures. Drugs that have been found to be useful in some cases include the dopamine agonists (bromocriptine, amantadine, or pergolide) and muscle relaxants (dantrolene sodium). Benzodiazepines are used for the management of agitation. Anticholinergic drugs are best avoided. Electroconvulsive therapy may be life-saving in severe cases, and the use of anesthetic agents and muscle relaxants (such as succinylcholine) is considered safe [33].

Tardive neuroleptic-induced movement disorders

The term dyskinesia (literally abnormal movement) is a generic term that refers to a range of movement abnormalities. In the case of TD, the movements are choreiform, athetoid, dystonic, stereotypic, or a combination of these. They most commonly involve the oro-buccal, lingual, and facial muscles, especially in older individuals. The lingual involvement in the form of fine vermicular movements of the tongue while it is sitting at the base of the oral cavity is a common and early feature. Dyskinetic blinking may be another early sign of TD. Lip smacking, puckering or pouting, chewing, jaw clenching or mouth opening, facial grimacing, blowing, blepharospasm, and frowning are also common features. The limbs and trunk often are involved, and the involvement of the respiratory muscles has been uncommonly reported. The fingers may display stereotypic movements, especially when held in extension, as if the patient is piano playing. Stereotypic leg movements are often present. Truncal movements are in the form of lateral, posterior or irregular neck movements, shoulder shrugging, twisting, flexion or extension of the trunk and pelvic rotation, or thrusting. Respiratory muscle involvement manifests in the form of irregular breathing, belching and grunting sounds, whistling or sucking, and aerophagia. Abdominal and pharyngeal muscles may be involved rarely [34].

The orobuccal-lingual-facial (OBLF) musculature is involved in three-quarters of affected individuals, the limbs in one-half and the trunk in up to a quarter, with all three groups being affected in about 10% [35]. The OBLF involvement is typical of the elderly, and limb-truncal (LT) involvement is more likely in the young. Although the movements are choreoathetoid, which are recognized to be characteristic of TD, neuroleptic-induced tardive movements may sometimes be dystonic, akathisic, tic-like, myoclonic, or tremorous in character. This has led to a debate between the 'lumpers' and 'splitters' (ie, those who include all these different movements within the rubric of TD, and those who make a distinction between TD and other tardive syndromes such as tardive dystonia [TDt], tardive akathisia, tardive tics, or Tourette's syndrome) (Box 2).

The movements of TD typically fluctuate in intensity over time, increase with emotional arousal, decrease with relaxation, and disappear during sleep. They also decrease when the affected muscles are used for voluntary activity. Distracting tasks, such as finger tapping or mental arithmetic, tend to exaggerate the movements and bring out movements that may otherwise be latent. Poor dental status may exaggerate oral movements in some patients. In mild cases, the patient may be unaware of the movements. The movements of TD have a variable response to medication. Neuroleptics, with the possible exception of clozapine, are recognized to suppress the movements. Increasing the dose of the offending drugs may, therefore, suppress the movements. Anticholinergic drugs, on the other hand, usually aggravate TD. These responses are, however, often unpredictable.

Tardive dyskinesia develops after a person has been on neuroleptics for months to years. The *Diagnostic and Statistical Manual of Mental Disorders, Fourth Edition* requires exposure of at least 3 months, but TD may occur as early as one month in elderly individuals. The onset may be while the patient is still on neuroleptics or within a few weeks of their withdrawal. The latter (withdrawal-emergent dyskinesia) may remit spontaneously or go on to become persistent. The onset is usually gradual, and the disorder is mild except for withdrawal dyskinesias, which can be severe from the early stages.

Box 2. Neuroleptic-induced tardive subsyndromes

Movement disorders
Tardive dyskinesia (TD)
- Oro-buccal-lingual-facial (OBLF) syndrome
- Limb-truncal (LT) syndrome
- Mixed

Tardive akathisia (TA)
Tardive dystonia (TDt)
Tardive tics and Tourette's syndrome (TTS)
Tardive myoclonus (TMyo)
Tardive tremor (TTrem)
Tardive parkinsonism (TPark)

*Behavioral syndromes**
Supersensitivity psychosis (SP)
Tardive dysmentia (TDem)
Tardive dysbehavior (TBeh)

---

* The status of the behavioral syndromes is uncertain.

Spontaneous dyskinesias

Dyskinesias, in particular oro-facial movements, have been reported to occur in some individuals with no exposure to neuroleptics and no neuroleptic disorder. They are more common in the elderly, with one study reporting prevalence rates of 0.8%, 6.0%, and 7.8% in the sixth, seventh, and eighth decades of life of otherwise healthy subjects [36]. Kane et al [37] reported a rate of 4.0% in healthy elderly (mean age 73 years) subjects. The prevalence is higher in psychogeriatric patients and those in institutions who have not received neuroleptics. It is particularly high in patients with dementia [38].

Is dyskinesia a feature of schizophrenia?

The occurrence of "peculiar, sprawling, irregular, choreiform, out-spreading movements" in schizophrenic patients were noted by Kraepelin [39]. Many studies have investigated neuroleptic-naive schizophrenic patients and reported rates of dyskinesia that vary from nil [40] to as high as 53% [41], with rates of 1% to 7.6% reported in first-episode schizophreniform psychosis. These movements usually are described as grimacing, tic-like, or stereotypic, but oro-facial dyskinesias and choreiform movements are observed less commonly. These findings have raised the argument that dyskinesias may be intrinsic to the pathophysiology of schizophrenia, and that neuroleptics serve to enhance the process.

Epidemiology

The prevalence of TD has been investigated extensively, and 76 published studies were reviewed by Yassa and Jeste [42]. The rates ranged from 3% to 70%, with a median rate of about 24% in patients on chronic neuroleptic treatment. The higher rates likely were reported in the elderly. Most TD is mild. The study by Woerner et al [43] is noteworthy for its attempt to address some of the methodological issues. The overall prevalence in neuroleptic-treated individuals was 23.4%, of which 3.8% had another neuro-medical illness that might have had an etiological role, thus giving a conservative prevalence rate of 19.6%. In the same study, when a group of patients with no evidence of TD was withdrawn from neuroleptic drugs and examined weekly for 3 weeks, 34% developed emergent dyskinesia. Rates of withdrawal-emergent dyskinesia of 8% [44] and 51% [45] have been reported in two studies of children on long-term neuroleptics. High rates have been reported in elderly patients on neuroleptics [46,47]. High rates also have been reported in neuroleptic-treated individuals with mental retardation [48,49].

Given the difficulties inherent in prevalence estimates, it has been much more rewarding to examine the incidence of TD in newly medicated patients followed longitudinally (Tables 1, 2). These studies suggest that the

Table 1
Summary of longitudinal studies of incidence of tardive dyskinesia in schizophrenia patients

Authors	N	Years	Risk/year	5-year risk
Gibson, 1981 [68]	343	3	5.6%	24.4%
Kane et al, 1984 [69]	554	7	3.9%	17.8%
Yassa & Nair, 1984 [70]	108	2	3.9%	17.8%
Chouinard et al, 1986 [71]	131	5	8.7%	35.1%
Morgenstern & Glazer, 1993 [72]	398	5	8.7%	35.1%
Jeste et al, 1995[a] [73]	266	3	20%	>60%
Chakos et al, 1996[b] [74]	118	4	5.2%	19.5%
Caligiuri et al, 1997[c] [75]	378	3	7.6%	22.9%
Woerner et al, 1998[a] [76]	261	3	17.6%	53%

[a] Elderly neuropsychiatric patients.
[b] First-onset schizophrenic patients followed-up.
[c] Severe tardive dyskinesia only.

cumulative incidence of TD increases with increasing duration of neuroleptic treatment, at a rate of about 3% to 5% per year for the first several years, to reach a plateau at about 20% to 25%, but new cases continue to occur many years after drug initiation. It is difficult to identify a point of time after which the risk decreases. The incidence is much higher in elderly individuals [50].

Natural history

For most people, TD does not become progressively worse, and when it does get worse, it generally tends to show a fluctuating course with some spontaneous remissions. In a 5-year follow-up study of Bergen et al [51], 24% showed a fluctuating course; 11% improved, and 7% worsened. From 5 to 10 years, about 50% of patients demonstrate a reduction in symptoms of at least 50%. The outcome is more favorable in the young, and if drug treatment can be stopped [52]. Improvement can be expected to continue for many years after neuroleptics have been ceased. The prognosis of withdrawal-emergent dyskinesia is more favorable, with over 75% showing improvement in 3 months [35].

Risk factors

Advancing age is the most consistently established risk factor for TD, and there appears to be a linear correlation between age and both the prevalence and severity of TD [53]. Although female gender has not emerged consistently as a risk factor in recent studies, there may be a female excess in elderly TD sufferers. Some ethnic differences, with higher rates in African Americans and lower rates in Chinese and other Asian populations, have been reported, the basis for which is not understood clearly.

Several investigators have commented on a higher relative incidence of TD in patients with affective disorder treated long-term with neuroleptics,

Table 2
Comparative studies on risk of tardive dyskinesia among various neuroleptics

Authors	Studies	Population	N	Duration	Outcome
Rosenheck et al, 1997 [77]	Randomised, double-blind comparative study of clozapine versus haloperidol	Treatment-refractory schizophrenia	423	1 year	Significant reduction in AIMS in clozapine-treated group
Beasley et al, 1999 [78]	Double blind maintenance phases of three acute studies of olanzapine versus haloperidol	Schizophrenia, schizoaffective and schizophreniform psychosis	174	2.6 years	Pooled data analysis: 1-year risk for tardive dyskinesia with olanzapine (0.52%) versus haloperidol (7.45%)
Tran et al, 1997 [79]	Randomised, double-blind study of olanzapine versus risperidone	Schizophrenia, schizoaffective and schizophreniform psychosis	339	28 weeks	Tardive dyskinesia as according to Schooler and Kane criteria: olanzapine (4.6%) versus risperidone (10.7%)
Jeste et al, 1999 [80] Copolov et al, 2000 [81]	Risperidone versus haloperidol Randomised double-blind study of quetiapine versus haloperidol	Chronic and subchronic schizophrenia	122 448	9 months 6 weeks	Significant improvement in AIMS score in quetiapine-treated group
Conley et al, 2001 [82]	Randomised double-blind study of olanzapine versus risperidone	Schizophrenia and schizoaffective disorder	337	8 weeks	No significant difference in dyskinesia item total score of the Extrapyramidal Symptom Rating Scale

Abbreviation: AIMS, Abnormal Involuntary Movements Scale.

but this finding is inconsistent, and may apply to early- and not late-onset TD. Kane et al [54] reported incidence figures of 26% for affective and schizoaffective disorders and 18% for schizophrenia. In schizophrenic patients, a family history of affective illness is reported to increase the risk. Depression may, furthermore, produce a state-dependent exacerbation of TD [55], while mania may lead to the reverse. Whether schizophrenia increases or decreases the risk for TD is not known. Within schizophrenia, those with the negative syndrome, or evidence of cognitive impairment and neurological deficits, are reported to be more at risk [56], and the presence of TD indicates a poorer prognosis for schizophrenia. The presence of brain damage (as evidenced by epilepsy, head trauma, or dementia) has been suggested as a risk factor, but the evidence is inconsistent. TD is known to develop in Tourette's syndrome patients treated with neuroleptics, but the prevalence rate, though not well-studied, is likely to be lower than that seen in schizophrenia, possibly because of the youth of the patients and the small neuroleptic doses used [57]. There has been recent interest in variables such as smoking, alcohol abuse, and diabetes as risk factors. A recent study found that alcohol/drug abuse increased the risk of TD by threefold [58]. Diabetics have an increased risk of spontaneous dyskinetic movements (21% in the study by Ganzini et al [59]) and TD (79% in diabetics versus 53% in nondiabetics) [59]. Woerner et al [60] reported a risk ratio of 2.3 for diabetics exposed to neuroleptic compared with nondiabetics, with the risk greater in aged diabetics. Alcoholics and smokers have an increased prevalence of spontaneous dyskinesias and TD [61]. It has been suggested that patients who are more prone to develop acute extrapyramidal adverse effects with neuroleptics are also at a higher risk of TD [62]. Genetic factors have been studied. An intriguing finding is that heterozygous carriers of mutated alleles of the CYP2D6 gene have an increased susceptibility to TD [63]. An association between TD and a dopamine D3 receptor gene variant also has been reported [64].

Recent longitudinal studies have shown that drug dose and duration of exposure are very important. The prevalence increases with duration of exposure as new cases are added, but this may reach a plateau after about 5 years. Whether drug type is important has remained controversial. There is no convincing evidence that once drug dosage has been accounted for, any of the conventional neuroleptics presents a differentially smaller risk; nor is there empirical evidence that depot neuroleptics are more likely to cause TD [35]. The evidence in relation to the newer atypical drugs is still preliminary but suggests that these drugs may present a lower risk for TD. Although TD has been reported with risperidone, olanzapine, quetiapine, sulpiride, and amisulpride, there is no convincing report of TD with clozapine monotherapy, and this may indeed be the safest drug [35]. Anticholinergic drugs are known to exaggerate TD or make latent TD become manifest, but there is no convincing evidence they are risk factors for TD per se [35]. Lithium is not known to increase the risk.

Pathophysiology

The pathophysiology of TD is not understood completely. Much of the traditional conceptualization of the disorder has been guided by the causative role of antipsychotic and other dopamine (DA) antagonists. This resulted in the proposal of the dopamine supersensitivity hypothesis of TD [65], which states that the chronic administration of DA antagonists leads to the development of postsynaptic DA receptor supersensitivity, thereby producing the hyperkinetic state of TD. This hypothesis is compatible with many clinical and laboratory observations, but it has limitations. Observations in animal models do not parallel clinical observations, as DA supersensitivity in rats develops rapidly (often after a single injection) and persists for only a short period after cessation of the DA antagonist drug. Supersensitivity in animals declines after desensitization with DA agonists, but these drugs are not effective in treating TD. Moreover, supersensitivity in animals is almost invariable, whereas TD develops only in a fraction of patients. DA supersensitive rats do not exhibit a behavioral change, which has to be brought out by challenging them with dopaminomimetic drugs. Rats that do develop an analog of TD continue to show the movements after DA supersensitivity has disappeared. There is no direct evidence of DA supersensitivity in TD patients, either from postmortem studies, cerebrospinal fluid studies, or radioligand imaging studies using positron emission tomography. DA-mediated endocrine function is not different in TD subjects from non-TD controls. The effects of DA agonists and antagonists are also inconsistent in TD patients. Moreover, the DA hypothesis does not explain the spontaneous occurrence of dyskinesia in many schizophrenic and healthy subjects and the increased risk with age and many other host factors.

The inadequacy of the DA hypothesis has led to the consideration of many other pathophysiological models. In relation to other neurotransmitters that are affected by neuroleptics, some attention has been given to changes in norepinephrine (NE), serotonin (5HT), and acetylcholine (ACh), but changes in γ-amino butyric acid (GABA) are considered to be the most salient for the development of TD [66]. Reduced activity in a subgroup of striatal GABA neurones has been suggested as the basis of TD, and this is supported by evidence from work in animals and in people [67].

Finally, the neurodegeneration hypothesis of TD has been presented. Free radical and excitatory mechanisms are brought into place by the increased turnover of DA and related mechanisms because of neuroleptic action. These lead to neurotoxicity and cell death, particularly of the GABA-ergic striatal neurones, because of the high levels of catecholamine turnover and oxidative metabolism in the striatum. This leads to the disinhibition of the lateral pallidal neurones and consequently the hyperkinetic state of TD, the manifestation of which is influenced by the prevalent dopaminergic tone. Withdrawal of DA antagonism will lead to the expression of a latent hyperkinetic state, whereas DA blockade produces the reverse. The DA receptor antagonism of neuroleptics is therefore important in the pathogenesis of TD, but the mediating mechanisms are multiple and DA receptor supersensitivity may be only one, and not the pre-eminent, aspect of this (Fig. 1).

Management

No effective treatment for TD is available, although several drugs have been tried, based on the still preliminary understanding of its pathophysiology. The primary strategy in its management remains preventative. Once TD becomes established, attempts are made to minimize its symptoms and reduce ongoing risk factors for the worsening of the disorder over time. The treatment strategies are summarized in Box 3.

Future directions

There are many lacunae in our understanding of TD, which explains why rational therapy or effective preventative strategies are not available. The increasing use of atypical neuroleptics has made it necessary that the epidemiology of TD be revisited, with the expectation that the newer drugs

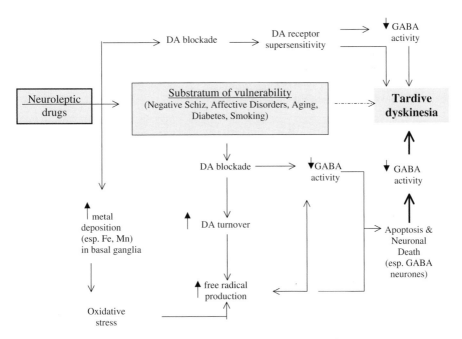

Fig. 1. Pathogenetic mechanisms for tardive dyskinesia.
Abbreviations: DA, dopamine; GABA, gamma amino butyric acid; Fe, iron; Mn, manganese.

Box 3. Drugs used in the treatment of tardive dyskinesia*

Dopaminergic:
• Antagonists:
Catecholamine depleters
Atypical neuroleptics: clozapine, risperidone, olanzapine
Other catecholamine depleters: AMPT
Classical neuroleptics: agonists–bromocriptine, L-dopa,
    apomorphine, piribedil, amphetamine, L-deprenyl

GABA-ergic drugs
Benzodiazepines, valproate, gamma-vinyl GABA, baclofen

Antinoradrenergic drugs
Propranolol, clonidine

Cholinergic drugs
Physostigmine
Deanol, choline, lecithin

Serotonergic drugs
L-tryptophan, 5-hydroxy tryptophan, cyproheptadine

Other
Lithium carbonate
Ca channel antagonists: verapamil, diltiazem, nifedipine

---

* Catecholamine depleters (eg, tetrabenazine) and GABA-ergic drugs (eg,
valproate, baclofen, clonazepam) are used most frequently. Dopamine agonists,
cholinergic drugs and serotonergic drugs are usually ineffective. Antiadrenergic
drugs have only a small role.

---

will provide new insights into its pathophysiology. TD, therefore, continues to present itself as a natural experiment to study the pathophysiology of movement disorders. Its careful study also may provide a window on the underlying neurobiology of schizophrenia. Longitudinal studies of patients who receive atypical neuroleptics as their primary treatment from the first episode of psychosis onwards are necessary to assess the incidence of TD with these drugs. The current hypotheses for its pathogenesis need further empirical support and refinement so that they can be translated into treatment strategies. The subsyndromes of TD should be investigated further for their risk factors and pharmacological properties. More antipsychotic drugs need to be developed that are devoid of extrapyramidal adverse effects and carry little or no risk of producing an irreversible neurological disorder.

Acknowledgments

Angie Russell assisted with manuscript preparation.

References

[1] Pohl R, Yeragani VK, Ortiz A. Response of tricyclic-induced jitteriness to a phenothiazine in two patients. J Clin Psychiatry 1986;47:427.

[2] Lapierre YD, Anderson K. Dyskinesia associated with amoxapine antidepressant therapy: a case report. Am J Psychiatry 1983;140:493–4.

[3] Arya DK. Extrapyramidal symptoms with selective serotonin reuptake inhibitors. Br J Psychiatry 1994;165:728–33.

[4] Sethi KD, editor. Drug-induced movement disorders. New York: Marcel Dekker; 2003.

[5] Jankovic JJ, Tolosa E, Scott-Conner CEH, editors. Parkinson's disease and movement disorders. New York: Lippincott Williams & Wilkins; 2002.

[6] Owens DCG. A guide to the extrapyramidal side-effects of antipsychotic drugs. Cambridge (UK): Cambridge University Press; 1999.

[7] Obeso JA, Rothwell JC, Lang AE, et al. Myoclonic dystonia. Neurology 1983;33:825–30.

[8] Sachdev P, Tang WM. Psychotic symptoms preceding ocular deviation in a patient with tardive oculogyric crises. Aust N Z J Psychiatry 1992;26:324–31.

[9] Ayd FJ. A survey of drug-induced extrapyramidal reactions. JAMA 1961;175:1054–60.

[10] Boyer WF, Bakalar NH, Lake CR. Anticholinergic prophylaxis of acute haloperidol-induced dystonic reactions. J Clin Psychopharmacol 1990;13:565–8.

[11] Marsden CD, Jenner P. The pathophysiology of extrapyramidal side effects of neuroleptic drugs. Psychol Med 1980;10:55–72.

[12] Sachdev P. Akathisia and restless legs. New York: Cambridge University Press; 1995.

[13] Sachdev P, Kruk J. Clinical characteristics and risk factors for acute neuroleptic-induced akathisia. Arch Gen Psychiatry 1994;51:963–74.

[14] Stahl SM. Akathisia and tardive dyskinesia. Changing concepts. Arch Gen Psychiatry 1985; 42:915–7.

[15] Sachdev P. Research diagnostic criteria for drug-induced akathisia: a proposal. Psychopharmacology (Berl) 1994;114:181–6.

[16] Van Putten T, Crumpton E, Yale C. Drug refusal in schizophrenia and the wish to be crazy. Arch Gen Psychiatry 1976;33:1443–6.

[17] Keckich WA. Neuroleptics. Violence as a manifestation of akathisia. JAMA 1978;240:2185.

[18] Shear MK, Frances A, Weiden P. Suicide associated with akathisia and depot fluphenazine treatment. J Clin Psychopharmacol 1983;3:235–6.

[19] Van Putten T, May PR, Marder SR. Akathisia with haloperidol and thiothixene. Arch Gen Psychiatry 1984;41:1036–9.

[20] Bruun RD. Subtle and under-recognized side effects of neuroleptic treatment in children with Tourette's disorder. Am J Psychiatry 1988;145:621–4.

[21] Sachdev P. Acute and tardive akathisia. In: Sethi KD, editor. Drug-induced movement disorders. New York: Marcel Dekker; 2003. p. 129–64.

[22] Freyhan FA. Psychomotility and parkinsonism in treatment with neuroleptic drugs. Arch Neurol Psychiatry 1957;78:465–72.

[23] Stephen PJ, Williamson J. Drug-induced parkinsonism in the elderly. Lancet 1984;2(8411): 1082–3.

[24] Nyberg S, Farde L, Halldin C. A PET study of 5HT2 and D2 dopamine receptor occupancy induced by olanzapine in healthy subjects. Neuropsychopharmacology 1997;16:1–7.

[25] Kapur S, Zipurski R, Remington G, et al. PET evidence that loxapine is an equipotent blocker of 5HT2 and D2 receptors: implications for the therapeutics of schizophrenia. Am J Psychiatry 1997;154:1525–9.

[26] Addonizio G, Sussman VL, Roth SD. Neuroleptic malignant syndrome: review and analysis of 115 cases. Biol Psychiatry 1987;22:1004–20.

[27] Sachdev P, Mason C, Hadzi-Pavlovic H. A case controlled study of neuroleptic malignant syndrome. Am J Psychiatry 1997;154:1156–8.

[28] Adityanjee MD, Singh S, Singh G, et al. Spectrum concept of neuroleptic malignant syndrome. Br J Psychiatry 1988;313:1293.

[29] Keck PE, Pope HG, Cohen BM, et al. Risk factors for neuroleptic malignant syndrome: a case-controlled study. Arch Gen Psychiatry 1989;46:914–8.

[30] Keck PE, Pope HG, McElroy SL. Frequency and presentation of neuroleptic malignant syndrome: a prospective study. Am J Psychiatry 1987;144:1344–6.

[31] Gelenberg AJ, Bellingham B, Wojcik JD, et al. A prospective survey of neuroleptic malignant syndrome in short-term psychiatric hospital. Am J Psychiatry 1988;145:517–8.

[32] Henderson VW, Wooten GF. Neuroleptic malignant syndrome: a pathogenetic role for dopamine receptor blockade? Neurology 1981;31:132–7.

[33] Trollor J, Sachdev P. Electroconvulsive treatment of neuroleptic malignant syndrome: review and report of cases. Aust N Z J Psychiatry 1999;33(5):650–9.

[34] Jeste DV, Wyatt RJ. Understanding and treating tardive dyskinesia. New York: Guildford Press; 1982.

[35] Kane JM, Jeste DV, Barnes TRE, et al. Tardive dyskinesia: a task force report of the American Psychiatric Association. Washington (DC): American Psychiatric Press; 1992.

[36] Klawans HL, Barr A. Prevalence of spontaneous lingual-facial-buccal dyskinesias in the elderly. Neurology 1982;32:558–9.

[37] Kane JM, Weinhold P, Kinon B, et al. Prevalence of abnormal involuntary movements (spontaneous dyskinesias) in the normal elderly. Psychopharmacology (Berl) 1982;77:105–8.

[38] Waddington JL, Crow TJ. Abnormal involuntary movements and psychosis in the preneuroleptic era and in unmedicated patients: implications for the concept of tardive dyskinesia. In: Wolf ME, Mosnaim A, editors. Tardive dyskinesia: biological mechanisms and clinical aspects. Washington (DC): American Psychiatric Press; 1988. p. 49–66.

[39] Kraepelin EP. Dementia praecox and paraphrenia. Edinburgh: E&S Livingston; 1919.

[40] Chorfi M, Moussaoui D. Les schizophrenes jamais traites n'ont pas de movements anormaux type dyskinesie tardive. Encephale 1985;11:263–5.

[41] Owens DGC, Johnstone EC, Frith CD. Spontaneous disorders of involuntary movement. Arch Gen Psychiatry 1982;39:643–50.

[42] Yassa R, Jeste DV. Gender differences in tardive dyskinesia: a critical review of the literature. Schizophr Bull 1992;18:701–15.

[43] Woerner M, Kane JM, Lieberman J, et al. The prevalence of tardive dyskinesia. J Clin Psychopharmacol 1991;11:34–42.

[44] McAndrew JB, Case Q, Treffert DA. Effects of prolonged phenothiazine intake on psychotic and other hospitalized children. J Autism Child Schizophr 1972;2:75–91.

[45] Polizos P, Engelhardt D. Dyskinetic prehomena in children treated with psychotropic medications. Psychopharmacol Bull 1978;14:65–8.

[46] Paulsen JS, Caligiuri MP, Palmer B, et al. Risk factors for orofacial and lmtruncal tardive dyskinesia in older patients: a prospective longitudinal study. Psychopharmacology (Berl) 1996;123:307–14.

[47] Byne W, White L, Parella M, et al. Tardive dyskinesia in a chronically institutionalized population of elderly schizophrenic patients: prevalence and association with cognitive impairment. Int J Geriatr Psychiatry 1998;13:473–9.

[48] Gualtieri CT, Schroeder SR, Hicks RE, et al. Tardive dyskinesia in young mentally retarded individuals. Arch Gen Psychiatry 1986;43:335–40.

[49] Sachdev PS. Drug-induced movement disorders in institutionalized adults with mental retardation: clinical characteristics and risk factors. Aust N Z J Psychiatry 1992;26:242–8.

[50] Jeste DV, Caliguiri MP, Paulsen JS, et al. Risk of tardive dyskinesia in older patients: a prospective longitudinal study of 266 patients. Arch Gen Psychiatry 1995;52:756–65.

[51] Bergen JA, Eyland EA, Campbell JA, et al. The course of tardive dyskinesia in patients with long-term neuroleptics. Br J Psychiatry 1989;154:523–8.

[52] Casey DE, Gardos G. Tardive dyskinesia: outcome at 10 years. Schizophr Res 1990;3:11 [abstract].

[53] Smith JM, Baldessarini RJ. Changes in prevalence, severity and recovery in tardive dyskinesia with age. Arch Gen Psychiatry 1980;37:1368–73.

[54] Kane JM, Woerner M, Weinhold P, et al. Incidence of tardive dyskinesia: five-year data from a prospective study. Psychopharmacol Bull 1984;20:39–40.

[55] Sachdev PS. Depression-dependent exacerbation of tardive dyskinesia. Br J Psychiatry 1989; 155:253–5.

[56] Waddington JL, Youssef HA, Dolphin C, et al. Cognitive dysfunction, negative symptoms, and tardive dyskinesia in schizophrenia. Arch Gen Psychiatry 1987;44:907–12.

[57] Glazer VM. Clinical outcomes of pharmacotherapy for schizophrenia and implications for health economics. Journal of Clinical Psychiatry Monographs 1997;15:22–3.

[58] van Os J, Fahy T, Jones P, et al. Tardive dyskinesia: who is at risk? Acta Psychiatr Scand 1997;6:206–16.

[59] Ganzini L, Heintz RT, Hoffman WF, et al. The prevalence of tardive dyskinesia in neuroleptic-treated diabetics. Arch Gen Psychiatry 1991;48:259–63.

[60] Woerner MG, Saltz BL, Kane JM, et al. Diabetes and development of tardive dyskinesia. Am J Psychiatry 1993;150:966–8.

[61] Nilsson A, Waller L, Rosengren A, et al. Cigarette smoking is associated with abnormal involuntary movements in the general male population—a study of men born in 1933. Biol Psychiatry 1997;41:717–23.

[62] Kane J, Woerner M, Borenstein M. Integrating incidence and prevalence of tardive dyskinesia. Psychopharmacol Bull 1986;22:254–8.

[63] Andreassen OA, MacEwen T, Gulbrandsen AK, et al. Nonfunctional CYP2D6 alleles and risk for neuroleptic-induced movement disorders in schizophrenic patients. Psychopharmacology (Berl) 1997;131:174–9.

[64] Steen VM, Lovlie R, MacEwan T, et al. Dopamine D3-receptor gene variant and susceptibility to tardive dyskinesia in schizophrenia. Mol Psychiatry 1997;2:139–45.

[65] Klawans HL, Goetz CG, Perlik S. Tardive dyskinesia: review and update. Am J Psychiatry 1980;137:900–8.

[66] Gerlach J, Casey DE. Tardive dyskinesia. Acta Psychiatr Scand 1988;77:369–78.

[67] Gunne LM, Haggstrom JE, Sjokvist B. Association with persistent neuroleptic-induced dyskinesia of regional changes in the brain GABA synthesis. Nature 1984;309:347–9.

[68] Gibson AC. Incidence of tardive dyskinesia in patients receiving depot neuroleptic injection. Acta Psychiatr Scand 1981;297:111–6.

[69] Kane JM, Woerner M, Weihold P, Wegner J, Kinon B, Borenstein M. Incidence of tardive dyskinesia: five-year data from a prospective study. Psychopharmacol Bull 1984;20: 387–9.

[70] Yassa R, Nair V, Schwartz G. Tardive dyskinesia: a two-year follow-up study. Psychosomatics 1984;25:852–5.

[71] Chouinard G, Annable L, Mercier P, et al. A five-year follow-up study of tardive dyskinesia. Psychopharmacol Bull 1986;22:259–63.

[72] Morgenstern H, Glazer WM. Identifying risk factors of tardive dyskinesia among long-term outpatients maintained with neuroleptic medications. Results of the Yale Tardive Dyskinesia Study. Arch Gen Psychiatry 1993;50:723–33.

[73] Jeste DV, Caliguiri MP, Paulsen JS, et al. Risk of tardive dyskinesia in older patients: A prospective longitudinal study of 266 patients. Arch Gen Psychiatry 1995;52:756–65.

[74] Chakos MH, Alvir JMJ, Woerner MG, et al. Incidence and correlates of tardive dyskinesia in first episode of schizophrenia. Arch Gen Psychiatry 1996;53:313–9.

[75] Caligiuri MP, Lacro JP, Rockwell E, et al. Incidence and risk factors for severe tardive dyskinesia in older patients. Br J Psychiatry 1997;171:148–53.

[76] Woener MG, Alvir JMJ, Saltz BL, et al. Prospective study of tardive dyskinesia in the elderly: rates and risk factors. Am J Psychiatry 1998;155:1521–8.

[77] Rosenheck R, Cramer J, Xu W, et al. A comparison of clozapine and haloperidol in hospitalized patients with refractory schizophrenia. N Engl J Med 1997;12:809–15.

[78] Beasley CM, Dellva MA, Tamura RN, et al. Randomised double-blind comparison of the incidence of tardive dyskinesia in patients with schizophrenia during long-term treatment with olanzapine or haloperidol. Br J Psychiatry 1999;174:23–30.

[79] Tran PV, Hamilton SH, Kuntz AJ, et al. Double-blind comparison of olanzapine versus risperidone in the treatment of schizophrenia and other psychotic disorders. J Clin Psychopharmacol 1997;17:407–18.

[80] Jeste DV, Lacro JP, Bailey A, et al. Lower incidence of tardive dyskinesia with risperidone compared with haloperidol in older patients. J Am Geriatr Soc 1999;47:716–9.

[81] Copolov DL, Link CGG, Kowalcyk B. A multi-centre, double-blind, randomised comparison of quetiapine (ICI 204,636, 'Seroquel') and haloperidol in schizophrenia. Psychol Med 2000;30:95–105.

[82] Conley RR, Mahmoud R. A randomized double-blind study of risperidone and olanzapine in the treatment of schizophrenia or schizoaffective disorder. Am J Psychiatry 2001;158: 765–74.

ELSEVIER
SAUNDERS

Psychiatr Clin N Am 28 (2005) 275–290

PSYCHIATRIC
CLINICS
OF NORTH AMERICA

Huntington's Disease and Related Disorders

Karen E. Anderson, MD

*Department of Psychiatry; Maryland Parkinson's and Movement Disorders Center,
Movement Disorders Division, University of Maryland, School of Medicine,
Room N4W49A, 22 South Greene Street, Baltimore, MD 21201, USA*

Disorders affecting movement long have been of interest to neurologists because of the often dramatic disturbances of normal coordination, gait, abnormal movements, and other physical symptoms seen with these conditions. The behavioral symptoms associated with these conditions, however, have received relatively little study. As those who study behavior have become more involved in working with these patients, it has become apparent clinically that behavioral symptoms are often as severe, or more so, than motor impairment. This article provides an overview of these conditions, focusing on behavioral symptoms, along with review of other pertinent clinical data. Huntington's disease (HD), a disorder caused by expanded trinucleotide repeats that has received the most clinical and investigative attention, is discussed in detail. Other conditions that should be considered in the differential diagnosis of a patient with chorea and behavioral symptoms are reviewed, including the autosomal dominant spinocerebellar ataxias, Wilson's disease, and neuroacanthocytosis. Several other conditions, some of which have associated psychiatric and cognitive symptoms, should be considered in the workup of a patient with chorea of unknown etiology, perhaps accompanied by psychiatric or cognitive changes. These include: cerebral palsy, medication-related chorea, lupus, chorea gravidarum, Sydenham's chorea, polycythemia vera, hyperthyroidism, chorea following toxin exposure, and cerebral vascular accidents leading to acute hemi–chorea/ballismus, which generally are caused by an infarct of the subthalamic nucleus. Basic tests for the work-up of chorea of undetermined cause are shown in Box 1.

E-mail address: kanderson@psych.umaryland.edu

0193-953X/05/$ - see front matter © 2005 Elsevier Inc. All rights reserved.
doi:10.1016/j.psc.2004.10.001   *psych.theclinics.com*

Box 1. Tests commonly used in evaluation of chorea of unknown origin

Complete blood cell count with differential
Urine toxin screen
Electrolytes, liver function tests
Ceruloplasmin level
Thyroid function tests
Genetic testing, including Huntington's, spinocerebellar ataxias*
Antinuclear antibodies, antistreptolysin O antibodies, reactive
   plasma reagin

---

 * Genetic counseling is important in cases where these disorders are suspected.

Huntington's disease

Huntington's disease, an inherited, progressive neurodegenerative disorder, is probably the best known of the trinucleotide repeat diseases. Symptoms of HD include abnormal movements, cognitive impairment leading to dementia, and psychiatric illness. Its autosomal dominant pattern of inheritance was recognized first by George Huntington in his classic paper describing the disorder [1]. Prevalence of HD is estimated at approximately 5 cases per 100,000 people. The disorder is seen less commonly among those of non-European ancestry [2]. Typically, onset is in the 30s or 40s, although onset as early as age 2 and well into the 80s has been reported [3,4].

Clinical features

Neurological abnormalities include involuntary movements (chorea and dystonia) and disorders of voluntary movement (gait disorders, impairment of saccades and smooth pursuit, dysarthria, and swallowing impairment). These symptoms worsen gradually over the course of 10 to 15 years, leading in most cases to severe disability. Chorea, the rapid and involuntary movements that are the hallmark of the disease, tends to worsen in the middle stages of the illness and then decreases as the patient becomes more debilitated. Dystonia, contraction of large muscle groups, worsens as the disease progresses. Later symptoms of HD include bradykinesia and rigidity (see Box 2). Patients with juvenile-onset HD, sometimes called the Westphal variant, with onset of symptoms before age 20, may have a differing clinical picture. These patients have Parkinsonism, increased frequency of seizures and myoclonus, and little chorea, making diagnosis challenging in the absence of family history. Progression of disease in juvenile-onset cases is extremely rapid. Those patients with onset later in life generally have

---

Box 2. Progression of neurological symptoms in Huntington's disease

Early
Chorea
Abnormal saccades, impaired smooth pursuit
Impairment of fine motor coordination

Mid to Late
Dystonia
Rigidity
Dysarthria
Gait impairment
Swallowing abnormalities

---

a slowly progressive course of illness with cognition relatively spared. These patients sometimes are misdiagnosed as having a Parkinsonian syndrome [5].

Genetics and disease mechanism

HD is caused by an abnormal expansion of trinucleotide repeats coding for glutamine at the N-terminus of the huntingtin protein [6]. The increase occurs in sequences of cytosine, adenine, and guanine (CAG) in exon 1 of the HD gene on chromosome 4. The gene, known as IT 15, which regulates production of huntingtin, is found throughout the body [7]. The normal function of huntingtin is unknown, but it may include protective effects for neurons, or antiapoptosis [8]. Several theories exist as to how neuronal damage and death occur in HD. Excitotoxic effects of glutamatergic transmission, mitochondrial dysfunction, and dysregulation of CREB-binding protein-mediated gene expression have been proposed [9–11]. The role of the nuclear inclusions, protein aggregates that are found in the neuronal intranuclear spaces in HD, is also unclear. The neuronal inclusions may represent attempts by the neuron to degrade abnormal huntingtin, or could be part of a protective response [12–14].

The HD gene is transmitted as an autosomal dominant trait, so that each child of an affected individual has a 50% chance of inheriting the gene. Normal individuals have between 9 and 29 CAG repeats on IT15. Those who develop HD have a higher number of repeats, usually greater than 40. The CAG repeat number is correlated inversely with age of disease onset. Those with juvenile-onset HD have a repeat size of 50 or more [15]. Rate of disease progression increases with higher repeat number [16]. No individual with 35 or fewer CAG repeats has been known to develop HD symptoms.

Those who have an HD gene with 36 to 39 repeats may develop the symptoms of HD, and they generally have a later onset if symptoms do become clinically apparent. They are, however, at risk of transmitting the disorder to subsequent generations, because the repeats expand in each successive generation. Paternal transmission tends to produce greater CAG expansion than maternal transmission [17]. Research is ongoing regarding the risk of those with 26 to 35 repeats passing on an expanded trinucleotide repeat to their offspring. Rare cases of pedigrees with disorders phenotypically similar to HD but deriving from a different CAG expansions have been reported recently [18–20].

Genetic counseling at a certified testing program is recommended by the Huntington's Disease Society of America (HDSA) for those seeking presymptomatic testing for the HD gene [21]. The HDSA also recommends that minors not be tested, except in extenuating circumstances. During counseling, individuals should be urged to explore the impact of positive or negative genetic test results on decisions regarding marriage, childbearing, and also the potential impact on other family members who may be at risk for HD. Adverse outcomes, including precipitation of major psychiatric illness, have occurred following genetic testing for HD [22]. Patients who have clinically apparent symptoms of HD but seek genetic testing for confirmation of the diagnosis also can benefit from genetic counseling before testing, as can family members.

Neuropathology

The characteristic neuropathology in HD is the decline in the number of medium spiny neurons in the striatum [23,24]. Caudate changes are the most impressive, but cell death also occurs in the globus pallidus. Volumetric MRI studies have demonstrated that degree of striatal degeneration correlates significantly with CAG repeat number [25]. Receptor studies of HD patients have found reductions in striatal dopamine receptor binding [26,27]. As the disease advances, widespread atrophy occurs in the caudate, frontal lobes, putamen, and other regions [28,29].

Cognitive symptoms

Deficits are generally reported to occur in visuospatial, memory, and executive task performance in detailed neuropsychological studies of HD patients. Visuospatial problems may be some of the earliest changes [30–32]. Deficits in recall and slowed rates of learning are also reported [33–36]. Free recall improves with cued recall and recognition [33,37,38]. Retention is relatively normal in HD; this is often cited as a useful method with which to differentiate HD from cortical dementia, such as Alzheimer's Disease (AD), on neuropsychological testing [33,37,39]. HD patients show a decrease in use of strategies such as semantic clustering to enhance memory performance [33,40]. Executive dysfunction also is reported consistently in studies of HD patients on various types of tasks, including planning and sequencing [41,42], working memory [43], and set shifting [30,34]. Procedural memory also is impaired, as is seen in tests of skill and motor learning [44].

Psychiatric symptoms

Psychiatric symptoms may occur in early, middle, or late stages of HD; they can thus predate the onset of motorical impairment. Unlike the somewhat predictable progression of memory and functional impairment, they have not been shown to follow a clear time course [45], with severity of these symptoms varying throughout the course of illness in individual patients. CAG repeat length has not been shown to correlate positively with age of onset of psychiatric symptoms or with presence of psychiatric disorders [46,47]. Psychiatric symptoms add greatly to the burden of caregivers, distress suffered by patients, and they often contribute to decisions to institutionalize patients [48]. The impairment in executive function probably contributes greatly to psychiatric morbidity in HD by resulting in decreased flexibility and problems in changing behavior to suit an evolving environment. Dysfunction of fronto–striatal pathways are implicated in the development of many psychiatric symptoms in HD, including impulsivity, apathy, depression, and obsessive–compulsive disorder (OCD) [49]. There is some work suggesting that apathy may correlate with progression of cognitive and motor symptoms [50]. Other symptoms that have received extensive study in HD, such as depression and irritability, have not been shown reliably to correlate with progression of the disease [45,46]. Many HD patients with psychiatric symptoms respond to standard pharmacotherapy; lower dosing ranges generally are recommended when starting treatment. A review by Anderson and Marder summarizes the limited research on treatment of behavioral symptoms in HD [51].

Over half of all HD patients will display irritable behavior at some point in the illness, making it a common symptom. This often is accompanied by aggression [49,52,53]. A study of HD patients and caregivers at centers across the United States, found that over 60% reported aggressive behavior on the part of the patient [53]. Over a third of HD patients in nursing homes were found to be aggressive in a retrospective study [54]. Irritability responds to pharmacotherapy in many cases, and behavioral interventions also may prove helpful.

Apathy is reported in over 50% of HD patients [52], and it has been shown to increase with duration of illness [55,56]. It also may be correlated positively with progression of cognitive and motor impairment, which could be related to fronto–striatal changes affecting cognition, especially in planning and sequencing tasks [50]. Apathy is often difficult to differentiate from depression, especially as the disease progresses and communication becomes challenging because of dysarthria or cognitive impairment.

Generally, apathy is more distressing to caregivers than to patients. There is little treatment that has been found to be effective for apathy, although structuring daily activities may be useful. Education of family members to promote reasonable expectations of patient behavior is often the most beneficial intervention.

Up to 50% of HD patients have an affective disorder at some point in the illness, with depression as the predominant condition. Depression may occur at any point in the illness, including prodromally. Brain imaging data suggest this could be because of disruption of frontal–striatal circuitry [57]. Suicide rates in HD are elevated compared with the general population. Rates from 3% to 7% have been reported, with over 25% of patients making suicide gestures [58].

The prevalence of mania and hypomania also are increased in HD. From the limited data available, mania appears to be found at a frequency of 5% [59]. Folstein et al reported episodes of mania or hypomania in 10% of patients [3].

Anxiety disorders have received relatively little study in HD. Older studies report anxiety as a frequent prodromal symptom [60]. Obsessive and compulsive symptoms have been found to occur with high frequency in HD patients. Twenty percent to 50% of HD patients have been reported to have obsessive or compulsive symptoms, depending on the measure used for assessment [53,61]. The possible relationship of obsessive and compulsive symptoms to frontal–striatal changes in HD is supported by positron emission tomography (PET) studies in primary OCD showing orbitofrontal or caudate hypermetabolism, which decreases in response to successful treatment [62]. Obsessions and compulsions also are seen with increased frequency in other illnesses affecting basal ganglia, including Tourette's syndrome, basal ganglia lesions, and Sydenham's chorea [63–65].

Psychotic symptoms are seen in 3% to 12% of patients [59]. High rates of psychosis and actual schizophrenia reported in older studies of patients in psychiatric hospitals may have been misleading, and newer work suggests the frequency of psychosis is probably closer to 3% [66,67]. Some data suggest psychotic symptoms result from hyperdopaminergic states interacting with abnormal basal ganglia circuitry [48].

Treatment

There is no proven treatment to prevent HD symptom onset or slow disease progression. Animal models being used to investigate possible therapeutic agents include transgenic mice and models created with *Drosophilia* and *C elegans* [67]. Research is underway to investigate agents that have shown a potential neuroprotective effect in animal models. These agents include creatine, which has been shown to slow disease progression in mice [68,69], and minocycline, a caspase inhibitor with beneficial effects in mouse models [70]. Coenzyme Q10, remacimide, and lamotrigene, have been studied for their potential to reduce oxidative stress [71,72]. None of these agents has been proven to be clinically useful in people. Treatment of chorea is not recommended, unless the chorea is extremely disabling, because the dopamine blocking agents used to suppress chorea may worsen other symptoms of HD. Treatment of psychiatric symptoms is extremely important and can greatly improve quality of life in these patients and their caregivers. Other measures to improve quality of life and maintain function in HD patients include physical therapy, speech and swallowing assessments and therapy, and dietary interventions, including increase in calories to maintain weight and modification of food to prevent choking.

Spinocerebellar ataxias

Autosomal dominant spinocerebellar ataxias (SCAs) are estimated to occur in the general population with an incidence of 5 in 100,000 [73,74]. Other hereditary ataxias show autosomal recessive (including Friedreich ataxia) or X-linked inheritance. The autosomal dominant SCAs, which originally were classified by associated symptoms, now increasingly are grouped by genetic etiology. Similar to HD, several of the spinocerebellar ataxias (SCAs) with autosomal transmission are caused by expanding CAG repeats that code for polyglutamines. SCAs characterized by abnormal protein polyglutamine expansions include SCAs 1,2,3 (Machado-Joseph disease), 7, and 17 [75]. As with HD, expansions of the repeat may occur in successive generations, leading to earlier onset of disease. There is a question in these SCAs, as in HD, of whether polyglutamine expansion causes gain or loss of function leading to disease pathology [76]. All of these SCAs are caused by abnormal CAG repeats, which manifest a threshold effect of polyglutamine expansion dose necessary to cause disease. Common brain areas affected include basal ganglia, brainstem nuclei, cerebellum, and spinal motor nuclei, along with distinct regions in each condition. There are other SCAs with differing mechanisms of pathogenesis, including channelopathies, gene expression disorders, which occur when repeat expansions occur outside of coding regions and may affect gene products, and those of unknown etiology [75].

Genetic counseling for autosomal dominant SCAs follows a model similar to that described for HD, understanding the limited ability of any genetic test to predict disease course [77]. There is no treatment to slow progression or prevent onset of symptoms in any of the SCAs. The hope is that future treatments developed for HD also will prove useful in similar neurodegenerative disorders, including the SCAs, and especially those caused by abnormal trinucleotide repeat expansions.

General clinical manifestations of the various autosomal dominant SCAs include ataxia, dysarthria, difficulty with fine motor tasks, Parkinsonism, ocular abnormalities, rigidity, and spasticity. Motor and behavioral signs and symptoms differ across the different SCAs, as do rates of disease progression [78]. SCA-3, Machado-Joseph disease, is the most common ataxia in the world with an autosomal dominant pattern of inheritance. First reported in Portuguese families, it has been described in diverse ethnic groups [74,79].

Dementia is reported in several of the SCAs, and psychiatric symptoms are seen in some patients, although this area has received little attention clinically or from researchers. In the most extensive study of behavioral symptoms in SCAs to date, Leroi et al [80] compared 31 patients with degenerative cerebellar disease with 21 HD patients. The degenerative cerebellar disease group included patients with sporadic and hereditary cerebellar disease. There were 20 SCA patients in the cerebellar group, including 11 sporadic cases and nine with a familial pattern of inheritance. The remaining patients with cerebellar degeneration had multi-system atrophy (five patients) or SCA with unknown etiology. Almost 80% of patients with cerebellar degeneration had psychiatric disorders, a frequency similar to that seen in the HD group, although the symptoms tended to be less severe in the cerebellar patients. Mood disorders and personality change were prominent symptoms in both patient groups. Cognitive impairment, including dementia, was seen in almost 20% of patients with cerebellar degeneration, compared with over 70% of HD patients. Mild dementia, resembling that seen in HD, has been reported in other work with hereditary ataxia patients [81]. Psychotic disorders were seen in 10% of patients with cerebellar degeneration, but not in the HD group. The authors noted that animal and human data suggest the cerebellum may modulate cognitive and emotional behavior [82,83]. These data confirm results from an older study of hereditary ataxia of all types, which found psychiatric disorders in 23% of patients [84]. Thus, although research has not focused specifically on autosomal dominant SCAs, data suggest that at the very least mild psychiatric symptoms and signs of cognitive impairment occur in a substantial number of these patients.

Wilson's disease

Wilson's disease, hepatolenticular degeneration, is one of the better known hereditary conditions that cause a movement disorder and behavioral symptoms. It may be confused with HD if the initial symptoms are neurological, although chorea is not a common neurological manifestation of Wilson's disease. Despite its relatively low prevalence, estimated at 17 cases per million of the population [85], it is an important disorder to consider in patients with unexplained movements and behavioral change, because, unlike the other disorders reviewed here, symptoms can be arrested and even reversed with early treatment. Inheritance of Wilson's disease is in an autosomal recessive pattern, and it is caused by mutations of the gene ATP7B on chromosome 13q14.3. This leads to a dysfunction in hepatic copper metabolism, with excess copper deposition throughout the body, especially in the liver and basal ganglia [86]. Because multiple mutations of the gene have been reported, genetic testing is not commercially available for Wilson's disease. Presentation of Wilson's disease may be hepatic, neurological, or psychiatric, with a diverse array of symptoms. Kayser-Fleischer rings from corneal copper deposition are only present in a few patients who manifest hepatic disease, but they are seen in most patients with neurological disease [87].

The diagnosis of Wilson's disease is made by measurement of ceruloplasmin, which is low, and 24-hour urinary cooper levels, which are elevated. These changes do not occur in all cases, and a liver biopsy to test for hepatic copper levels should be obtained for confirmation of the diagnosis [88]. Wilson's disease is treated with anticopper agents. Neurological, hepatic, and behavioral symptoms should be addressed during treatment. Early diagnosis and treatment are vital to ensure optimal benefits [89,90]. Penicillamine is the treatment of choice, but other agents may be used if penicillamine is not tolerated because of adverse effects or toxicity [91,92].

Early neurological manifestations of Wilson's disease include tremor and dysarthria, both of which are generally mild. As the disease progresses, other symptoms include bradykinesia, Parkinsonism, or ataxia [87,88]. Chorea is seen in childhood-onset cases, but it is not a common symptom in adults [93]. Hepatic changes include hepatomegaly, hepatitis, and cirrhosis. Several secondary systematic symptoms also may occur in patients with hepatic symptoms. If left untreated, patients become bedridden and completely dependent on others for care. Death occurs anywhere from a few months to 5 years following onset of symptoms in untreated cases.

Patients with Wilson's disease often have behavioral changes as part of the illness, sometimes predating the development of other symptoms. In a third of patients, behavioral changes are the major initial symptom. Personality changes, including irritability, cognitive impairment, and affective disorders are the most commonly seen behavioral symptoms in Wilson's disease [89,90,94]. Many other symptoms have been reported, including psychosis, aggression, catatonia, and anxiety [95]. The risk of suicide in these patients is elevated, and suicide gestures have been reported to occur in up to 16% of patients [96]. Psychiatric symptoms may improve with anticopper therapies. Psychotropic medications may be helpful, but they should be used cautiously because of hepatic abnormalities, which may affect their metabolism.

Neuroacanthocytosis

Neuroacanthocytosis is a broad term for several rare multi-system hereditary conditions associated with neurological symptoms and behavioral abnormalities. Because of the combination of chorea, behavioral changes, and also striatal degeneration seen on imaging in these patients, diagnostic confusion with HD may occur in cases where a family history is questionable or incomplete. Acanthocytosis is a term derived from the Greek word for thorn, referring to the distinctive appearance of erythrocytes seen in these disorders. The clinical manifestations, genetics, and molecular pathology of these conditions are discussed in detail in a recent review by Rampoldi et al [97]. There are three major classes of neuroacanthocytosis: chorea–acanthocytosis, abetalipoproteinemia, and McLeod syndrome, although acanthocytosis may be seen in other neurological disorders. Dysarthria, areflexia, and neuropathy are clinical symptoms of all three of the major classes of neuroacanthocytosis, while only chorea–acanthocytosis and McLeod syndrome have associated hyper- and hypo-kinetic movements. All three conditions show striatal degeneration on radiological studies, which may be misinterpreted as HD [97].

Chorea–acanthocytosis is an autosomal recessive disorder characterized by progressive chorea, dysphagia, orofaciolingual dyskinesia, dysarthria, areflexia, seizures, and dysarthria [98]. Elevated serum creatine kinase levels and myopathy are common, although these abnormalities, along with areflexia caused by peripheral neuropathy, also are seen in McLeod syndrome. Motor tics also may occur, and later in the disorder, the movement symptoms may evolve into Parkinsonism [99]. Among reported behavioral symptoms are dementia, executive impairment, and psychiatric symptoms [100]. The small studies to date have found that cognitive impairment is seen in 70% of patients, and psychiatric symptoms affect 60% of patients [101]. Psychiatric symptoms may include affective disorders, lability, anxiety disorders, and paranoia. In a study of neuropsychiatric symptoms in 10 patients, symptoms similar to those seen in HD were found, including apathy and impairment of executive function, suggesting frontal lobe dysfunction [102].

McLeod syndrome is an X-linked disorder. Female carriers, however, may show mild symptoms. Chorea, peripheral neuropathy, and areflexia are common clinical manifestations of the disorder. In some cases, the condition may resemble chorea–acanthocytosis. Abnormal expression of Kell blood group antigens and a permanent hemolytic state are seen in patients with this form of neuroacanthocytosis [100]. Behavioral changes are reported to occur in almost half of these patients. These are similar to those seen in HD and chorea–acanthocytosis and may include impairment of memory and executive function, emotional lability, depression, and hallucinations. Additionally, anxiety symptoms, including compulsions, have been reported to occur in patients with this condition, although these symptoms usually are seen later in the disorder, and this estimate is based on a small number of cases [103]. The similarities between HD, chorea–acanthocytosis, and McLeod syndrome have led some authors to suggest that dysfunction in these diseases may be caused by damage to a final common pathway [100].

The final major class of neuroacanthocytosis is abetalipoproteinemia. Patients with this autosomal recessive condition show a fat-soluble vitamin deficiency and fat intolerance, because of missing serum lipoproteins containing apolipoprotein B [104]. It is associated with a progressive spinocerebellar ataxia, with peripheral neuropathy. Retinopathy with loss of vision also may occur. Chorea and other indications of striatal involvement are not reported in these patients, despite PET studies indicating striatal degeneration, which is caused by vitamin E deficiency in this condition [105]. Behavioral changes are not generally characteristic of this disorder.

Summary

Numerous conditions are known to produce movement abnormalities, including chorea, along with cognitive and psychiatric symptoms. HD has received the most clinical and research attention, in part because of the availability of precise genetic testing, but commercial genetic tests are available for several other conditions, including SCAs. Genetic testing is helpful in some trinucleotide repeat disorders, but the impact of testing on the patient and family should be assessed. Degeneration of the basal ganglia is seen in several of these conditions, and may account for some of the behavioral changes, especially deficits in impulse control, motivation, and executive function, along with motor symptoms. Because many of the conditions discussed can present with similar motor and behavioral symptoms, a careful family history, examination, and select use of laboratory tests may be needed if the diagnosis is in question. Psychiatric symptoms are common in these disorders, and may cause comparable disability to that caused by the movement disorder itself. There is little research on treatment of psychiatric conditions in these disorders, but standard therapies may be useful and should be tried if necessary.

References

[1] Huntington G. On chorea. Medical Surgical Reports 1872;26:320–1.
[2] Folstein SE, Chase GA, Wahl WE, et al. Huntington's disease in Maryland: clinical aspects of racial variation. Am J Hum Genet 1987;41:168–79.
[3] Folstein SE, editor. Huntington disease: a disorder of families. 1st edition. Baltimore (MD): The Johns Hopkins Press; 1989.
[4] Gilstad J, Reich SG. Chorea in an octogenarian. Neurologist 2003;9(3):165–6.
[5] Reuter I, Hu MTM, Andrew TC, et al. Late onset levodopa responsive Huntington's disease with minimal chorea masquerading as Parkinson plus syndrome. J Neurol Neurosurg Psychiatry 2000;68:238–41.
[6] Huntington's Disease Collaborative Research Group. A novel gene containing a trinucleotide repeat that is expanded and unstable on Huntington's disease chromosomes. Cell 1993;72:971–83.
[7] Strong TV, Tagle DA, Valdes JM, et al. Widespread expression of the human and rat Huntington's disease gene in brain and non-neural tissues. Nat Genet 1993;5:259–65.
[8] Rigamonti D, Bauer JH, De-Fraja C, et al. Wild-type huntingtin protects form apoptosis upstream of caspase-3. J Neurosci 2000;20:3705–13.

[9] Difiglia M. Excitotoxic injury of the neostriatum is a model for Huntington's disease. Trends Neurosci 1990;13:286–9.

[10] Beal MF. Does impairment of energy metabolism result in excitotoxic neuronal death in neurodegenerative illnesses? Ann Neurol 1992;31:119–30.

[11] Nucifora FC Jr, Sasaki M, Peters MF, et al. Interference by huntingtin and atrophin-1 with cbp-mediated transcription leading to cellular toxicity. Science 2001;291(5512):2423–8.

[12] Davies SW, Turmaine M, Cozens BA, et al. Formation of neuronal intranuclear inclusions underlies the neurological dysfunction in mice transgenic for HD mutation. Cell 1997;90: 537–48.

[13] Ferrigno P, Silver PA. Polyglutamine expansions: proteolysis, chaperones, and the dangers of promiscuity. Neuron 2000;26:9–12.

[14] Ordway JM, Tallaksen-Greene S, Gutekunst CA, et al. Ectopically expressed CAG repeats caused intranuclear inclusions and a progressive late onset neurological phenotype in the mouse. Cell 1997;91:753–63.

[15] Duyao M, Ambrose C, Myers R, et al. Trinucleotide repeat length instability and age of onset in Huntington's disease. Nat Genet 1993;4:387–92.

[16] Furtado S, Suchowersky O, Rewcastle NB, et al. The relationship of the trinucleotide repeat sequences and neuropathological changes in Huntington's disease. Ann Neurol 1996;39: 132–6.

[17] Zuhlke C, Riess O, Bockel B, et al. Mitotic stability and meiotic variability of the (CAG) n repeat in the Huntington disease gene. Hum Mol Genet 1993;2:2063–7.

[18] Margolis RL, O'Hearn E, Rosenblatt A, et al. A disorder similar to Huntington's disease is associated with novel CAG repeat expansion. Ann Neurol 2001;50:373–80.

[19] Richfield EK, Vonsattel JP, MacDonald ME, et al. Selective loss of striatal preprotachykinin neurons in a phenocopy of Huntington's disease. Mov Disord 2002;17:327–32.

[20] Stevanin G, Camuzat A, Holmes SE, et al. CAG/CTG repeat expansions at the Huntington's disease-like 2 locus are rare in Huntington's disease patients. Neurol 2002; 58:965–7.

[21] Hersch S, Jones R, Koroshetz W, et al. The neurogenetics genie: testing for the Huntington's disease mutation. Neurology 1994;44:1369–73.

[22] Almqvist EW, Bloch M, Brinkman R, et al. A worldwide assessment of the frequency of suicide, suicide attempts or psychiatric hospitalization after predictive testing for Huntington disease. Am J Hum Genet 1999;64:1293–304.

[23] Hersch SM, Ferrante RJ. Neuropathology and pathophysiology of Huntington's disease. In: Watts RL, Koller WC, editors. Movement disorders: neurologic principles and practice. New York: McGraw-Hill; 1997.

[24] Hedreen JC, Folstein SE. Early loss of neostriatal striosome neurons in Huntington's disease. J Neuropathol Exp Neurol 1995;54:105–20.

[25] Rosas HD, Goodman J, Chen YI, et al. Striatal volume loss in HD as measured by MRI and the influence of CAG repeat. Neurology 2001;57:1025–8.

[26] Turjanski N, Weeks R, Dolan R, et al. Striatal D1 and D2 receptor binding in patients with Huntington's disease and other choreas: a PET study. Brain 1995;118:689–96.

[27] Ginovart N, Lundin A, Farde L, et al. PET study of pre and postsynaptic dopaminergic markers for the neuordegenerative process in Huntington's disease. Brain 1997;120:503–14.

[28] Vonsattel JM, Myers RH, Stevens TJ, et al. Neuropathological classification of Huntington's disease. J Neuropathol Exp Neurol 1985;44:559–77.

[29] Hedreen JC, Peyser CE, Folstein SE, et al. Neuronal loss in layers V and VI of cerebral cortex in Huntington's disease. Neurosci Lett 1991;133:257–61.

[30] Josiassen RC, Curry LM, Mancall EL. Development of neuropsychological deficits in Huntington's disease. Arch Neurol 1983;40:791–6.

[31] Hodges JR, Salmon DP, Butters N. Differential impairment of semantic and episodic memory in Alzheimer's and Huntington's diseases: a controlled prospective study. J Neurol Neurosurg Psychiatry 1990;53:1089–95.

[32] Pillon B, Dubois B, Lhermitte F, et al. Heterogeneity of cognitive impairment in progressive supranuclear palsy, Parkinson's disease, and Alzheimer's disease. Neurology 1986;36: 1179–85.

[33] Massman PJ, Delis DC, Butters N, et al. Are all subcortical dementias alike? Verbal learning and memory in Parkinson's and Huntington's disease patients. J Clin Exp Neuropsychol 1990;12:729–44.

[34] Pillon B, Dubois B, Ploska A, et al. Severity and specificity of cognitive impairment in Alzheimer's, Huntington's and Parkinson's diseases and progressive supranuclear palsy. Neurology 1991;41:634–43.

[35] Weingartner H, Caine ED, Ebert MH, et al. Imagery, encoding, and retrieval of information from memory: some specific encoding-retrieval changes in Huntington's disease. J Abnorm Psychol 1979;88:52–8.

[36] Butters N. The clinical aspects of memory disorders: contributions from experimental studies of amnesia and dementia. J Clin Neuropsychol 1984;6:17–36.

[37] Butters N, Salmon DP, Cullum CM, et al. Differentiation of amnesic and demented patients with the Wechsler Memory Scale-Revised. Clin Neuropsychol 1988;2:133–48.

[38] Pillon B, Deweer B, Michon A, et al. Are explicit memory disorders of progressive supranuclear palsy related to damage to striato–frontal circuits? Comparison with Alzheimer's, Parkinson's, and Huntington's diseases. Neurology 1994;44:1264–70.

[39] Savage CR. Neuropsychology of subcortical dementias. Psychiatr Clin North Am 1997; 20(4):911–31.

[40] Wilson RS, Como PG, Garron DC, et al. Memory failure in Huntington's disease. J Clin Exp Neuropsychol 1987;9:147–54.

[41] Lange KW, Paul GM, Robbins TW, et al. L-DOPA and frontal cognitive function in Parkinson's disease. Adv Neurol 1993;60:475–8.

[42] Brandt J. Cognitive impairments in Huntington's disease: insights into the neuropsychology of the striatum. In: Corkin S, Grafman J, Boller F, editors. Handbook of neuropsychology. Volume 5. Amsterdam: Elsevier; 1991.

[43] Lange KW, Sahakian BJ, Quinn NP, et al. Comparison of executive and visuospatial memory function in Huntington's disease and dementia of Alzheimer type matched for degree of dementia. J Neurol Neurosurg Psychiatry 1995;58:598–606.

[44] Knopman D, Nissen MJ. Procedural learning is impaired in Huntington's disease: evidence from the serial reaction time task. Neuropsychologia 1991;29:245–54.

[45] Huntington Study Group. Unified Huntington's disease rating scale: reliability and consistency. Mov Disord 1996;11:136–42.

[46] Zappacosta B, Monza D, Meoni C, et al. Psychiatric symptoms do not correlate with cognitive decline, motor symptoms, or CAG repeat length in Huntington's disease. Arch Neurol 1996;53:493–7.

[47] Weigel-Weber M, Schmid W, et al. Psychiatric symptoms and CAG expansion in Huntington's disease. Am J Med Genet 1996;67:53–7.

[48] Cummings JL. Behavioral and psychiatric symptoms associated with Huntington's disease. In: Weiner WJ, Lang AE, editors. Behavioral neurology of movement disorders. New York: Raven Press; 1995. p. 179–86.

[49] Paulsen JS, Ready RE, Hamilton JM, et al. Neuropsychiatric aspects of Huntington's disease. J Neurol Neurosurg Psychiatry 2001;71(3):310–4.

[50] Thompson JC, Snowden JS, Craufurd D, et al. Behavior in Huntington's disease: dissociating cognition-based and mood-based changes. J Neuropsychiatry Clin Neurosci 2002;14:1:37–43.

[51] Anderson KE, Marder KS. An overview of psychiatric symptoms in Huntington's disease. Curr Psychiatry Rep 2001;3:379–88.

[52] Pflanz S, Besson JAO, Ebmeier KP, et al. The clinical manifestation of mental disorder in Huntington's disease: a retrospective case record study of disease progression. Acta Psychiatr Scand 1991;83:53–60.

[53] Marder K, Zhao H, Myers RH, et al. Rate of functional decline in Huntington's disease. Huntington Study Group. Neurology 2000;54(2):452–8.

[54] Nance MA, Sanders G. Characteristics of individuals with Huntington disease in long-term care. Mov Disord 1996;11(5):542–8.

[55] Paulsen JS, Butter N, Sadek JR, et al. Distinct cognitive profiles of cortical and subcortical dementia in advanced illness. Neurology 1995;45:951–6.

[56] Levy ML, Cummings JL, Fairbanks LA, et al. Apathy is not depression. J Neuropsychiatry Clin Neurosci 1998;10:314–9.

[57] Mayberg HS, Starkstein SE, Peyser CE, et al. Paralimbic frontal lobe hypometabolism in depression associated with Huntington's disease. Neurology 1992;42(9):1791–7.

[58] Farrer LA. Suicide and attempted suicide in Huntington disease: implications for preclinical testing of persons at risk. Am J Med Genet 1986;24(2):305–11.

[59] Mendez MF. Huntington's disease: update and review of neuropsychiatric aspects. Int J Psychiatry Med 1994;24:189–208.

[60] Dewhurst K, Oliver JE, McKnight AL. Socio–psychiatric consequences of Huntington's disease. Br J Psychiatry 1970;116:255–8.

[61] Anderson KE, Louis ED, Stern Y, et al. Cognitive correlates of obsessive and compulsive symptoms in Huntington's disease. Am J Psychiatry 2001;158(5):799–801.

[62] Benkelfat C, Nordahl TE, Semple WE, et al. Local cerebral glucose metabolic rates in obsessive-compulsive disorder. Patients treated with clomipramine. Arch Gen Psych 1990; 47(9):840–8.

[63] Cath DC, Spinhoven P, van Woerkom TC, et al. Gilles de la Tourette's syndrome with and without obsessive–compulsive disorder compared with obsessive–compulsive disorder without tics: which symptoms discriminate? J Nerv Ment Dis 2001;189(4):219–28.

[64] Laplane D, Levasseur M, Pillon B, et al. Obsessive–compulsive and other behavioural changes with bilateral basal ganglia lesions. A neuropsychological, magnetic resonance imaging and positron tomography study. Brain 1989;112:699–725.

[65] Swedo SE, Leonard HL, Garvey M, et al. Pediatric autoimmune neuropsychiatric disorders associated with streptococcal infections: clinical description of the first 50 cases. Am J Psych 1998;155(2):264–71.

[66] Jensen P, Sorenson SA, Fenger K, et al. A study of psychiatric morbidity in patients with Huntington's disease, their relatives, and controls: admissions to psychiatric hospitals in Denmark from 1969–1991. Br J Psychiatry 1993;163:790–7.

[67] SuttonBrown M, Suchowerdky O. Clinical and research advances in Huntington's disease. Can J Neurol Sci 2003;30(Suppl 1):S45–52.

[68] Ferrante RJ, Andreassen OA, Jenkins BG, et al. Neuroprotective effects of creatine in transgenic mouse model of Huntington's disease. J Neurosci 2000;20:4389–97.

[69] Andreassen OA, Dedeoglu A, Ferrante RJ, et al. Creatine increases survival and delays motor symptoms in a transgenic animal model of Huntington's disease. Neurobiol Dis 2001;8(3):479–91.

[70] Chen M, et al. Minocycline inhibits caspase-1 and caspase-3 expression and delays mortality in a transgenic mouse model of Huntington disease. Nat Med 2000;6:797–801.

[71] Huntington Study Group. A randomized, placebo-controlled trial of coenzyme Q10 and remacemide in Huntington's disease. Neurology 2001;57:397–404.

[72] Kremer B, Clark CM, Almqvist EW, et al. Influence of lamotrigine on progression of early Huntington's disease: a randomized clinical trial. Neurology 1999;53:1000–11.

[73] Harding AE. The clinical features and classification of the late onset autosomal dominant cerebellar ataxias: a study of 11 families, including descendants of the Drew family of Walworth. Brain 1982;105:1–28.

[74] Campanella G, Filla A, De Michele G. Classifications of hereditary ataxias: a critical overview. Acta Neurol 1992;14:408–19.

[75] Margolis RL. The spinocerebellar ataxias: order emerges from chaos. Curr Neurol Neurosci Rep 2002;2:447–56.

[76] Ross CA. Polyglutamine pathogenesis: emergence of unifying mechanisms for Huntington's disease and related disorders. Neuron 2002;35(5):819–22.

[77] Tan E, Ashizawa T. Genetic testing in spinocerebellar ataxias: defining a clinical role. Arch Neurol 2001;58:191–5.

[78] Evidente VGH, Gwinn-Hardy KA, Caviness JN, Gilman S. Hereditary ataxias. Mayo Clin Proc 2000;75:475–90.

[79] Durr A, Stevanin G, Cancel G, et al. Spinocerebellar ataxia 3 and Machad-Joseph disease: clinical, molecular, and neuropathological features. Ann Neurol 1996;39:490–9.

[80] Leroi I, O'Hearn E, Marsh L, et al. Psychopathology in patients with degenerative cerebellar diseases: a comparison to Huntington's disease. Am J Psychiatry 2002;159:1306–14.

[81] Kish SJ, El-Awar M, Stuss D, et al. Neuropsychological test performance in patients with dominantly inherited spinocerebellar ataxia: relationship to ataxia severity. Neurology 1994;44:1738–46.

[82] Berman AJ. Amelioration of aggression: response to selective cerebellar lesions in the rhesus monkey. Int Rev Neurobiol 1997;41:111–9.

[83] Liotti M, Mayberg HS, Brannan SK, et al. Differential limbic–cortical correlates of sadness and anxiety in healthy subjects: implications for affective disorders. Biol Psychiatry 2000; 48:30–42.

[84] Skre H. A study of certain traits accompanying some inherited neurological disorders. Clin Genet 1975;8:117–35.

[85] Reilly M, Daly L, Hutchinson M. An epidemiological study of Wilson's disease in the Republic of Ireland. J Neurol Neurosurg Psychiatry 1993;56(3):298–300.

[86] Roelofsen H, Wolters H, Van Luyn MJ, et al. Copper-induced apical trafficking of ATP7B in polarized hepatoma cells provides a mechanism for billiary copper excretion. Gastroenterology 2000;119:782–93.

[87] Oder W, Grimm G, Kollegger H, et al. Neurological and neuropsychiatric spectrum of Wilson's disease: a prospective study of 45 cases. J Neurol 2001;238:281–7.

[88] Lauterbach EC. Wilson's disease (hepatolenticular degeneration). In: Lauterbach EC, editor. Psychiatric management in neurological disease. Washington (DC): American Psychiatric Press; 2000. p. 93–136.

[89] Akil M, Brewer GJ. Psychiatric and behavioral abnormalities in Wilson's disease. Adv Neurol 1995;65:171–8.

[90] Denning TR, Berrios GE. Wilson's disease: a longitudinal study of psychiatric symptoms. Biol Psychiatry 1990;28:255–65.

[91] Walshe JM. Penicillamine: the treatment of first choice for patients with Wilson's disease. Mov Disord 1999;14(4):545–50.

[92] Brewer GJ. Penicillamine should not be used as initial therapy in Wilson's disease. Mov Disord 1999;14(4):551–4.

[93] Arendt G, Hefter H, Stremmel W, et al. The diagnostic value of multi-modality evoked potentials in Wilson's disease. Eltromyogr Clin Neurophysiol 1994;34:137–48.

[94] Lauterbach EC. Wilson's disease. Psychiatr Ann 2002;32:114–20.

[95] Akil M, Schwartz JA, Dutchak D, et al. The psychiatric presentations of Wilson's disease. J Neuropsychiatry Clin Neurosci 1991;3(4):377–82.

[96] Lauterbach EC, Cummings JL, Duffy J, et al. Neuropsychiatric correlates and treatment of lenticulostriatal diseases: a review of the literature and overview of research opportunities in Huntington's, Wilson's, and Fahr's diseases. J Neuropsychiatry Clin Neurosci 1998;10: 249–66.

[97] Rampoldi L, Danek A, Monaco AP. Clinical features and molecular bases of neuro-acanthocytosis. J Mol Med 2002;80:475–91.

[98] Hardie RJ, Pullon HW, Harding AE, et al. Neuroacanthocytosis. A clinical, haematological and pathological study of 19 cases. Brain 1991;114:13–49.

[99] Spitz MC, Jankovic J, Killian JM. Familial tic disorder, Parkinsonism, motor neurone disease, and acanthocytosis: a new syndrome. Neurology 1985;35:366–70.

[100] Danek A, Rubio JP, Rampoldi L, et al. McLeod neuroacanthocytosis: genotype and phenotype. Ann Neurol 2001;50:755–64.

[101] Rampoldi L, Dobson-Stone C, Rubio JP, et al. A conserved sorting-associated protein is mutant in chorea-acanthocytosis. Nat Genet 2001;28(2):119–20.

[102] Kartsounis LD, Hardie RJ. The pattern of cognitive impairments in neuroacanthocytosis. Arch Neurol 1996;53:77–80.

[103] Danek A, Tierney M, Sheesley L, et al. Cognitive findings in patients with chorea-acanthocytosis. Mov Disord 2001;16:S30.

[104] Kane JP, Havel RJ. Disorders of the biogenesis and secretion of lipoproteins containing the B apolipoproteins. In: Scrivner CR, Beaudet AL, Sly WS, et al, editors. The metabolic bases of inherited disease, 7th edition. New York: McGraw-Hill; 1995. p. 1853–85.

[105] Dexter DT, Brooks DJ, Harding AE, et al. Nigrostriatal function in vitamin E deficiency: clinical, experimental, and positron emission tomographic studies. Ann Neurol 1994;35: 298–303.

ELSEVIER
SAUNDERS

PSYCHIATRIC
CLINICS
OF NORTH AMERICA

Psychiatr Clin N Am 28 (2005) 291–299

Index

Note: Page numbers of article titles are in **boldface** type.

A

Abetalipoproteinemia, 284–285

Adolescents, depression in, obesity and, 45
low-glycemic index diets in, studies of,
133–134
obesity in, health risks of, 14–15

Affective disorders, in Huntington's disease,
180

Agouti-related protein (AgRP), in energy
balance regulation, 28–30, 29–30

Akathisia, acute neuroleptic-induced,
aspects of, 257
causes of, 257
characterization of, 257–258
diagnosis of, 257–258
pharmacologic treatment of, 259

Alpha-melanocyte-stimulating hormone, in
energy balance regulation, 28

Anticholinergics, movement disorders and,
255

Anticonvulsants, movement disorders with,
255

Antidepressants, weight gain with, 50–51
monitoring for, 51

Antipsychotics, atypical (second-
generation), metabolic abnormalities
with, 48
weight gain with, 47–48
diabetes mellitus, type 2, and
dyslipidemia and, 49
risk for, 49
first-generation, movement disorders
with, 47
obesity and, 47–50
weight gain with, 47–48
monitoring for, 49–50

Anxiety disorders, binge eating disorder
and, 108–109
in Huntington's disease, 180

Apathy, in Huntington's disease, 279–280

B

Bariatric surgery, body image and,
improvement of, 81
candidates for, 170–171
development of, 220
effects on comorbid conditions in
metabolic syndrome, 229–232
indications and evaluation for, 220
laparoscopy and, 228
malabsorptive procedures, 223
biliopancreatic diversion (with
and without duodenal
switch), 223–224
restrictive procedures, adjustable
gastric band, 226–228
gastric bypass, 225
vertical banded gastroplasty,
225–226, 228
Roux en Y gastric bypass, 220–223,
226

Behavioral treatment, of obesity,
characteristics of, goal-orientation, 153
process orientation, 153
small versus large changes,
153–154
cognitive restructuring in, 155
group versus individual,
156–157
long-term results of, 160–162
with telephone and mail
contact, 161
practice of key behaviors in,
162–163
principles of, 152–153
self-monitoring in, 154
short-term weight loss with, 157
dietary option with,
158–160
stimulus control in, 154–155
structure of, 155–156
summary of studies, 157
with Internet and e-mail,
161–162

Behavioral weight loss programs, for binge
eating disorder, 59

Changing Your Address?

Make sure your subscription changes too! When you notify us of your new address, you can help make our job easier by including an exact copy of your Clinics label number with your old address (see illustration below.) This number identifies you to our computer system and will speed the processing of your address change. Please be sure this label number accompanies your old address and your corrected address—you can send an old Clinics label with your number on it or just copy it exactly and send it to the address listed below.

We appreciate your help in our attempt to give you continuous coverage. Thank you.

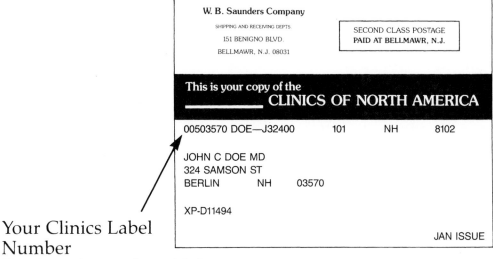

Your Clinics Label Number

Copy it exactly or send your label along with your address to:
W.B. Saunders Company, Customer Service
Orlando, FL 32887-4800
Call Toll Free 1-800-654-2452

Please allow four to six weeks for delivery of new subscriptions and for processing address changes.

Order your subscription today. Simply complete and detach this card and drop it in the mail to receive the best clinical information in your field.

Please Print:

Name _____

Address _____

City _____ State _____ ZIP _____

Method of Payment

❏ Check (payable to **Elsevier**; add the applicable sales tax for your area)

❏ VISA   ❏ MasterCard   ❏ AmEx   ❏ Bill me

Card number _____ Exp. date _____

Signature _____

Staple this to your purchase order to expedite delivery

Adolescent Medicine Clinics
- ❏ Individual $95
- ❏ Institutions $133
- ❏ *In-training $48

Anesthesiology
- ❏ Individual $175
- ❏ Institutions $270
- ❏ *In-training $88

Cardiology
- ❏ Individual $170
- ❏ Institutions $266
- ❏ *In-training $85

Chest Medicine
- ❏ Individual $185
- ❏ Institutions $285

Child and Adolescent Psychiatry
- ❏ Individual $175
- ❏ Institutions $265
- ❏ *In-training $88

Critical Care
- ❏ Individual $165
- ❏ Institutions $266
- ❏ *In-training $83

Dental
- ❏ Individual $150
- ❏ Institutions $242

Emergency Medicine
- ❏ Individual $170
- ❏ Institutions $263
- ❏ *In-training $85
- ❏ Send CME info

Facial Plastic Surgery
- ❏ Individual $199
- ❏ Institutions $300

Foot and Ankle
- Individual $160
- Institutions $232

Gastroenterology
- ❏ Individual $190
- ❏ Institutions $276

Gastrointestinal Endoscopy
- ❏ Individual $190
- ❏ Institutions $276

Hand
- ❏ Individual $205
- ❏ Institutions $319

Heart Failure (NEW in 2005!)
- ❏ Individual $99
- ❏ Institutions $149
- ❏ *In-training $49

Hematology/Oncology
- ❏ Individual $210
- ❏ Institutions $315

Immunology & Allergy
- ❏ Individual $165
- ❏ Institutions $266

Infectious Disease
- ❏ Individual $165
- ❏ Institutions $272

Clinics in Liver Disease
- ❏ Individual $165
- ❏ Institutions $234

Medical
- ❏ Individual $140
- ❏ Institutions $244
- ❏ *In-training $70
- ❏ Send CME info

MRI
- ❏ Individual $190
- ❏ Institutions $290
- ❏ *In-training $95
- ❏ Send CME info

Neuroimaging
- ❏ Individual $190
- ❏ Institutions $290
- ❏ *In-training $95
- ❏ Send CME info

Neurologic
- ❏ Individual $175
- ❏ Institutions $275

Obstetrics & Gynecology
- ❏ Individual $175
- ❏ Institutions $288

Occupational and Environmental Medicine
- ❏ Individual $120
- ❏ Institutions $166
- ❏ *In-training $60

Ophthalmology
- ❏ Individual $190
- ❏ Institutions $325

Oral & Maxillofacial Surgery
- ❏ Individual $180
- ❏ Institutions $280
- ❏ *In-training $90

Orthopedic
- ❏ Individual $180
- ❏ Institutions $295
- ❏ *In-training $90

Otolaryngologic
- ❏ Individual $199
- ❏ Institutions $350

Pediatric
- ❏ Individual $135
- ❏ Institutions $246
- ❏ *In-training $68
- ❏ Send CME info

Perinatology
- ❏ Individual $155
- ❏ Institutions $237
- ❏ *In-training $78
- ❏ Send CME info

Plastic Surgery
- ❏ Individual $245
- ❏ Institutions $370

Podiatric Medicine & Surgery
- ❏ Individual $170
- ❏ Institutions $266

Primary Care
- ❏ Individual $135
- ❏ Institutions $223

Psychiatric
- ❏ Individual $170
- ❏ Institutions $288

Radiologic
- ❏ Individual $220
- ❏ Institutions $331
- ❏ *In-training $110
- ❏ Send CME info

Sports Medicine
- ❏ Individual $180
- ❏ Institutions $277

Surgical
- ❏ Individual $190
- ❏ Institutions $299
- ❏ *In-training $95

Thoracic Surgery (formerly Chest Surgery)
- ❏ Individual $175
- ❏ Institutions $255
- ❏ *In-training $88

Urologic
- ❏ Individual $195
- ❏ Institutions $307
- ❏ *In-training $98
- ❏ Send CME info

BUSINESS REPLY MAIL

FIRST-CLASS MAIL   PERMIT NO 7135   ORLANDO FL

POSTAGE WILL BE PAID BY ADDRESSEE

PERIODICALS ORDER FULFILLMENT DEPT
ELSEVIER
6277 SEA HARBOR DR
ORLANDO FL 32821-9816